THE PSYCHOLOGICAL QUEST FOR MEANING

The Psychological Quest for Meaning

Edited by

Kentaro Fujita
Ayelet Fishbach
Nira Liberman

THE GUILFORD PRESS
New York London

A Division of Guilford Publications, Inc.
www.guilford.com

Printed in the United States of America

This book is printed on acid-free paper.

For product and safety concerns within the EU, please contact *GPSR@taylorandfrancis.com*, Taylor & Francis Verlag GmbH, Kaufingerstraße 24, 80331 München, Germany.

Last digit is print number: 9 8 7 6 5 4 3 2 1

Library of Congress Cataloging-in-Publication Data is available from the publisher.

ISBN 978-1-4625-5856-8 (cloth)

About the Editors

Kentaro Fujita, PhD, is Professor of Psychology at The Ohio State University (OSU), where he studies social psychology, decision making, and consumer behavior. His work seeks to help people achieve their goals to live a fuller, healthier, and more productive life. Dr. Fujita is an elected Fellow of the Association for Psychological Science, the Society for Personality and Social Psychology, the Society of Experimental Social Psychology, and the Midwestern Psychological Association. He is a recipient of numerous awards for his research and mentoring/teaching, including the Sage Young Scholars Award from the Foundation for Personality and Social Psychology and the Susan M. Hartmann Mentoring and Leadership Award from OSU. Dr. Fujita has published over 100 articles and chapters.

Ayelet Fishbach, PhD, is the Eric J. Gleacher Distinguished Service Professor of Behavioral Science and Marketing at The University of Chicago Booth School of Business, where she studies social psychology, management, and consumer behavior. She also studies self-control, intrinsic motivation, feedback, patience, and promoting a healthy lifestyle. Dr. Fishbach's work shows how people can live up to their highest aspirations. She is past president of the Society for the Science of Motivation and the International Social Cognition Network. Dr. Fishbach is a recipient of the Best Dissertation Award and the Career Trajectory Award from the Society of Experimental Social Psychology, the Distinguished Scientific Contribution Award from the Society for Consumer Psychology, and the Fulbright Educational Foundation Award.

Nira Liberman, PhD, is Professor of Social Psychology at Tel Aviv University in Israel and an International Faculty member in the area of Behavioral Economic Engineering and Social Cognition at the University of Cologne, Germany. She studies mental representation, motivation, self-control, decision making, and psychological distance. Dr. Liberman also studies obsessive–compulsive behavior, in particular how it may reflect deficient access to internal states. She is a Fellow of the Association for Psychological Science and the Society of Experimental Social Psychology, from which she received the Career Trajectory Award. An elected member of the Israel Academy of Sciences and Humanities, Dr. Liberman is a recipient of the Kadar Family Award for Outstanding Research from Tel Aviv University and of the Rothschild Prize.

Contributors

Daniel N. Albohn, PhD, The University of Chicago Booth School of Business, Chicago, Illinois

Emily Balcetis, PhD, Department of Psychology, New York University, New York, New York

Shannon Burns, PhD, Psychology Department, Pomona College, Claremont, California

Jessica J. Carnevale, PhD, Purchase College, State University of New York, Purchase, New York

Jordan S. Daley, PhD, Department of Psychology, New York University, New York, New York

Emily B. Falk, PhD, Annenberg School for Communication, University of Pennsylvania, Philadelphia, Pennsylvania

Melissa J. Ferguson, PhD, Department of Psychology, Yale University, New Haven, Connecticut

Ayelet Fishbach, PhD, The University of Chicago Booth School of Business, Chicago, Illinois

Kentaro Fujita, PhD, Department of Psychology, The Ohio State University, Columbus, Ohio

Ran R. Hassin, PhD, Psychology Department and the Federmann Center for the Study of Rationality, The Hebrew University of Jerusalem, Jerusalem, Israel

E. Tory Higgins, PhD, Department of Psychology, Columbia University, New York, New York

Tali Kleiman, PhD, Department of Psychology, The Hebrew University of Jerusalem, Jerusalem, Israel

Arie W. Kruglanski, PhD, Department of Psychology, University of Maryland, College Park, Maryland

Jenna P. Landy, PhD, Psychology Department, New York University, New York, New York

Nira Liberman, PhD, School of Psychological Sciences, Tel Aviv University, Tel Aviv, Israel

Sam J. Maglio, PhD, Department of Management, University of Toronto Scarborough, Toronto, Ontario, Canada

Sophia Moskalenko, PhD, Department of Communications, Georgia State University, Atlanta, Georgia

Laetitia Mwilambwe-Tshilobo, PhD, Department of Psychology, Princeton University, Princeton, New Jersey

Emily Nakkawita, PhD, Department of Psychology, Columbia University, New York, New York

Constantine Sedikides, PhD, School of Psychology, University of Southampton, Southampton, United Kingdom

Sebastian Speer, PhD, Department of Psychology, Princeton University, Princeton, New Jersey

Diana I. Tamir, PhD, Department of Psychology, Princeton University, Princeton, New Jersey

Alexander Todorov, PhD, The University of Chicago Booth School of Business, Chicago, Illinois

Yaacov Trope, PhD, Department of Psychology, New York University, New York, New York

Lily Tsoi, PhD, Department of Psychology, Caldwell University, Caldwell, New Jersey

Cheryl Wakslak, PhD, Department of Management and Organization, Marshall School of Business, University of Southern California, Los Angeles, California

Jiabi Wang, MA, MS, The University of Chicago Booth School of Business, Chicago, Illinois

Abigail S. Weber, MA, The Jewish Theological Seminary, New York, New York

Tim Wildschut, PhD, Department of Psychology, University of Southampton, Southampton, United Kingdom

Contents

CHAPTER 1

Introduction

The Psychology of Creating Meaning

Ayelet Fishbach, Kentaro Fujita, and Nira Liberman

The quest for psychological meaning is one of the most profound and defining aspects of human life, shaping how we make sense of the world, pursue our ambitions, and construct our identities. This book takes a deep dive into the psychological forces behind meaning making, weaving together insights from perception, motivation, and emotion. How do we transform scattered experiences into a coherent narrative? What drives us to seek patterns, purpose, and understanding? The essays in this collection unpack the mechanisms that structure our reality and govern our actions.

Although the quest for psychological meaning runs through much of the research in psychology and spans various subdisciplines, it has not been systematically defined and studied until recently. In fact, this is the first collection of essays that is explicitly devoted to the processes and consequences of creating psychological meaning. Although the evidence was scattered through the journals of our discipline, the story has not been told. At least not until now.

But before we dive in, what exactly is *psychological meaning*? Why do humans seek to create it?

Psychological meaning arises from a mental connection between stimuli or between a stimulus and a concept. This connection is not formed through some self-evident features of the stimuli but is actively created or constructed by the person. By forming this mental link, a person places a stimulus within a broader context. They may recognize that an item is part of a group, that an action has caused an effect, that a behavior reflects intention, or that an object serves a purpose. A meaning is created, for example, when a person concludes that a rock is a paperweight (or art) or that their action conveyed generosity (or fear). They may reflect on their life's work, believing it advanced science or strengthened their legacy and impact. In either case, when the stimulus is perceived as part of a larger context, it is understood, fostering the experience of psychological meaning.

Indeed, the world does not reveal itself in an orderly fashion. The broader picture is rarely announced. For example, effects do not immediately follow causes, and finding the cause of something is often a difficult endeavor. Actions occur without the actor explicitly declaring their purpose. Objects typically lack labels indicating their potential use. People may belong to groups whose members may not appear near one another. Causal associations, intentions, usages, category memberships, and group affiliations must be inferred.

Without the psychological process of "meaning making," the world would present itself as a stream of unrelated stimuli, much like the static between stations on a radio dial. The social world, in particular, would be what William James (1890/1981) described as "a blooming, buzzing confusion" (p. 462). Information would feel scattered, fragmented, and piecemeal. Thanks to meaning making, however, this is not our experience of the world. Instead of chaos, humans perceive order. Instead of getting stuck in the concrete, they can abstract. The process of creating psychological meaning can take many forms. For example, basic perception is largely a top-down process—one in which meaning is actively created from what people see, hear, and otherwise experience. Further, people construct narratives about their lives.

Yaacov Trope argues that the process of creating meaning is fundamental to human experiences and involves "reducing mental entropy by transforming irregular and disconnected elements into coherent, interconnected, and stable cognitive and conative structures" (this volume). The quest for meaning happens in all processing modes (e.g., automatic or controlled, conscious or unconscious, fast or slow; Gawronski, Sherman, & Trope, 2014; Ferguson & Hassin, this volume). By forming connections that embed stimuli in context, humans perceive the world as organized and purposeful—a world governed by rules and order, where we can operate with ease.

This collection of essays on the quest for meaning is inspired by Yaacov Trope's seminal work in experimental psychology, and it is authored by many of his colleagues, friends, and students—categories that often overlap. Contributors explore a wide range of topics within psychological science that, at first glance, may seem unrelated: The book highlights recent research on emotion, perception, social interaction, and motivation—subjects typically covered in separate chapters of an introductory psychology textbook. Despite working within distinct subdisciplines, the common thread uniting these authors is their focus on the basic question of how psychological meaning is created. They all explore how we come to understand our world and ourselves, how we imbue the world around us with meaning, and how we imbue our lives with meaning.

We thus study the quest for meaning in cognition, or what people believe exists, and in motivation, or what people desire to exist. We investigate meaning seeking as both an intrapersonal process and an interpersonal one because social networks shape meaning, and individuals bond over shared understandings of the world. Additionally, we examine how humans make sense of the world and how they find meaning in their lives. The search for meaning is fundamental to self-knowledge, often emerging through reflection and self-observation. After all, the self is both familiar and unknown. It is a source of endless curiosity as people seek the meaning of their lives through art, culture, science, and most critically, through the everyday psychological processes that we describe here.

A BRIEF HISTORICAL CONTEXT

Is the quest for meaning a new topic in psychological research? Yes and no. Starting with a clear "no," we noted earlier that in classic texts, William James observed that human psychology imbues meaning in a world that might otherwise appear chaotic. Consistent with his thoughtful observation, much of early experimental work in psychology uncovered the principles underlying the perception of connections, context, and hence, meaning making.

Consider, for example, the discoveries of Gestalt psychology in studying low-level perceptual processes (Koffka, 1935). These researchers identified key principles that explain how we perceive visual elements as parts of a unified whole rather than as isolated fragments. The Gestalt principles—proximity, similarity, closure, continuity, figure–ground, and common fate—demonstrate how we group nearby or similar objects and how our brains fill in missing information to create shapes out of disjoint elements (closure). These principles describe how we perceive continuous lines despite interruptions (continuity), how we distinguish objects from their backgrounds (figure–ground), and how we infer that stimuli that travel together in space form a unit (common fate). These principles are all about ways of creating meaning. They illustrate how perception is shaped by the quest for understanding a stimulus within a broader context.

Beyond cognition, early research documented the creation of meaning to motivate action. For example, Bruner and Goodman (1947) found that children from lower socioeconomic backgrounds overestimated the size of coins compared with wealthier children. The need for financial resources shaped these low-income children's visual perception, making a desirable object seem bigger and perhaps closer, consistent with their motivation to seek out money. Bluma Zeigarnik's early research on the need for closure—the "Zeigarnik effect"—documented that people remember unfinished or interrupted tasks better than completed ones (Zeigarnik, 1927). Why does the mind "get stuck" on incomplete tasks, finding it hard to let go? Possibly because the meaning of these tasks has not been realized yet.

Early psychological research also recognized that people seek meaning in their lives. They want to understand themselves. Atkinson's achievement theory (Atkinson, 1957) posited that people set goals to gather information about themselves based on their performance. Specifically, people wish to succeed and fear failure. Those with high achievement motivation set challenging goals where the probability of success is moderate because this offers the greatest potential for personal satisfaction. Conversely, those with a higher fear of failure opt for very easy or very hard tasks, such that success will be granted or, alternatively, failure will be nondiagnostic. According to Atkinson, humans choose tasks to make their lives meaningful.

The field's seminal cognitive dissonance (Festinger, 1957) and self-perception (Bem, 1972) theories further documented the desire to understand behavior within the context of a person's overall sense of self. Individuals seek to interpret the meaning of their actions in relation to who they are or might be and how they should understand themselves.

The essays in this collection explore the quest for meaning as an everyday pursuit rather than a response to unusual circumstances. Humans engage in meaning making not only when they perceive a lack of meaning. These processes are not solely designed to solve problems. As such, the pursuit of meaning is not just a response to perceived chaos, nor is it abandoned once order is achieved. For example, although a conflict between one's actions and cognitions may require resolution (e.g., through dissonance reduction), people strive to identify and categorize their actions even in the absence of conflict. They may infer that they have a goal or a trait, and they may perceive purpose and continuity. In either case, they imbue their actions with meaning.

MAJOR THEMES

The essays in this book explore three areas of research on psychological meaning: creating meaning to understand the world (perception), to find direction in personal striving (motivation), and to make sense of the self and one's life (meaning in life). The authors point out new discoveries on how humans seek and create meaning in the world around us. Some of the main insights from their research agendas are summarized next.

Creating Meaning to Understand the World

The quest for psychological meaning is universal, yet its manifestation is highly individualistic. When evaluating the same stimulus, different people see different things. Todorov and Albohn explore this heterogeneity in meaning making, demonstrating that people's evaluations of stimuli are not universally shared. Evaluations of complex stimuli, such as faces or art, reveal significant *idiosyncratic preferences*, suggesting that subjective factors heavily influence how people derive meaning from their environment.

How individuals intuitively evaluate *distance*—whether spatial, temporal, social, or probabilistic—is essential to their understanding of the world. Maglio explores this process. Building on construal-level theory (Liberman & Trope, 2008; Trope & Liberman, 2010; Trope, Ledgerwood, Liberman, & Fujita, 2021), he argues that psychological assessment of distance (e.g., how close a travel destination feels) explains how individuals move from perceiving their environment to making sense of it and ultimately finding meaning. In this way, the perception of distance influences subsequent actions, decisions, and feelings.

Meaning making happens both within the person and between persons. Meaning as an interpersonal process occurs whenever people seek to understand each other and form a shared meaning of the world. Moving to the social context of meaning making, Speer et al. explore how people come to understand themselves and others through *conversations*. Conversations contribute to a sense of belonging, self-worth, and identity. However, not all conversations yield these benefits equally. Successful conversations balance psychological closeness (through alignment and empathy) with distance (through exploration and diverse viewpoints), enabling deeper connections and collective cohesion.

Further exploring interpersonal meaning making, Wakslak explores *communication*. She finds that the way people communicate is shaped by their audience's distance, size, and diversity. Communicating with distant or diverse audiences often prompts speakers to use more abstract language. The reason is that abstraction facilitates understanding across differences. This dynamic is not only functional—allowing messages to resonate more broadly—but also reciprocal because abstract communication can shape perceptions of the speaker, signaling power or competence.

Creating Meaning to Find Direction in Personal Striving

Much of the research on meaning making addresses its functionality in enabling and facilitating personal striving. Landy, Daley, and Balcetis study *motivated perception*. Like Todorov and Albohn, they demonstrate that perception is idiosyncratic, and they explain these variations by noting that people see the world through a motivated lens. Their perceptions are a function not just of what is actually presented to them but also of their goals, expectations, identities, and experiences. By "filling in the gaps," people create meaning at the earliest levels of information processing. This motivated perception, or "wishful seeing," allows people to create a desired meaning of the world around them.

Next, Nakkawita and Higgins explore a particular context where meaning making influences motivation: *multitasking*. They demonstrate that how people structure their engagement in multiple activities affects the inferences they draw about their enjoyment of and interest in those activities. Through the lens of activity engagement theory (Higgins, Lee, Kwon, & Trope, 1995), they explain that switching between tasks—especially those that are enjoyable—can undermine perceived interest in the primary task because the act of switching signals that the initial activity might not have been sufficiently engaging. Conversely, switching between tasks that are initially unattractive can enhance perceived interest in those activities.

Staying on the theme of juggling *multiple goals*, Fishbach and Wang explore how our various ambitions—whether career, family, or health—can either fuel one another or create tension. Research reveals that when people perceive their goals as harmonious, they feel more intrinsically motivated, making long-term pursuits feel rewarding and engaging. In contrast, when goals seem to clash, self-control kicks in as a necessary tool to resist short-term temptations and stay on course. Ultimately, these authors suggest that effectively navigating multiple goals often depends on the perceived relationships between goals and the resulting meaning of their pursuits.

Kleiman argues that in the course of pursuing meaningful outcomes, cognitive control—the ability to regulate attention and behavior in alignment with goals—can transfer across different domains. When tasks are motivationally meaningful, people can leverage a general *control readiness* mechanism that enables cross-domain conflict resolution: Prior engagement in cognitive control can reduce stereotypical biases, influence attention allocation, and enhance decision-making flexibility. When meaning connects two previously unrelated tasks, mechanisms engaged in one may "carry over" to the next.

Finally, metamotivation matters for creating meaning. *Metamotivation* refers to the beliefs and processes that support people's ability to regulate their motivational states to attain desired outcomes. For example, whereas some tasks demand being sensitive to more distant priorities (e.g., delay of gratification), others demand being sensitive to more immediate concerns (e.g., proofreading). According to Carnevale and Fujita, metamotivation allows people to flexibly construct new meanings for tasks to motivate themselves to perform at their best.

Creating Meaning in Life

How do people find meaning in their lives? How does research on the quest for psychological meaning explain self-perceptions?

First, Ferguson and Hassin challenge the view that finding meaning in life is mainly a conscious process, arguing instead that *non-conscious* and *implicit cognitive processes* play a crucial role. They explore difficult, life-changing decisions that reshape our sense of self (e.g., having a child or getting divorced), arguing that what is considered "thinking" and "deciding" in these decisions is often governed by non-conscious processes. More broadly, their approach suggests that implicit cognition is not rigid and simplistic but flexible, capable of updating beliefs, integrating relational information, and even engaging in causal reasoning.

Next, Sedikides and Wildschut explore *nostalgia* as an emotion that bridges gaps between disjointed aspects of the self, fostering a sense of self-continuity, which in turn enhances meaning in life. When individuals experience self-discontinuity—feeling disconnected from their past selves—nostalgia acts as a psychological resource that reconnects them to their past to promote emotional resilience and reinforce identity. In this way, nostalgia mitigates discomfort, reduces existential anxiety, and provides meaning (in this case, coherence) to one's life narrative.

Ultimately, meaning making is the process by which a stimulus is evaluated within a broader context. Applying this principle to the self, Liberman explains that the experience of meaning in life arises from the interplay between engagement with reality and the creation of *abstract mental constructs* such as narratives and purpose. According to this analysis, meaning emerges when individuals feel a sense of continuity across time, space, social connections, and possibilities. Such continuity must align with higher-level abstractions that organize experiences into coherent narratives and purposeful goals.

Finally, Moskalenko and Kruglanski distinguish between two systems of meaning in life, based on two complementary motivational states: a need for significance and a need for awe. *Need for significance* refers to the desire to feel important and to matter; it prioritizes status, competition, achievement, aggression, and clear and firm answers to questions or problems (need for closure). By contrast, *need for awe* is a desire to contemplate vast and incomprehensible phenomena that make one feel insignificant by comparison, such as God, beauty, and nature; it prioritizes harmony, equality, connectedness, and questions rather than answers. Although the need for awe and the need for significance are both essential, individuals and cultures often focus on one over the other, resulting in different "default" interpretations and meanings assigned to the same events.

CLOSING REMARKS

The last chapter in this book is authored by Yaacov Trope, and we would not blame our readers if they read it first. In it, Trope teaches us that meaning making is a fundamental psychological process that reduces entropy by connecting elements into a coherent structure. Drawing from cognitive and social psychology, he explains that meaning emerges from integrating beliefs, behaviors, and goals into unified frameworks, both at the individual and collective levels. This process not only provides individuals with a sense of predictability, agency, and self-worth but also expands the regulatory scope of collectives, enabling societies to extend their influence across time, space, and social contexts.

As a final note, this introduction would not be complete without sharing with you, the reader, another main reason this group of authors got together to write about the quest for psychological meaning. Our collective work is a tribute to our friend and mentor, Yaacov, and it was inspired by his scholarship. Each of the authors was deeply influenced by him on personal and intellectual levels. Yaacov taught us to pay close attention to people and to how they see the world. We learned to look carefully, to find patterns and rules in the messy data on human thought and actions. Yaacov has shaped the field of social psychology, and many researchers have been personally influenced. We count ourselves among those fortunate scholars. His guidance continues to inspire us to seek meaning and understand how people find it in every facet of life.

REFERENCES

Atkinson, J. W. (1957). Motivational determinants of risk-taking behavior. *Psychological Review, 64*(6, Pt.1), 359–372.

Bem, D. J. (1972). *Self-perception theory.* In L. Berkowitz (Ed.), *Advances in experimental social psychology* (Vol. 6, pp. 1–62). Academic Press.

Bruner, J. S., & Goodman, C. C. (1947). Value and need as organizing factors in perception. *Journal of Abnormal and Social Psychology, 42*(1), 33–44.

Festinger, L. (1957). *A theory of cognitive dissonance.* Stanford University Press.

Higgins, E. T., Lee, J., Kwon, J., & Trope, Y. (1995). When combining intrinsic motivations undermines interest: A test of activity engagement theory. *Journal of Personality and Social Psychology, 68*(5), 749–767.

James, W. (1981). *The principles of psychology* (Vol. 1, p. 462). Harvard University Press. (Original work published 1890)

Koffka, K. (1935). *Principles of Gestalt psychology.* Harcourt.

Liberman, N., & Trope, Y. (2008). The psychology of transcending the here and now. *Science, 322*(5905), 1201–1205.

Sherman, J. W., Gawronski, B., & Trope, Y. (Eds.). (2014). *Dual-process theories of the social mind.* Guilford Press.

Trope, Y., Ledgerwood, A., Liberman, N., & Fujita, K. (2021). Regulatory scope and its mental and social supports. *Perspectives on Psychological Science, 16*(2), 204–224.

Trope, Y., & Liberman, N. (2010). Construal-level theory of psychological distance. *Psychological Review, 117*(2), 440–463.

Zeigarnik, B. (1927). Über das Behalten von erledigten und unerledigten Handlungen, *Psychologische Forschung, 9*, 1–85.

PART I

CREATING MEANING TO UNDERSTAND THE WORLD

CHAPTER 2

The Idiosyncratic Nature of Evaluation

Alexander Todorov and Daniel N. Albohn

Whether we are looking at abstract geometric patterns, novel three-dimensional objects, abstract art, or human faces, we immediately evaluate these stimuli. That is, we derive meaning from them. We know whether we like the stimuli or not, whether we find them dangerous or beautiful. Such evaluative meaning-making processes are remarkably efficient, occur after minimal exposure to visual stimuli (Ballew & Todorov, 2007; Bar, Neta, & Linz, 2006; Colombatto, Uddenberg, & Scholl, 2021; Rule, Ambady, & Adams, 2009; Oh, Shafir, & Todorov, 2020; Todorov, Loehr, & Oosterhof, 2010; Todorov, Pakrashi, & Oosterhof, 2009; Willis & Todorov, 2006), and can be made without any explicit intention to evaluate the stimuli (Klapper, Dotsch, van Rooij, & Wigboldus, 2016; Siddique et al., 2023; Swe et al., 2020, 2022; Verosky, Zoner, Marble, Sammon, & Babarinsa, 2020). At the same time, these evaluations need not be simple and can be characterized by a rapid integration of the available visual cues, even if people are instructed (and incentivized) to ignore particular cues (Aviezer, Trope, & Todorov, 2012a, 2012b; Oh et al., 2020; Todorov et al., 2010). In short, extracting meaning from visual stimuli appears obligatory.

Importantly, these evaluations are also statistically reliable. That is, if people are asked to evaluate the same stimuli on repeated occasions, their evaluations are positively correlated. These correlations imply that there is a consistent mapping from perceptual features of stimuli to specific evaluations. Finding this mapping has been the primary objective of data-driven computational models of face evaluation (Oosterhof & Todorov, 2008; Peterson, Uddenberg, Griffiths, Todorov, & Suchow, 2022; Todorov, Dotsch, Wigboldus, & Said, 2011; Todorov & Oosterhof, 2011; Todorov & Oh, 2021). These models have been successful in identifying configurations of features that drive a variety of different evaluations. But how consistent is the mapping of perceptual features to evaluations across people?

The modeling approach, as well as the standard experimental approach, typically aggregates across participants, implicitly assuming that individual variation in evaluations is unimportant. As it turned out, this assumption is demonstrably false. Consider judgments of facial trustworthiness, which we have extensively studied (Oh, Wedel, Labbree, & Todorov, 2023; Oosterhof & Todorov, 2008; Todorov, 2008; Todorov, Oh, Uddenberg, & Albohn, 2025; Todorov, Said, Engell, & Oosterhof, 2008). Models of trustworthiness judgments consistently show that feminine features and features resembling happy expressions increase evaluations of trustworthiness. But these models of aggregated judgments are models of stimulus features. Variance-partitioning approaches (Martinez, Funk, & Todorov, 2020), which are discussed later in the chapter, show that stimulus features contribute surprisingly little to trustworthiness judgments. As shown in Figure 2.1, across four different datasets, stimulus features account for less than 20% of the meaningful variance of judgments.[1] In fact, for standardized images of faces, they account for less than 5% of the variance. Aggregating across participants essentially hides the diversity of complex evaluations.

The same issues arise in the standard theory-driven experimental approach. Suppose you are testing whether the angularity (vs. roundness) of features increases threat evaluations (e.g., Aronoff, Barclay, & Stevenson, 1988; Aronoff, Woike, & Hyman, 1992; Bar & Neta, 2006). Ideally, you would manipulate the same visual stimuli to have more angular versus rounder features and compare the mean threat evaluations of these two types of stimuli. Observing the predicted main effect would be interpreted as indicating that people find visual objects with angular features more threatening. But chances are that there is tremendous individual variation in the evaluation of these stimuli. This variation is typically ignored, implicitly assuming that it is just statistical noise. But if the same participants were to repeat the experiment, you may find out that their preferences are quite consistent. Hence, we have failed to understand evaluations at the individual level and overstated the generality of our findings.

The premise of this chapter is that the amount of interrater agreement—indicating similar interpretations of stimulus features across people—has been greatly exaggerated in the experimental literature because of inaccurate assumptions, standard research practices, and

[1]Data and analysis scripts for the results presented in this chapter are available at *osf.io/wx6f8*.

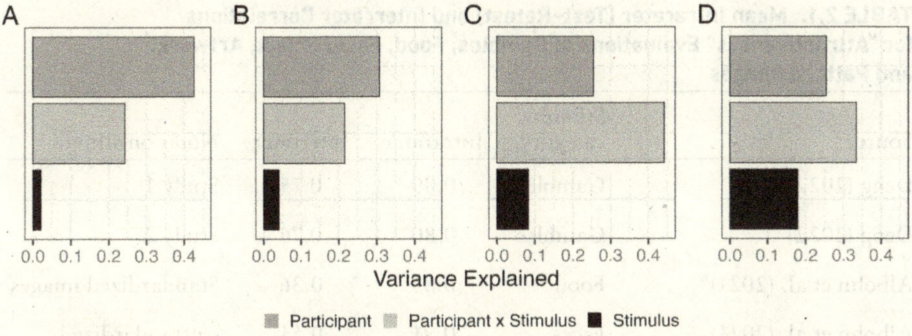

FIGURE 2.1. Variance accounted for by stimulus and idiosyncratic components for trustworthiness evaluations of face images across four different datasets and participants: (A and B) 120 neutral faces from the Chicago Face Database (Ma, Correll, & Wittenbrink, 2015), (C) 120 neutral "in-the-wild" faces, and (D) 100 hyperrealistic images generated by StyleGAN2 (Karras, Laine, & Aila, 2018). The stimulus variance component is the amount of variance accounted for by stimulus features. The participant and participant × stimulus components represent the amount of variance that is attributable to individual participants. The rest of the variance is due to a measurement error (not plotted).

misleading analyses (Hönekopp, 2006; Martinez et al., 2020). In Section I, using a range of visual stimuli, we show that although evaluative responses are highly consistent within individuals, they need not be consistent across individuals. We describe methods for variance partitioning, which identifies the contributions of stimulus features (shared contributions) and participants' contributions (idiosyncratic contributions) to evaluations, and show that for complex evaluations, idiosyncratic contributions trump shared ones. In Section II, we discuss the factors that affect the relative share of stimulus and idiosyncratic contributions to evaluations. In Section III, we discuss the implications of the findings and showcase a method for building models of idiosyncratic evaluations.

I. MEASURING STIMULUS AND IDIOSYNCRATIC CONTRIBUTIONS TO EVALUATION

In Table 2.1, we have assembled descriptive correlational data from multiple studies conducted in our lab, in which participants rated the attractiveness, beauty, or appeal of a variety of stimuli: gambles (e.g., 75% probability of winning $5 and 25% probability of losing $6), food items, different types of faces (e.g., standardized, nonstandardized "in

TABLE 2.1. Mean Intrarater (Test–Retest) and Interrater Correlations for "Attractiveness" Evaluations of Gambles, Food, Face, Object, Artwork, and Pattern Images

Source	Stimulus category	Intrarater	Interrater	Notes on stimuli
Deng (2022)	Gambles	0.80	0.75	Study 1
Deng (2022)	Gambles	0.80	0.76	Study 2
Albohn et al. (2021)^	Food	0.83	0.36	Standardized images
Albohn et al. (2021)	Faces	0.91	0.51	Unstandardized "in-the-wild" faces
Albohn et al. (2024)	Faces	0.71	0.47	Unstandardized "in-the-wild" faces
Deng (2022)	Faces	0.80	0.51	Study 1; Hyper-realistic faces
Martinez et al. (2020)*	Faces	0.62	0.34	Study 1; Standardized faces
Martinez et al. (2020)*#	Faces	0.54	0.40	Study 3; Standardized faces
Albohn et al. (2024)	Faces	0.51	0.25	Standardized faces
Specker et al. (2024)*	Faces	0.74	0.48	Study 1; Standardized faces
Specker et al. (2024)*	Faces	0.69	0.50	Study 2; Standardized faces
Specker et al. (2024)*	Faces	0.62	0.43	Study 3; Standardized faces
Kurosu & Todorov (2017)*	Objects	0.50	0.02	Study 2; Family-X novel objects
Kurosu & Todorov (2017)*	Objects	0.61	0.38	Study 2; Family-Y novel objects
Kurosu & Todorov (2017)*	Objects	0.57	0.19	Study 2; Family-Z novel objects
Martinez et al. (2020)*	Objects	0.49	0	Study 1; Family-X novel objects
Martinez et al. (2020)*#	Objects	0.57	0.03	Study 3; Family-X novel objects

(continued)

TABLE 2.1. *(continued)*

Source	Stimulus category	Intrarater	Interrater	Notes on stimuli
Deng (2022)	Artwork	0.63	0.18	Study 2
Specker et al. (2024)*	Artwork	0.68	0.10	Study 1
Specker et al. (2024)*	Artwork	0.62	0.14	Study 2
Specker et al. (2024)*	Artwork	0.63	0.15	Study 3
Martinez et al. (2020)*	Patterns	0.07	0	Study 1

Note. Intrarater correlations are computed for each participant between their repeated judgments of the same stimuli. Interrater correlation represents the average correlation between each participant's judgments and every other participant's judgments. ^ corresponds to studies where the judgment was "appealing"; * corresponds to studies where the judgment was "beautiful"/"beauty"; # is a reanalysis of Kurosu and Todorov (2017) Study 1.

the wild," hyperrealistic synthetic), art images, novel three-dimensional objects, and highly complex patterns.

With the exception of extremely complex and meaningless patterns (e.g., matrices of 100 × 100 square blocks, where the color of each block was randomly generated), the intraparticipant correlations are positive and generally high. The range of correlations, excluding the meaningless patterns, is from .49 to .91, with a median of .63. Notice that the magnitude of these correlations is not determined by the category of evaluated stimuli. For example, although the intrarater correlations appear to be higher for faces than art images, this is not true for judgments of standardized faces (i.e., the ones typically used in psychology research). Thus, irrespective of the stimulus category, evaluative responses to meaningful stimuli are consistent within individuals.

In contrast to the intrarater correlations, there is much higher variation for the interrater correlations. Excluding the complex meaningless patterns, the range is from 0 to .76, with a median of .36. Although these correlations are high for relatively simple stimuli (e.g., gambles, where people seem to be approximating their expected values), they are low for most complex stimuli and are essentially zero for some categories of stimuli. Thus, although evaluations are consistent within individuals, there is very large variation in the agreement between individuals.

The fact that interrater correlations are lower than intrarater correlations is not surprising. The latter sets the limit of the magnitude of meaningful correlations, and one of the arguments in favor of aggregation is the gain in increased reliability of the measured responses. Rather than relying on descriptive statistics, a better approach is to partition the variance of judgments (Hönekopp, 2006). We have discussed this approach in detail elsewhere (Martinez et al., 2020). Briefly, the approach requires repeated evaluations of the same stimuli. Having this repeated measurement, it is possible to partition the meaningful variance after accounting for noise or measurement error.

The three variance components of theoretical interest are stimulus, participant, and participant × stimulus. Stimulus variance represents how stimulus features influence judgments—for instance, when certain objects are consistently rated as more beautiful than others across all participants. In essence, models of aggregated judgments are models of stimulus variance. The participant and participant × stimulus variance components represent idiosyncratic variance, or how individual differences influence judgments, although the interpretation of these two components is different.

Participant variance reflects consistent individual differences in how people respond across all stimuli. Although technically a form of idiosyncratic variance, its interpretation can be ambiguous (Cronbach, 1955; Hönekopp, 2006). If a participant consistently gives higher beauty ratings than another participant across all stimuli, it could reflect either differences in scale use (e.g., some participants always provide higher ratings) or actual meaningful variation in evaluation (e.g., some participants truly find the objects more beautiful).

In contrast to the participant variance component, the participant × stimulus variance unambiguously represents idiosyncratic variance. This component captures true idiosyncratic variance that cannot be explained solely by either stimulus features or participants' general rating tendencies (e.g., participant 1 likes stimulus A more than stimulus B, but participant 2 likes stimulus B more than stimulus A). One way to think of this component is that it captures the extent to which the relative ranking of the stimuli differs across participants.

Table 2.2 shows the variance attributed to these three components—stimulus, participant, and participant × stimulus variance—for the same stimuli from Table 2.1.

The only category of stimuli for which the stimulus variance exceeds the idiosyncratic variance is gambles. Ignoring the participant's variance because of the ambiguities in its interpretation, for evaluation of faces, the stimulus and participant × stimulus contributions are comparable. That is, about half of the variance in attractiveness judgments of faces is idiosyncratic, a finding first reported and discussed by Hönekopp (2006) almost 20 years ago. For the remaining stimuli, the idiosyncratic contributions tend to be larger than the stimulus contributions. In some cases, the stimulus contributions are essentially zero. Clearly, focusing on aggregated judgments is missing most of the contributions to evaluation.

TABLE 2.2. Variance Accounted for by Stimulus and Idiosyncratic Components for "Attractiveness" Evaluations of Gambles, Food, Face, Object, Artwork, and Pattern Images

Source	Stimulus category	Stimulus	Participant	Participant × Stimulus
Deng (2022)	Gambles	0.56	0.14	0.15
Deng (2022)	Gambles	0.59	0.12	0.12
Albohn et al. (2021)^	Food	0.27	0.17	0.43
Albohn et al. (2021)	Faces	0.31	0.29	0.23
Albohn et al. (2024)	Faces	0.32	0.22	0.25
Deng (2022)	Faces	0.30	0.31	0.25
Martinez et al. (2020)*	Faces	0.17	0.44	0.20
Martinez et al. (2020)*#	Faces	0.15	0.44	0.15
Albohn et al. (2024)	Faces	0.10	0.42	0.18
Specker et al. (2024)*	Faces	0.30	0.22	0.27
Specker et al. (2024)*	Faces	0.31	0.21	0.23
Specker et al. (2024)*	Faces	0.23	0.30	0.20
Kurosu & Todorov (2017)*	Objects	0	0.29	0.41
Kurosu & Todorov (2017)*	Objects	0.20	0.34	0.20
Kurosu & Todorov (2017)*	Objects	0.09	0.56	0.19
Martinez et al. (2020)*	Objects	0	0.35	0.34
Martinez et al. (2020)*#	Objects	0.01	0.24	0.44
Deng (2022)	Artwork	0.09	0.34	0.32
Specker et al. (2024)*	Artwork	0.06	0.22	0.46
Specker et al. (2024)*	Artwork	0.08	0.20	0.41
Specker et al. (2024)*	Artwork	0.09	0.19	0.41
Martinez et al. (2020)*	Patterns	0	0.63	0.01

Note. The stimulus variance component is the amount of variance accounted for by stimulus features. The participant and participant-by-stimulus components represent the amount of variance that is attributable to individual participants. The rest of the variance is due to a measurement error. ^ corresponds to studies where the judgment was "appealing"; * corresponds to studies where the judgment was "beautiful"/"beauty"; # is a reanalysis of Kurosu and Todorov (2017) Study 1. See Table 2.1 for notes about the specific stimuli.

II. DETERMINANTS OF STIMULUS AND IDIOSYNCRATIC CONTRIBUTIONS TO EVALUATION

Although the variance-partitioning approach controls for measurement error, it is possible that the idiosyncratic components are less stable or more error prone than the stimulus component. However, the estimates of these components are not affected by the set size of the stimuli (from a set of 50 to a set of 500; Todorov & Oh, 2021, Figure 17) or cognitive load during the evaluation task (Specker, Albohn, Tinio, Leder, & Todorov, 2024). Thus, these estimates appear to be equally stable.

Inspecting Table 2.2, it is easy to assume that the relative share of stimulus and idiosyncratic variance is a function of the type of stimuli. For example, for art images and most novel objects, idiosyncratic variance trumps stimulus variance. However, this assumption is misleading, as illustrated in Figure 2.2.

For the spiky objects in Figure 2.2 (Family-X in Tables 2.1 and 2.2), the average interrater agreement in their beauty evaluation is essentially zero, and thus the stimulus contribution to this evaluation is zero, too. Some people find spiky objects beautiful, whereas others find them ugly. However, when the same objects are evaluated on danger, the stimulus variance trumps idiosyncratic variance. Most people find the spikier objects more dangerous. In contrast to the spiky objects, for the spherical objects (Family-Y in Tables 2.1 and 2.2), there is more consensus in their beauty evaluations than in their danger evaluations. As noted in the introduction, the statistical reliability of evaluation implies that there is a consistent mapping from perceptual features to specific evaluations *within individuals*. When this mapping is consistent *across individuals*, most of the meaningful variance would be stimulus variance. This is the case for the danger evaluations of the spiky objects.

We can illustrate the same principle with different judgments of the same faces sampled from the Chicago Face Database (Ma et al., 2015). For masculinity/femininity judgments, we consistently find that stimulus contributions trump shared contributions (Albohn, Martinez, & Todorov, 2024), as shown in Figure 2.3. For this particular judgment, the mapping of features to judgments is consistent across individuals. However, this mapping is more heterogeneous for judgments of attractiveness, and even more so for judgments of trustworthiness. Thus, the relative share of stimulus and idiosyncratic variance is a function of both the type of stimulus and the specific judgment.

As a general rule, for judgments of attributes that are *read into* faces, there will be greater idiosyncratic variance compared with shared

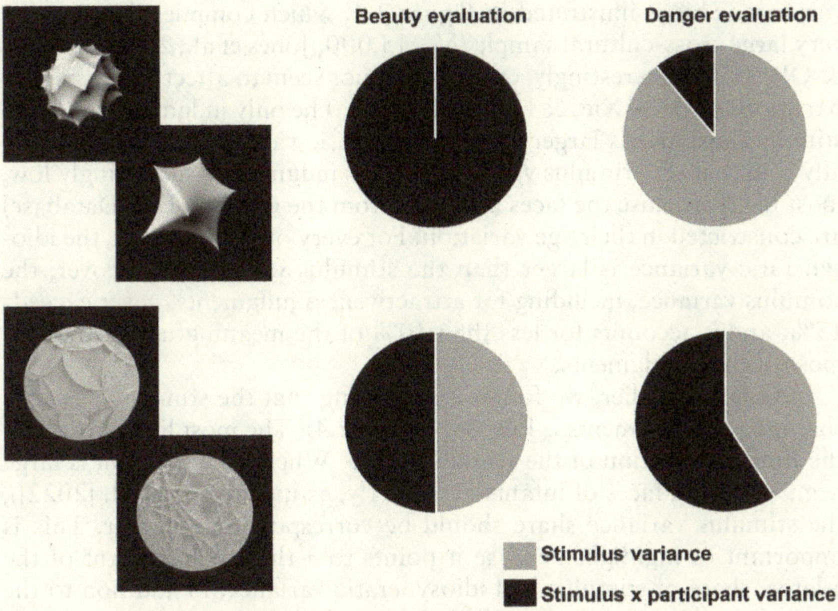

FIGURE 2.2. Relative share of stimulus and idiosyncratic (participant × stimulus) variance in beauty and danger evaluations of novel three-dimensional objects. Data from Kurosu and Todorov (2017).

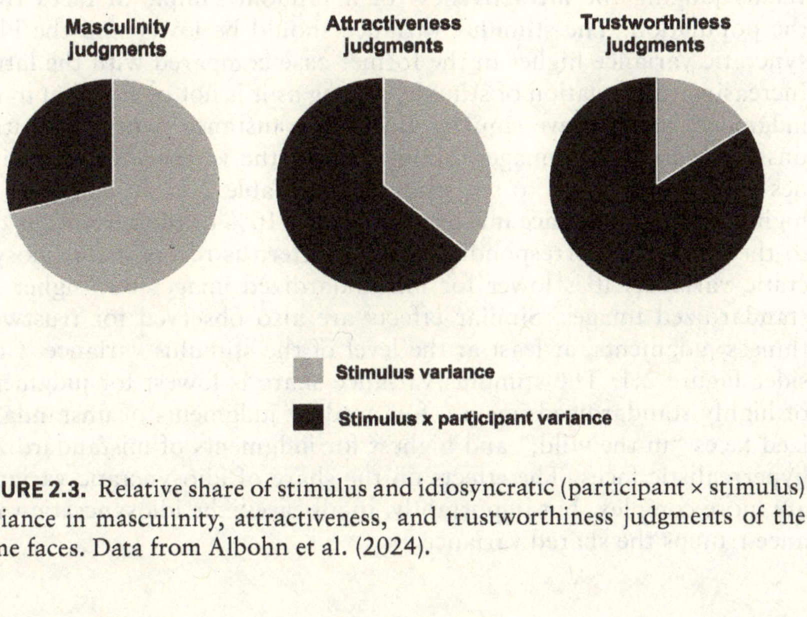

FIGURE 2.3. Relative share of stimulus and idiosyncratic (participant × stimulus) variance in masculinity, attractiveness, and trustworthiness judgments of the same faces. Data from Albohn et al. (2024).

variance. This is illustrated in Figure 2.4, which compiles data from a very large cross-cultural sample ($N > 15{,}000$; Jones et al., 2021; Todorov & Oh, 2021). Interestingly, culture does not seem to affect how variance partitions (Hester, Xie, & Hehman, 2021). The only judgment for which stimulus variance is larger than idiosyncratic variance is age. We actually find that the stimulus variance for this judgment is surprisingly low, most likely because the faces (sampled from the Chicago Face Database) are constricted in their age variation. For every other judgment, the idiosyncratic variance is larger than the stimulus variance. Moreover, the stimulus variance, including for attractiveness judgments, never exceeds 15%, and it accounts for less than 10% of the meaningful variance for most of these judgments.

As noted earlier, we found it surprising that the stimulus variance share for age judgments is low (see Figure 2.4). The most likely reason is the limited variation of the stimuli on age. When this variation is large (e.g., including faces of infants and elderly, as in Peterson et al. [2022]), the stimulus variance share should be correspondingly larger. This is important to highlight because it points to a third determinant of the relative share of stimulus and idiosyncratic variance, in addition to the type of stimulus and the specific judgment. When the relevant variation for the judgment at hand is restricted, this would reduce the share of stimulus variance and increase the share of idiosyncratic variance (cf. Hönekopp, 2006).

Consider the case of judging the attractiveness of supermodels versus judging the attractiveness of a random sample of faces from the population. The stimulus variance should be lower and the idiosyncratic variance higher in the former case compared with the latter. Increasing the variation of stimuli, as long as it is not orthogonal to the judgment, should have similar effects. For instance, when evaluating unstandardized face images, about 32% of the variance in attractiveness judgments is due to the stimulus (see Table 2.2). In contrast, for highly standardized face images, only about 10% of the variance is due to the stimulus. Correspondingly, this pattern is reversed for idiosyncratic variance: It is lower for unstandardized images but higher for standardized images. Similar effects are also observed for trustworthiness judgments, at least at the level of the stimulus variance. Consider Figure 2.1: The stimulus variance share is lowest for judgments of highly standardized images, followed by judgments of unstandardized faces "in the wild," and highest for judgments of unstandardized hyperrealistic faces. The effects on the share of idiosyncratic variance are more complex, but importantly, in all cases, the idiosyncratic variance trumps the shared variance.

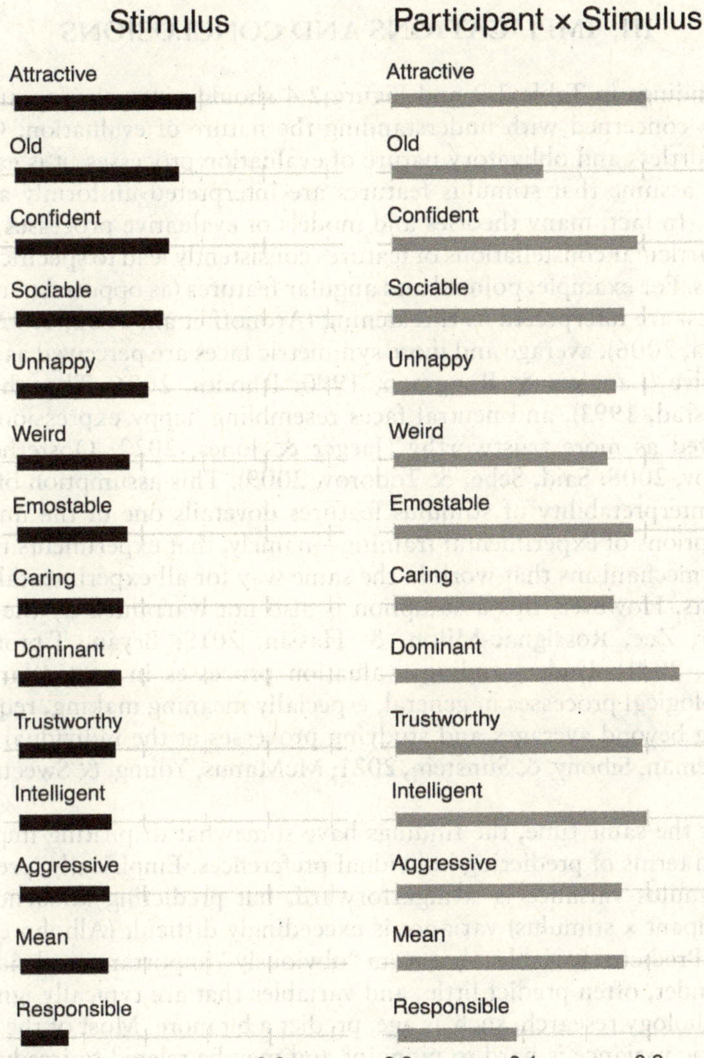

FIGURE 2.4. Variance accounted for by stimulus and idiosyncratic (participant × stimulus) contributions for 14 social judgments. Data from Jones et al. (2021).

III. IMPLICATIONS AND CONCLUSIONS

The findings in Table 2.2 and Figure 2.4 should give pause to anyone who is concerned with understanding the nature of evaluation. Given the effortless and obligatory nature of evaluation processes, it is easy to falsely assume that stimulus features are interpreted uniformly across people. In fact, many theories and models of evaluative processes posit that particular constellations of features consistently lead to specific evaluations. For example, pointed and angular features (as opposed to round features) are interpreted as threatening (Aronoff et al., 1988, 1992; Bar & Neta, 2006), average and more symmetric faces are perceived as more attractive (Langlois & Roggman, 1990; Rhodes, 2006; Thornhill & Gangestad, 1993), and neutral faces resembling happy expressions are perceived as more trustworthy (Jaeger & Jones, 2022; Oosterhof & Todorov, 2008; Said, Sebe, & Todorov, 2009). This assumption of uniform interpretability of stimulus features dovetails one of the implicit assumptions of experimental training—namely, that experiments reveal causal mechanisms that work in the same way for all experimental participants. However, this assumption is also not warranted by the data (Bolger, Zee, Rossignac-Milon, & Hassin, 2019; Bryan, Tipton, & Yeager, 2021). Understanding evaluation processes in particular and psychological processes in general, especially meaning making, requires moving beyond averages and studying processes at the individual level (Kahneman, Sibony, & Sunstein, 2021; McManus, Young, & Sweetman, 2023).

At the same time, the findings have somewhat dispiriting implications in terms of predicting individual preferences. Empirically, predicting stimulus variance is straightforward, but predicting idiosyncratic (participant × stimulus) variance is exceedingly difficult (Albohn et al., 2024). Predictor variables that seem "obviously" important, such as race and gender, often predict little, and variables that are typically ignored in psychology research, such as age, predict a bit more. Most of the idiosyncratic variance is hard to pinpoint and may be related to irreducible individual differences tied to the specific life histories of the individuals. We can formulate and test specific hypotheses about potential sources of these individual differences, such as face typicality as a function of one's experience with faces (Dotsch, Hassin, & Todorov, 2016; Sofer et al., 2017) and resemblance to personally familiar faces (Verosky & Todorov, 2010, 2013), but may not be able to predict specific individual differences *a priori*. The very first stages of meaning making—evaluating what individuals perceive—are already shaped by the individuals' histories.

Yet there is a way forward. For simple judgments where the mapping of perceptual features to evaluation is consistent across people, understanding how stimulus features contribute to evaluation is sufficient. For complex judgments where the mapping is inconsistent across people, we need to understand the different ways in which individuals use stimulus features to arrive at different evaluations of the same stimuli. Instead of (or rather, in addition to) building models of aggregated judgments, we need to build models of specific individuals (Albohn, Uddenberg, & Todorov, 2022, 2025). Advances in machine learning and the availability of large databases of images make this possible. Figure 2.5 shows an example of individual models for "appealing" judgments of art images. As evidenced across the individual participant models, the resulting images are quite different. Whereas some participants prefer figurative paintings, others prefer landscapes or abstract artwork.

Notice that the standard modeling approach of building models of aggregated judgments and the approach of building individual models represent the ends of a continuum. We can still build models of specific groups based on a prior theoretical interest (e.g., political affiliation; Uddenberg, Nguyen, Albohn, & Todorov, 2024) and inspect the individual variation in these models.

CONCLUSIONS

We started off this chapter by suggesting that evaluation is obligatory—when presented with a face, a piece of artwork, or a novel object, we cannot help but derive some sort of meaning. Although the focus of this chapter was primarily on evaluation, the implications of this work extend far beyond the very first stages of meaning making. Understanding meaning-making processes requires moving beyond averages and studying processes at the individual level (Bryan et al., 2021; McManus et al., 2023; Saqr, Vogelsmeier, & López-Pernas, 2024).

The shift toward a person-centric, "meaning-making" approach to psychological processes has the potential to reveal new insights that traditional research approaches have missed. Recent studies using within-person modeling have made important contributions to understanding complex psychological phenomena, such as situational experiences, personality maturation, and the effectiveness of interventions (e.g., Bryan et al., 2021; DiGiovanni, Vannucci, Ohannessian, & Bolger, 2021; Kuper et al., 2024; Saqr et al., 2024; Seifert, Rohrer, & Schmukle, 2024).

Ultimately, our understanding of evaluation and meaning making must move beyond studying aggregated data and pretending that such data are representative of individuals. By recognizing the importance

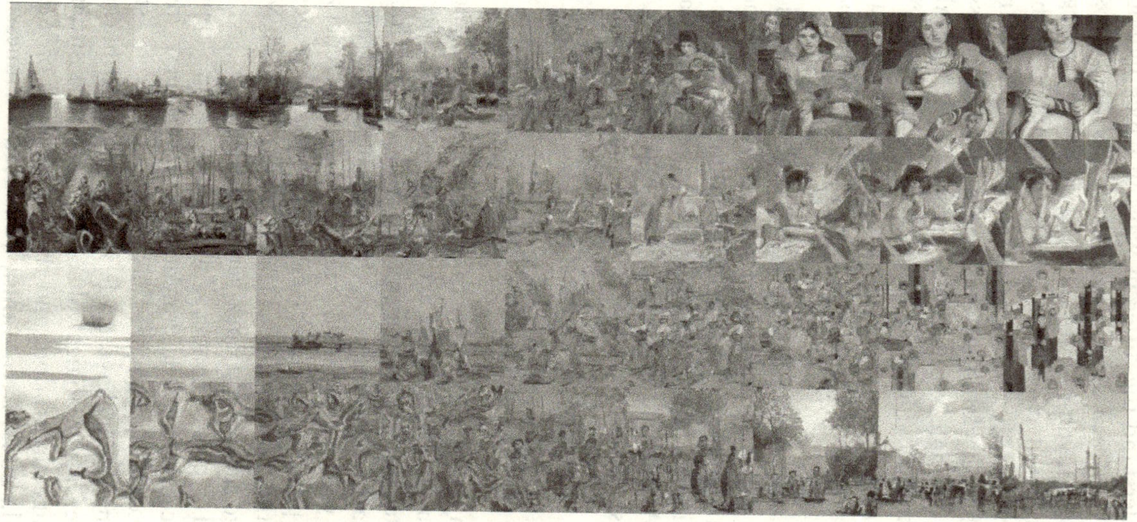

FIGURE 2.5. Example novel images generated from individual participants' models of appealing art images. Each row represents an individual participant. The center image in each row represents the average of all images that participants evaluated as "neutral." Images to the left and right of the center image in each row represent ±2 standard deviations from the mean. Thus, images to the right of center represent what participants evaluated as appealing, and images to the left of center represent what participants evaluated as unappealing.

of individual variation, we can gain a more accurate and nuanced understanding of human behavior. However, this shift requires a fundamental change in how we approach research, moving from a focus on shared stimulus features to embracing the complexities of individual differences.

REFERENCES

Albohn, D. N., Martinez, J. E., & Todorov, A. (2024). Determinants of shared and idiosyncratic contributions to judgments of faces. *Journal of Experimental Psychology: Human Perception and Performance, 50*(11), 1117–1130.

Albohn, D. N., Uddenberg, S., & Todorov, A. (2022). A data-driven, hyper-realistic method for visualizing individual mental representations of faces. *Frontiers in Psychology, 13*, Article 997498.

Albohn, D. N., Uddenberg, S., & Todorov, A. (2025). Individualized models of social judgments and context-dependent representations. *Scientific Reports, 15*(1), Article 4208.

Aronoff, J., Barclay, A. M., & Stevenson, L. A. (1988). The recognition of threatening facial stimuli. *Journal of Personality and Social Psychology, 54*(4), 647–655.

Aronoff, J., Woike, B. A., & Hyman L. M. (1992). Which are the stimuli in facial displays of anger and happiness? Configurational bases of emotion recognition. *Journal of Personality and Social Psychology, 62*(6), 1050–1066.

Aviezer, H., Trope, Y., & Todorov, A. (2012a). Body cues, not facial expressions, discriminate between intense positive and negative emotions. *Science, 338*(6111), 1225–1229.

Aviezer, H., Trope, Y., & Todorov, A. (2012b). Holistic person processing: Faces with bodies tell the whole story. *Journal of Personality and Social Psychology, 103*(1), 20–37.

Ballew, C. C., & Todorov, A. (2007). Predicting political elections from rapid and unreflective face judgments. *Proceedings of the National Academy of Sciences of the USA, 104*(46), 17948–17953.

Bar, M., & Neta, M. (2006). Humans prefer curved visual objects. *Psychological Science, 17*(8), 645–648.

Bar, M., Neta, M., & Linz, H. (2006). Very first impressions. *Emotion, 6*(2), 269–278.

Bolger, N., Zee, K. S., Rossignac-Milon, M., & Hassin, R. R. (2019). Causal processes in psychology are heterogeneous. *Journal of Experimental Psychology: General, 148*(4), 601–618.

Bryan, C. J., Tipton, E., & Yeager, D. S. (2021). Behavioural science is unlikely to change the world without a heterogeneity revolution. *Nature Human Behaviour, 5*(8), 980–989.

Colombatto, C., Uddenberg, S., & Scholl, B. J. (2021). The efficiency of demography in face perception. *Attention, Perception, & Psychophysics, 83*(8), 3104–3117.

Cronbach, L. (1955). Processes affecting scores on "understanding of others" and "assumed similarity." *Psychological Bulletin, 52*(3), 177–193.

Deng, X. (2022). *The idiosyncrasy of preferences across domains* [Master's thesis, University of Chicago]. *knowledge.uchicago.edu/record/4365/files/Deng%20MA%20Final%20Draft.pdf*

DiGiovanni, A. M., Vannucci, A., Ohannessian, C. M., & Bolger, N. (2021). Modeling heterogeneity in the simultaneous emotional costs and social benefits of co-rumination. *Emotion, 21*(7), 1470–1482.

Dotsch, R., Hassin, R. R., & Todorov, A. (2016). Statistical learning shapes face evaluation. *Nature Human Behaviour, 1*(1), 1–6.

Hester, N., Xie, S. Y., & Hehman, E. (2021). Little between-region and between-country variance when people form impressions of others. *Psychological Science, 32*(12), 1907–1917.

Hönekopp, J. (2006). Once more: Is beauty in the eye of the beholder? Relative contributions of private and shared taste to judgments of facial attractiveness. *Journal of Experimental Psychology: Human Perception and Performance, 32*(2), 199–209.

Jaeger, B., & Jones, A. L. (2022). Which facial features are central in impression formation? *Social Psychological and Personality Science, 13*(2), 553–561.

Jones, B. C., DeBruine, L. M., Flake, J. K., Tullio Liuzza, M., Antfolk, J., Arinze, N. C., et al. (2021). To which world regions does the valence-dominance model of social perception apply? *Nature Human Behaviour, 5*(1), 159–169.

Kahneman, D., Sibony, O., & Sunstein, C. R. (2021). *Noise: A flaw in human judgment.* William Collins.

Karras, T., Laine, S., & Aila, T. (2018). *A style-based generator architecture for generative adversarial networks.* arXiv. *arxiv.org/abs/1812.04948*

Klapper, A., Dotsch, R., van Rooij, I., & Wigboldus, D. H. (2016). Do we spontaneously form stable trustworthiness impressions from facial appearance? *Journal of Personality and Social Psychology, 111*(5), 655–664.

Kuper, N., von Garrel, A. S., Wiernik, B. M., Phan, L. V., Modersitzki, N., & Rauthmann, J. F. (2024). Distinguishing four types of person × situation interactions: An integrative framework and empirical examination. *Journal of Personality and Social Psychology, 126*(2), 282–311.

Kurosu, A., & Todorov, A. (2017). The shape of novel objects contributes to shared impressions. *Journal of Vision, 17*(13), 14.

Langlois, J. H., & Roggman, L. A. (1990). Attractive faces are only average. *Psychological Science, 1*(2), 115–121.

Ma, D. S., Correll, J., & Wittenbrink, B. (2015). The Chicago Face Database: A free stimulus set of faces and norming data. *Behavior Research Methods, 47*(4), 1122–1135.

Martinez, J. E., Funk, F., & Todorov, A. (2020). Quantifying idiosyncratic and shared contributions to judgment. *Behavior Research Methods, 52*(4), 1428–1444.

McManus, R. M., Young, L., & Sweetman, J. (2023). Psychology is a property of persons, not averages or distributions: Confronting the group-to-person generalizability problem in experimental psychology. *Advances in Methods and Practices in Psychological Science, 6*(3), Article 25152459231186615.

Oh, D., Shafir, E., & Todorov, A. (2020). Economic status cues from clothes affect perceived competence from faces. *Nature Human Behavior, 4*(3), 287–293.

Oh, D., Wedel, N., Labbree, B., & Todorov, A. (2023). Trustworthiness judgments without the halo effect: A data-driven computational modeling approach. *Perception, 52*(8), 590–607.

Oosterhof, N. N., & Todorov, A. (2008). The functional basis of face evaluation. *Proceedings of the National Academy of Sciences of the USA, 105*(32), 11087–11092.

Peterson, J. C., Uddenberg, S., Griffiths, T. L., Todorov, A., & Suchow, J. W. (2022). Deep models of superficial face judgments. *Proceedings of the National Academy of Sciences of the USA, 119*(17), Article E2115228119.

Rhodes, G. (2006). The evolutionary psychology of facial beauty. *Annual Review of Psychology, 57*, 199–226.

Rule, N. O., Ambady, N., & Adams, R. B. (2009). Personality in perspective: Judgmental consistency across orientations of the face. *Perception, 38*(11), 1688–1699.

Said, C., Sebe, N., & Todorov, A. (2009). Structural resemblance to emotional expressions predicts evaluation of emotionally neutral faces. *Emotion, 9*(2), 260–264.

Saqr, M., Vogelsmeier, L. V. D. E., & López-Pernas, S. (2024). Capturing where the learning process takes place: A person-specific and person-centered primer. *Learning and Individual Differences, 113*, Article 102492.

Seifert, I. S., Rohrer, J. M., & Schmukle, S. C. (2024). Using within-person change in three large panel studies to estimate personality age trajectories. *Journal of Personality and Social Psychology, 126*(1), 150–174.

Siddique, S., Sutherland, C. A. M., Jeffery, L., Swe, D. C., Gwinn, O. S., & Palermo, R. (2023). Children show neural sensitivity to facial trustworthiness as measured by fast periodic visual stimulation. *Neuropsychologia, 180*, Article 108488.

Sofer, C., Dotsch, R., Oikawa, M., Oikawa, H., Wigboldus, D. H. J., & Todorov, A. (2017). For your local eyes only: Culture-specific face typicality influences perceptions of trustworthiness. *Perception, 46*(8), 914–928.

Specker, E., Albohn, D. N., Tinio, P., Leder, H., & Todorov, A. (2024). *The importance of person-related variance for judgement* [Unpublished manuscript].

Swe, D. C., Palermo, R., Gwinn, O. S., Bell, J., Nakanishi, A., Collova, J., & Sutherland, C. A. M. (2022). Trustworthiness perception is mandatory: Task instructions do not modulate fast periodic visual stimulation trustworthiness responses. *Journal of Vision, 22*(11), 1–19.

Swe, D. C., Palermo, R., Gwinn, O. S., Rhodes, G., Neumann, M., Payart, S., & Sutherland, C. A. M. (2020). An objective and reliable electrophysiological marker for implicit trustworthiness perception. *Social Cognitive and Affective Neuroscience, 15*(3), 337–346.

Thornhill, R., & Gangestad, S. W. (1993). Human facial beauty: Averageness, symmetry, and parasite resistance. *Human Nature, 4*(3), 237–269.

Todorov, A. (2008). Evaluating faces on trustworthiness: An extension of systems for recognition of emotions signaling approach/avoidance behaviors. In A. Kingstone & M. Miller (Eds.), *The year in cognitive neuroscience 2008* (pp. 208–224). Blackwell.

Todorov, A., Dotsch, R., Wigboldus, D., & Said, C. P. (2011). Data-driven methods for modeling social perception. *Social and Personality Psychology Compass, 5*(10), 775–791.

Todorov, A., Loehr, V., & Oosterhof, N. N. (2010). The obligatory nature of holistic processing of faces in social judgments. *Perception, 39*(4), 514–532.

Todorov, A., & Oh, D. (2021). The structure and perceptual basis of social judgments from faces. *Advances in Experimental Social Psychology, 63*, 189–246.

Todorov, A., Oh, D., Uddenberg, S., & Albohn, D. N. (2025). Face evaluation: Findings, methods, and challenges. *Annals of the New York Academy of Science, 1545*(1), 28–37.

Todorov, A., & Oosterhof, N. N. (2011). Modeling social perception of faces. *IEEE Signal Processing Magazine, 28*(2), 117–122.

Todorov, A., Pakrashi, M., & Oosterhof, N. N. (2009). Evaluating faces on trustworthiness after minimal time exposure. *Social Cognition, 27*(6), 813–833.

Todorov, A., Said, C. P., Engell, A. D., & Oosterhof, N. N. (2008). Understanding evaluation of faces on social dimensions. *Trends in Cognitive Sciences, 12*(12), 455–460.

Uddenberg, S., Nguyen, Z., Albohn, D. N., & Todorov, A. (2024). Hyperrealistic reverse correlation reveals a gender bias in representations of leadership. *Journal of Vision, 24*(10), 418.

Verosky, S. C., & Todorov, A. (2010). Generalization of affective learning about faces to perceptually similar faces. *Psychological Science, 21*(6), 779–785.

Verosky, S. C., & Todorov, A. (2013). When physical similarity matters: Mechanisms underlying affective learning generalization to the evaluation of novel faces. *Journal of Experimental Social Psychology, 49*(4), 661–669.

Verosky, S. C., Zoner, K. A., Marble, C. W., Sammon, M. M., & Babarinsa, C. O. (2020). Implicit responses to face trustworthiness measured with fast periodic visual stimulation. *Journal of Vision, 20*(7), Article 29.

Willis, J., & Todorov, A. (2006). First impressions: Making up your mind after 100 ms exposure to a face. *Psychological Science, 17*(7), 592–598.

CHAPTER 3

Means and Meanings in Measurement

Sam J. Maglio

Actuaries must have an incredibly difficult time explaining what they do for a living. I certainly am not one, but I imagine their story going something like this. We start by taking mountains of data on the probabilities of thousands of possibilities. Then we put it all together into an overall sense of risk that some dreadful thing like a hurricane or a market crash or an untimely death will happen. At the end of all that, we advise firms, governments, and individuals on how to manage that risk. If I'm reasonably close, then the job of an actuary breaks down into two jobs. First, they perceive the odds of all those eventualities and boil them down to an overall summary. Second, based on that summary, they recommend the most advisable path forward.

All humans do an equally complex version of this two-stage job, without the tables and the spreadsheets, just by living. Perceiving and acting on the world require an understanding of the events that fill a life. To get from perceiving to acting, the mind first makes sense of what it has to work with. An actuary might incorporate family history and lifestyle factors to calculate a black-and-white probability that someone will remain healthy into their 80s; a commuter might incorporate meteorology reports with how the weather looks outside their window to estimate the chance that it will rain today. After making sense, the mind makes meaning. What price tag should the firm put on a life insurance policy? Should I take an umbrella to work? Tallying the pros and cons, a course of action presents itself and gets taken.

Actuaries predict the likelihood that what is currently hypothetical will eventually become real. In this sense, they trade in the measurement of psychological distance, appraising whether some event is a near certainty or a remote possibility. The more unlikely the event, the further it sits from immediate, egocentric reality. The construct of psychological distance suggests that distance is like ice cream, coming in many different flavors. Long odds have much in common with long physical expanses, long times ago and from now, and long-forgotten friends. How unlikely an event, how remote from a place, how removed in time, and how dissimilar to another person can all be answered in a universal language of near and far. Probability, geographical space, time, and social distance represent four distinct yet interrelated dimensions of psychological distance. This means that what holds true for one flavor of distance tends to hold true for the rest (Bar-Anan, Liberman, Trope, & Algom, 2007; Fiedler, Jung, Wänke, & Alexopoulos, 2012; Maglio, Trope, & Liberman, 2013a).

Non-actuaries also measure a variety of psychological distances as a first step in making sense of the world. Commuters gauge the distance of their trip when deciding between walking or driving. Sunday-morning layabouts consider how much time they have until a brunch date when deciding whether to tackle a load of laundry. Conversants take the temperature of how socially close they feel to the group before choosing whether to crack a risqué joke or stick to the weather. In all of these instances, the outside and inside worlds provide a wealth of perceptual information in need of measurement. That measurement makes sense of where things sit. Such distillation guides meaning making by providing a map for what to do next.

Two landmarks thus become crucial in order to understand how people consider psychological distance in working their way from perception to sense making to making meaning. First, what predicts how perceptual information gives rise to the measurement of distance needed to make sense of the world? What are the means by which measurement occurs, and what elements of the person and the situation collaborate to result in a solid grounding of sense making? Second, what does this measurement of distance predict? How do people take what they have concluded and fit it into a broader context in the service of making meaning?

Two points warrant consideration when working through these questions. The first is that measurement, even on its best day, is really estimation. The priciest mechanical Rolex on the market still loses about two minutes a month. A carpenter taking a ruler to a piece of wood doesn't bother going to three decimal places before making a cut. Any act of measuring leads to approximation and rounding off. This happens because the estimate proves good enough for the objective at hand: making sense in order to make meaning. The length of a trip or the time until an appointment gets measured in unambiguous terms, but there's still always some wiggle room around it. Human measurers take their perception and turn it into their own personal evaluation of the measurement that allows it to make sense. There's more wiggle room around more ambiguous or unknowable measurements, such as when an employee might get a promotion or the likelihood that a stock will hit. There, measurement turns all the more into estimation, taking given perceptions and converting them into a subjective feeling in order to make sense of them (Hu & Maglio, 2018; Loewenstein, Weber, Hsee, & Welch, 2001; Van Boven & Caruso, 2015).

The second is that the process from perception to meaning making to sense making easily works in reverse as well. Plenty of objects and phenomena in the world come precolored with meaning, triggering a sequence from meaning to sense making on down to perception itself. In distance, people prefer to pull good things closer and push bad things back (Landy, Daley, & Balcetis, this volume). For instance, thirst makes water bottles appear closer because the closer they are, the sooner thirst can be quenched. Rather than being a universal, unidirectional path, the relationship between perception, sense, and meaning operates recursively.

Distance therefore figures prominently in the translation from perception to sense making to meaning making. At its most basic, distance needs to be measured, with individuals estimating the distance between themselves and some other thing in the interest of making sense of it. Along the way, the body, the mind, and the outside world interact with perception before arriving at a subjective sense of understanding distance. At its most impactful, distance makes the leap from this felt understanding of measurement to a larger sense of why it matters for lived lives. For people to get there, measured distance informs the actions they take, the choices they make, and the feelings they feel.

WHAT PREDICTS MEASUREMENT?

The Body

Most bodies, unless they belong to Charlie Bucket's family, move. Even Grandpa Joe got out and jigged after Charlie scored his golden ticket to Willy Wonka's chocolate factory. A body in motion might tend to stay in motion, but the body thinks about motion even before taking a single step. Upcoming locomotion will move the body through physical space. As a result, measurement of that space proves especially sensitive to the state of the body. When the effort required to traverse distance looms large, the length of that distance subjectively elongates. For example, people saddled with heavy backpacks and eyeing steep hills overestimate the size of a given length of distance relative to those facing a less cumbersome—but equally long—stroll (Proffitt, Stefanucci, Banton, & Epstein, 2003; Stefanucci, Proffitt, Banton, & Epstein, 2005). Premotion people have a reasonably strong sense of not just what their body can do but also what it's about to do. In one experiment supporting this idea, Evan Polman and I recruited passengers at subway stations who were standing on either the westbound platform or the eastbound platform. Westbound passengers rated stations toward which their bodies were oriented—farther west along the line—as subjectively closer than eastbound passengers oriented away from those same stations. The pattern reversed for eastbound passengers, who rated stations to the east as relatively close and those to the west as relatively far (Maglio & Polman, 2014). Bodily feedback offers direct, relevant information that colors perception of the space through which it expects to move.

Even without any anticipated movement, people still take proprioceptive stock of their bodies, which in turn affects how they measure distances other than physical space. Consider the influence of elevation—not height per se, but how high up or low down the body has gone. A physically high vantage point necessarily allows people to observe remote locations. Less intuitively, it also makes them see time differently. The mind holds a fundamental association between vertical position and broad scope that goes beyond remote locations to include remote time as well (Nussinson et al., 2021; see also Nussinson et al., 2019). Accordingly, minds inside of bodies that happen to be standing on a high floor (relative to those relegated to the basement) more often opt to receive a larger reward in the future over a smaller reward sooner (Aggarwal & Zhao, 2015; Slepian, Masicampo, & Ambady, 2015). Like a train appearing no bigger than a tortoise from the vantage point of an ascending airplane, these results suggest that elevation may have made the time delay to the better outcome seem smaller and less painful to endure (Zauberman, Kim, Malkoc, & Bettman, 2009).

Bodies consult inward as much as outward, and there, too, the body finds cues that guide the measurement of time. The heart serves as one such guide. In a series of studies, Eugene Chan and I first found that thinking about coffee (like writing about its health benefits) speeds up the heart by an average of 6 beats per minute relative to participants thinking about tea (Chan & Maglio, 2019). In a later study, we again had participants think about either coffee or tea, then asked when they expected to perform three activities of their own choosing. Coffee participants believed that activities would happen sooner than tea participants. Arousal appears to truncate time, like that separating now from a future event (as does emotional intensity; Van Boven, Kane, McGraw, & Dale, 2010). This exemplifies how conditions of the body help the mind make sense of the goings-on outside it. In other instances, inasmuch as it can, the mind acts independently of the body.

The Mind

Ask anyone fresh off a round-trip journey about the time they spent traveling, and an irrational quirk of time estimation tends to emerge. Even though both legs—there and back—took approximately the same amount of time, people often say that the outbound trip seemed longer while the return trip passed quickly. Yes, travel puts bodies into motion, but this return-trip effect results less from the physical sensation of movement than how travelers think. Whereas homebound trips tend to bring people toward relatively familiar locations, outbound trips point toward destinations marked by more question marks, like what will happen there. Such a sense of uncertainty makes time drag. Research participants in one experiment, made to walk from one room to another and then back, reported a higher sense of this return-trip effect when they were not told what task they would perform in that other room than participants who knew what they'd be doing from the outset (Maglio & Kwok, 2016). Other effects in estimating time, such as how many changes happen during it, illustrate that characteristics of time make its duration seem longer or shorter (Zakay & Block, 1997). More broadly, they reflect the role of the mind in making sense of the distance it perceives.

The mind brings all manner of mindsets to the task of making sense. When sense needs to be made of distance, one frame of mind exerts perhaps the strongest influence: level of construal. Construal-level theory differentiates between two means of interpretation (Trope & Liberman, 2010). An abstract, high-level perspective attunes the mind toward the essential, invariant gist; a concrete, low-level perspective focuses on secondary, temporary details. A restaurant, from a high level, represents a place for nourishment, whereas that same restaurant from a low level becomes a building characterized by particular cuisine and décor. What's more, construal tracks with distance (Liberman, this volume). Hungry diners right now prioritize how easily they can get to food, but planning a future meal makes diners concern themselves with how good the food will be. Distance, in other words, shifts the level of construal.

Owing to the foundational link between distance and construal, the reverse also works. Abstract minds tend to estimate that things are distant, and concrete minds tend to estimate that things are nearby (Bar-Anan, Liberman, & Trope, 2006). Put people into an abstract mindset, and relative to those in a concrete mindset, they see objects in their field of vision as farther away, such as stickers on a desk in a research lab or shapes presented on a computer monitor (Chan & Maglio, 2023; Liberman & Förster, 2009). These findings showcase the role of construal level in distorting something as primary as visual perception. Even scaling beyond what people can touch and see, the effect of construal on making sense of distance persists. Abstraction additionally makes people estimate that places are farther away in geographical space (Alter & Oppenheimer, 2008; see also Mrkva, Travers, & Van Boven, 2018), that actions and events will happen later in time (Liberman, Trope, McCrea, & Sherman, 2007), that others share less in common with themselves (Rim, Min, Liu, Chartrand, & Trope, 2019; Stephan, Liberman, & Trope, 2011), and that events are less likely to happen at all (Wakslak & Trope, 2009).

How the mind thinks directly changes how the mind perceives. Furthermore, this higher-order process interacts with other means by which the mind makes sense. The previous section summarized how people rely on the body in making measurements. This happens in part because someone wearing a heavy backpack gets asked one question ("How long is the distance from here to there?") but answers a different question ("How far does the distance feel to me, in this body, right now?"). But the backpack, like so many bodily states, is a fleeting condition—the kind that matters a great deal right now but that will, eventually, change. Abstraction downweighs these kinds of temporary concerns. Accordingly, abstraction has a way of pulling people out of their bodies. One experiment recreated the backpack study, randomly assigning some participants to wear one while others did not. Separately, participants were led into an abstract or concrete frame of mind. When everyone estimated the length of a hallway, those thinking concretely showed the standard effect of a backpack making the hallway appear longer. Those thinking abstractly, however, made nearly identical judgments of visual distance whether they were carrying a heavy pack or not (Maglio & Trope, 2012). As also noted earlier, time warps as a function of how many changes happen during a given span of time, with more tending to add up to a longer felt duration. However, from a construal-level perspective, these changes can be minor and incidental, making them the exact kind of thing that an abstract mind overlooks. Because those changes go unseen, abstraction can make time feel slower and longer (Hansen & Trope, 2012). Through means both indirect and direct, mental states introduce a unique component in moderating the sense-making process.

The Outside World

Independent of where the body and mind have brought themselves, external forces compel them to measure distance in distinct ways. A starting question might ask what distance does to distance itself. A mile or a minute may represent straightforward spans of space and time, but they can have varying degrees of distance imposed on them. The first mile of a cross-country road trip appears longer than the last mile, just like exercisers evaluate the first minute of a workout as longer than the last minute. In both instances, an initial distance (hundreds of miles, dozens of minutes) makes farther distances in the same domain seem shorter (the final mile, the final minute). Combine this diminishing sensitivity within the same distance (space, time) with the tendency to think of all distances as interrelated, and a broader insight emerges: Situating some amount of any distance as already far in any distance should similarly make it appear smaller. Consider the possibility of going to a museum. Today, the 27 miles to get there might look like quite a ways to travel. But schedule that same visit for a year from now, and the same 27 miles come across as subjectively shorter. Similarly, 2 years of someone's own life seems significantly longer than the same 2 years in the life of a socially distant someone else (Maglio, Trope, & Liberman, 2013b). Regardless of which comes first and which comes second, any stretch of distance has a tendency to shorten when it is already far.

But what constitutes *far* in the first place? Boundaries provide an easy answer for this otherwise intractable question because boundaries conveniently chop the outside world into neat categories. And boundaries come in many forms. Place an object at a given distance away from people, and they evaluate the distance to it as shorter if they can reach it compared with people who cannot (Witt, Proffitt, & Epstein, 2005). Someone waiting in line for an automated teller machine (ATM) behaves as though the ATM is physically closer when grouped within the same boundary of people who are close to it, such as standing on the same carpet in front of the machine, with everyone ahead of them similarly having crossed that boundary marker (Zhao, Lee, & Soman, 2012). People even treat threats, such as disease, as farther away when those threats would have to cross a state line to get to them as compared with relatively greater worry for the same threats at the same objective but within the same state (Mishra & Mishra, 2010). A boundary necessarily, if arbitrarily, parses space, and people readily use boundaries to make sense of the distance on either side of them.

A boundary creates two big here-or-there chunks. That one chunk, holding actual distance constant, makes there feel farther than here. Beyond this binary distinction, the same rule of more chunks elongating distance applies as more and more get added to distance. Units of measurement create one means by which chunks become bountiful or scant. Ask people to measure distance in the smaller unit of feet, and they tend to overestimate its length, but measure in the larger unit of yards, and their estimates will likely fall short of how long it actually is (Maglio & Trope, 2011). Time measurement, too, proves susceptible to the effects of chunking. More discrete events make time feel longer, so thinking of how much happened in the past year makes a year ago recede further into the subjective past than thinking of how dull it was (Zauberman, Levav, Diehl, & Bhargave, 2010; but see Kaju and Maglio [2022] for how expected memory distorts time perception). Be it millimeters or milliseconds, measuring distance in more precise, more numerous units expands its length.

Just as any distance gets presented in some unit of measurement, any object from which someone may be close or far gets assigned a name. Although names, like chunked units, might appear arbitrary, their impact on perceptions of distance is anything but. Certain names go in and out of fashion, but look more closely at names—specifically, the sounds that make them up—and a universal pattern emerges. Name sounds fall into different categories, and people unwittingly use one particular category to judge the distance between themselves and named things: where the mouth makes the sound. The mouth produces some sounds toward the front (by the lips), like the *ee* sound in *green*, and others toward the back (by the throat), like the *oo* sound in *blue*. Put these sounds in a name, and they turn out to track with how far away people see the named object as being. Observers looking at an object named *koov* (with a back vowel) rate it as farther away in physical space than the same object, at the same distance, named *keev* (a front vowel; Rabaglia, Maglio, Krehm, Seok, & Trope, 2016). Going from physical to social distance, people judge others named with front vowels (like Tim) as more similar to themselves than others named with back vowels (like Tom; Maglio & Feder, 2017).

People usually have no say over their names, but they can control how fast they say them and every other word that comes out of their mouths. Under the same broad banner of language, the rate of another's speech influences the measurement of psychological distance in much the same way as their name (Nussinson et al., 2024). In one study, researchers created audio clips engineered to play at fast or slow speeds. After listening to them, participants estimated the psychological distance between the speaker and their audience. The slower-paced clips led participants to expect that speakers were spatially and socially farther away from their audience (and a larger audience size as well). A separate study found that slow speech seems particularly relevant for temporally distant consequences as well. Therefore, across different dimensions of psychological distance, both what is said (e.g., a name) and how it is said (e.g., speech rate) color how observers make sense of distances associated with the people responsible for those words.

This section reviewed the forces that govern how people incorporate relevant information into their measurement of distance. Each instance begins with simple perception, observing distance beyond the self or consulting within the self to make a measurement of distance. In the process, perceptual information undergoes a transformation. The body, the mind, and the outside world inject their own distinct effects during the transformation of information into something usable—in other words, perception begets sense making. Once individuals make sense of the distances surrounding themselves, they turn to the next task: converting that coherent interpretation into a narrative that makes meaning.

WHAT DOES MEASUREMENT PREDICT?

Doing

Measurement of distance serves as the sense-making precursor to acting on that measurement. Measurers go from static to dynamic, ready to contract, expand, or avoid the length of distance between themselves, here and now, and the removed, remote, over-there thing. For geographical space, the simplest resulting action comes in the form of moving through that distance—or not. When the physical distance to a location feels longer and more daunting, people are more inclined to stay put (Nelson & Simmons, 2009). Backpack-wearers seeing distance as especially long can be understood in the same way. Their burdened condition lets them know that it will be more of a formidable trek than a simple walk in the park. In the interest of economizing action given limited physical energy, their elongated measurements reflect a mind aware of the heightened physiological costs associated with hauling across it. Only with this big con listed alongside any pros can the person conclude whether to attempt the pass.

Measurement of geographical space gives people the option of *whether* and how to move through that physical distance. They do not have that same luxury of choice for time, which marches forward regardless of whether anybody wants it to. Over time, doing relates not to whether but *when* and how to act. Inaction is, of course, the opposite of action, and procrastinators might justify the former today by promising to tackle the latter tomorrow—then put the task off a little longer when tomorrow rolls around. Perpetual postponement indefinitely delays progress toward goals because getting things done demands that tasks be started before they can be middled and then finished. Measuring distance in the right way kick-starts the hard work of doing. Sensing a short distance to undertaking an activity, like joining a gym or signing up for piano lessons, spurs action and achieves goals (McCrea, Liberman, Trope, & Sherman, 2008). On the flip side of that coin, a sense of short time backfires when applied to the amount of time available to act rather than the urgency of acting. If the next hour or two feel particularly brief rather than particularly long, work gets left undone

(Tonietto, Malkoc, & Nowlis, 2019). The future never stops turning into the present, and measurement of the time between now and later predicts action across time.

This holds true for small-scale to-do lists and medium-range goals, as well as for the broad scope of an autobiographical narrative. From day to day, people track the progression of more immediate and pressing concerns, like opening an investment account or lowering their blood pressure. On a much larger scale, people track the progression of their lives. Their measurement of time in the grand sweep of life shifts their priorities today. Despite the many ways to organize the chapters of one's life, an easy default goes by decade: your 20s, 30s, all the way up to 80s, 90s, and beyond if you play your cards and genetics right. Ask anyone their age, and not only can they answer, but they'll also be keenly attuned to whether it ends in a 9. Being 29, 39, or 79 makes it clear that, as of your next birthday, a new chapter starts. For that reason, a degree of "What am I doing with my life?" panic sets in among people when their age ends in 9. More than at other ages, they concern themselves with finding meaning in their lives. Their behavior, for better or worse (running a marathon, looking for an extramarital affair), follows suit (Alter & Hershfield, 2014). So called 9-enders have a sense that time is limited before their next birthday in much the same way that getting older creates a sense that time on Earth is limited. When people (and not only older people) see the remaining time of their lives as limited, they pursue social goals that prioritize emotional fulfillment (like savoring bonds with meaningful people) in order to make the most of the time they have left (Carstensen, Isaacowitz, & Charles, 1999).

Deciding

Doing something is, of course, its own kind of deciding. Many other decisions involve choosing between options, with measurement of distance figuring prominently into what gets picked. There's one way of thinking about time that, although they may not ponder it all that often, people can readily answer: When does the present end and the future begin? Although a nebulous estimation, answers to this question reliably predict what people do now in the service of their future. Seeing the present as shorter and the future as starting sooner makes people more likely to save money for retirement rather than spending it on today (Hershfield & Maglio, 2020). It is worth noting that the majority of respondents report that the future starts within the next day, which suggests that the effect is not necessarily driven by their answer making far-off retirement seem closer. Rather, there appears to be something inherent to the measurement of time itself that makes people more patient.

The question of when the future begins measures ever-present time in and of itself. Decisions also depend on how choosers measure the distance to the options they consider. Spending or saving can be recast as choosing between a good time for the present self and financial security for the future self. All the power lies with the present self, whose choices affect both selves (Maglio & Hershfield, 2021). The future self stands a better shot of a comfortable retirement when the present self sees a close social connection between the now and later selves (Hershfield & Bartels, 2018). Accordingly, interventions designed to bridge the gap between selves over time make present selves more generous to the people they will one day become. For instance, when people mentally travel from the present to the future, the time to get there feels longer, and the connection to the future self feels weaker. But ask them to start in the future and travel back to the present ("The year is 2055. Rewind back to 2025. Save for 2055 you!"), the trip feels shorter, and the connection feels stronger, making people more likely to invest in their personal, long-term well-being (Christensen, Hershfield, & Maglio, 2024).

Future selves might feel like others, but they tend to be notoriously silent. Other others, encountered in the present, communicate in ways that guide the measurement of distance. As an obvious entry point, they use verbs marked with tenses that correspond directly to time: past tense (*was*) relates to the past, future tense (*will be*) relates to the future, and present tense (*is*) relates to the present. When people read claims written in the present tense, such as a favorable online product review, those claims feel closer and ultimately more helpful (Fang & Maglio, 2024; see also Hansen & Wänke, 2010). Supporting *ad nauseum* advice from writing coaches, the same goes for the active voice, which also makes readers more likely to find claims true than identical claims written in the passive voice (Chan & Maglio, 2020; see also Kaju & Maglio, 2018).

In these instances, language pulls ideas closer to readers, making readers decide to believe those ideas. Lacking a clearly stated chance, such as a 90% probability that the claim is accurate, they use cues to infer closeness. Should communicators put chances in these exact terms, people still convert the odds to a subjective sense of likelihood before making decisions. In an illustrative experiment, attendees at a farmers' market were offered the choice between two free bottles of wine: one with a retail value of $15 and another with a retail value of $40 but with a 15% chance of contamination, rendering it undrinkable. Half of the participants were told that the odds of contamination had been revised upward, from a prior 10% chance, while the other half were told that the odds had been revised downward, from a prior 20% chance. Those who learned about the downward revision, measuring the same 15% chance as less risky, were more likely to choose the more expensive wine than those who learned about an upward revision (Maglio & Polman, 2016). Whether measuring the distance to items in a consideration set or distance in and of itself, people make sense of distance in order to make meaning through their decisions.

Feeling

People feel feelings in the present, but the source of those feelings can come from the past, the present, and the future. Adding this temporal component introduces the possibility that measuring distance across time shapes affective experiences. Everyone has heard that time flies when you're having fun, and almost everyone believes it (Tonietto, VanEpps, Malkoc, & Maglio, 2022). That belief is so strong that it works even in reverse and when applied to the past: You're having fun when time flies (Sackett, Meyvis, Nelson, Converse, & Sackett, 2010). When experimenters went to great deceptive lengths to con participants into thinking that time had passed especially quickly, participants rated what they did during that time, such as listening to a favorite song, as especially enjoyable. This isn't the only way that measured time makes songs more pleasant. In another study, research participants listened to a favorite song enough times to get sick of it, then came back to the lab the next day. Before another listening session, participants measured the previous day as rather far away or rather recent. Those who saw yesterday's overexposure as belonging to the distant past liked the latest listen more than those seeing it as closer (Galak, Redden, Yang, & Kyung, 2014). A subjective sense of time helps people recover from hedonic adaptation in much the same way as actual, objective time.

Holding actual distance constant, shifting measurement of that distance reduces feelings of satiation. A similar process occurs for harder feelings like anger and sadness. Negative emotions may feel all-encompassing, but their experience belongs to the individual in the here and now. Emotional intensity should decrease the more that people get out of the visceral. The fly-on-the-wall vantage point looks at the self's emotions as if they belong to another person. Such self-distancing imposes categorical social distance, transforming from first-person self to third-person other. People can flip from the first- to the third-person view by simply changing how they refer to themselves. They stay immersed in emotions when thinking of themselves with first-person pronouns like *I*, *me*, and *mine*, but calling the self names like *you*, *her/him/them*, or even one's own name fosters a sense of distance (Kross et al., 2014). As a result, feelings feel less overwhelming, and actions follow suit, such as performing better on a stressful task (Kross & Ayduk, 2017)—an effect that generalizes across all varieties of distance (Moran

& Eyal, 2022). It might not be time that heals all wounds as much as the right measurement of distance that offers new meaning.

Time figures just as prominently into increasing positive emotions as it does into decreasing negative emotions. For desirable states like happiness, the focal question changes from "How do I get some distance on this?" to "How am I using the time I have?" The way people feel about their lives and how much time they have at their disposal remain closely intertwined. Someone might wake in the morning and wonder how they can possibly accomplish everything they hope to do. That same someone might head to bed that night wondering where the day went. The happiness-sapping culprit behind both experiences is a sense of time scarcity, the pressed-for-time feeling that one has too much to do and not enough time in which to do it. When time scarcity makes people feel unhappy, they often respond by trying to make themselves happier, and often to their own detriment. Although life, liberty, and the pursuit of happiness are seen as unalienable rights, people may do well to waive that last one. Trying to make oneself happier has been shown to backfire, ultimately undermining well-being in what has come to be known as the *happiness paradox* (Mauss, Tamir, Anderson, & Savino, 2011). To understand why, consider someone on a quest for greater happiness. They realize that happiness often comes from doing things, and doing things takes time, making yet more happiness one more burdensome task on an already long to-do list. The more people try to be happier, the less time they sense themselves having, which ends up making them that much more miserable (Kim & Maglio, 2018).

Sure, people can solve this problem by increasing the actual amount of time they have, such as by spending money to outsource less-than-fulfilling tasks (Whillans, Dunn, Smeets, Bekkers, & Norton, 2017). Perhaps more productively, they can also have less actual time while simultaneously feeling as if time is more plentiful. One way to have it both ways comes from giving away time, like volunteering to help others (Mogilner, Chance, & Norton, 2012). Spending time on these kinds of tasks makes people feel more in control of their time, which creates a feeling of time affluence (the opposite of feeling hamstrung by commitments in pursuing happiness). Although donating time may remedy the pervasive, exhausting sense of time famine, one indeed can have too much of what's widely considered to be a good thing. Recent research suggests that there's a sweet spot when it comes to how much time one has at their disposal. To be sure, overcommitment leads to frazzled unhappiness. At the same time, being underbooked also undermines well-being (Sharif, Mogilner, & Hershfield, 2021). The surest path to a good life seems to include both enough important obligations to feel meaningful and flex time sprinkled in between for the freedom to explore.

WHAT IT ALL MEANS

The world is noisy, the human mind is limited, and the scattered bits the former throws at the latter need to gel. This process isn't easy. Perception brings information about psychological distance into the system, which undergoes a transformation from an incoherent jumble into something that ultimately comes to make some semblance of sense. Perception becomes perspective. Measurement of distance gives people a solid grounding in evaluating how big, long, or far distance feels. The ability to work with distance is crucial to finding and making meaning (Waytz, Hershfield, & Tamir, 2015). Once the mind has made sense of the distance it measures, it scaffolds this conclusion to construct a road map for what comes next. Distance becomes something to move through, to work with, to savor, or to change. In so doing, distance becomes a launchpad to understanding how the self relates to everything beyond. Conceptualized in this way, the self stands a chance of figuring out what it all means.

ACKNOWLEDGMENTS

Preparation of this chapter was supported by the Social Sciences and Humanities Research Council of Canada.

REFERENCES

Aggarwal, P., & Zhao, M. (2015). Seeing the big picture: The effect of height on the level of construal. *Journal of Marketing Research, 52*(1), 120–133.

Alter, A. L., & Hershfield, H. E. (2014). People search for meaning when they approach a new decade in chronological age. *Proceedings of the National Academy of Sciences, 111*(48), 17066–17070.

Alter, A. L., & Oppenheimer, D. M. (2008). Effects of fluency on psychological distance and mental construal (or why New York is a large city, but *New York* is a civilized jungle). *Psychological Science, 19*(2), 161–167.

Bar-Anan, Y., Liberman, N., & Trope, Y. (2006). The association between psychological distance and construal level: Evidence from an implicit association test. *Journal of Experimental Psychology: General, 135*(4), 609–622.

Bar-Anan, Y., Liberman, N., Trope, Y., & Algom, D. (2007). Automatic processing of psychological distance: Evidence from a Stroop task. *Journal of Experimental Psychology: General, 136*(4), 610 622.

Carstensen, L. L., Isaacowitz, D. M., & Charles, S. T. (1999). Taking time seriously: A theory of socioemotional selectivity. *American Psychologist, 54*(3), 165–181.

Chan, E. Y., & Maglio, S. J. (2019). Coffee cues elevate arousal and reduce level of construal. *Consciousness and Cognition, 70*, 57–69.

Chan, E. Y., & Maglio, S. J. (2020). The voice of cognition: Active and passive voice influence distance and construal. *Personality and Social Psychology Bulletin, 46*(4), 547–558.

Chan, E. Y., & Maglio, S. J. (2023). Seeing far: Abstract construal and visual distance judgments. *Psychonomic Bulletin & Review, 30*(6), 2196–2202.

Christensen, K. L., Hershfield, H. E., & Maglio, S. J. (2024). Back to the present: How direction of mental time travel affects perceptions of similarity over time and saving behavior. *Journal of Consumer Research, 51*(1), 761–774.

Fang, D., & Maglio, S. J. (2024). Time perspective and helpfulness: Are communicators more persuasive in the past, present, or future tense? *Journal of Experimental Social Psychology, 110*, 1–9.

Fiedler, K., Jung, J., Wänke, M., & Alexopoulos, T. (2012). On the relations between distinct aspects of psychological distance: An ecological basis of construal-level theory. *Journal of Experimental Social Psychology, 48*(5), 1014–1021.

Galak, J., Redden, J. P., Yang, Y., & Kyung, E. J. (2014). How perceptions of temporal distance influence satiation. *Journal of Experimental Social Psychology, 52*, 118–123.

Hansen, J., & Trope, Y. (2012). When time flies: How abstract and concrete mental construal affect the perception of time. *Journal of Experimental Psychology: General, 142*(2), 336–347.

Hansen, J., & Wänke, M. (2010). Truth from language and truth from fit: The impact of linguistic concreteness and level of construal on subjective truth. *Personality and Social Psychology Bulletin, 36*(11), 1576–1588.

Hershfield, H. E., & Bartels, D. M. (2018). The future self. In G. Oettingen, A. Sevincer, & P. Gollwitzer (Eds.), *The psychology of thinking about the future* (pp. 89–109). Guilford Press.

Hershfield, H. E., & Maglio, S. J. (2020). When does the present end and the future begin? *Journal of Experimental Psychology: General, 149*(4), 701–718.

Hu, J., & Maglio, S. J. (2018). When soon feels far and later looms imminent: Decoupling absolute and relative timing estimates. *Journal of Experimental Social Psychology, 76*(6), 169–174.

Kaju, A., & Maglio, S. J. (2018). Urgently yours: Temporal communication norms and psychological distance. *Journal of Consumer Psychology, 28*(4), 665–672.

Kaju, A., & Maglio, S. J. (2022). Yesterday's great expectations: Metamemory and retrospective subjective duration. *Journal of Experimental Social Psychology, 98*, Article 104242.

Kim, A., & Maglio, S. J. (2018). Vanishing time in the pursuit of happiness. *Psychonomic Bulletin & Review, 25*(4), 1337–1342.

Kross, E., & Ayduk, O. (2017). Self-distancing: Theory, research, and current directions. In J. M. Olson (Ed.), *Advances in experimental social psychology* (Vol. 55, pp. 81–136). Elsevier.

Kross, E., Bruehlman-Senecal, E., Park, J., Burson, A., Dougherty, A., Shablack, H., et al. (2014). Self-talk as a regulatory mechanism: How you do it matters. *Journal of Personality and Social Psychology, 106*(2), 304–324.

Liberman, N., & Förster, J. (2009). Distancing from experienced self: How global-versus-local perception affects estimation of psychological distance. *Journal of Personality and Social Psychology, 97*(2), 203–216.

Liberman, N., Trope, Y., McCrea, S. M., & Sherman, S. J. (2007). The effect of level of construal on the temporal distance of activity enactment. *Journal of Experimental Social Psychology, 43*(1), 143–149.

Loewenstein, G., Weber, E. U., Hsee, C. K., & Welch, N. (2001). Risk as feelings. *Psychological Bulletin, 127*(2), 267–286.

Maglio, S. J., & Feder, M. (2017). The making of social experience from the sounds in names. *Social Cognition, 35*(6), 663–674.

Maglio, S. J., & Hershfield, H. E. (2021). Pleas for patience from the cumulative future self. *Behavioral & Brain Sciences, 44*, e46.

Maglio, S. J., & Kwok, C. Y. N. (2016). Anticipating ambiguity prolongs the present: Evidence of a return trip effect. *Journal of Experimental Psychology: General, 145*(11), 1415–1419.

Maglio, S. J., & Polman, E. (2014). Spatial orientation shrinks and expands psychological distance. *Psychological Science, 25*(7), 1345–1352.

Maglio, S. J., & Polman, E. (2016). Revising probability estimates: Why increasing likelihood means increasing impact. *Journal of Personality and Social Psychology, 111*(2), 141–158.

Maglio, S. J., & Trope, Y. (2011). Scale and construal: How larger measurement units shrink length estimates and expand mental horizons. *Psychonomic Bulletin & Review, 18*(1), 165–170.

Maglio, S. J., & Trope, Y. (2012). Disembodiment: Abstract construal attenuates the influence of contextual bodily state in judgment. *Journal of Experimental Psychology: General, 141*(2), 211–216.

Maglio, S. J., Trope, Y., & Liberman, N. (2013a). The common currency of psychological distance. *Current Directions in Psychological Science, 22*(4), 278–282.

Maglio, S. J., Trope, Y., & Liberman, N. (2013b). Distance from a distance: Psychological distance reduces sensitivity to any further psychological distance. *Journal of Experimental Psychology: General, 142*(3), 644–657.

Mauss, I. B., Tamir, M., Anderson, C. L., & Savino, N. S. (2011). Can seeking happiness make people unhappy? Paradoxical effects of valuing happiness. *Emotion, 11*(4), 807.

McCrea, S. M., Liberman, N., Trope, Y., & Sherman, S. J. (2008). Construal level and procrastination. *Psychological Science, 19*(12), 1308–1314.

Mishra, A., & Mishra, H. (2010). Border bias: The belief that state borders can protect against disasters. *Psychological Science, 21*(11), 1582–1586.

Mogilner, C., Chance, Z., & Norton, M. I. (2012). Giving time gives you time. *Psychological Science, 23*(10), 1233–1238.

Moran, T., & Eyal, T. (2022). Emotion regulation by psychological distance and level of abstraction: Two meta-analyses. *Personality and Social Psychology Review, 26*(2), 112–159.

Mrkva, K., Travers, M., & Van Boven, L. (2018). Simulational fluency reduces feelings of psychological distance. *Journal of Experimental Psychology: General, 147*(3), 354–376.

Nelson, L. D., & Simmons, J. P. (2009). On southbound ease and northbound fees: Literal consequences of the metaphoric link between vertical position and cardinal direction. *Journal of Marketing Research, 46*(6), 715–724.

Nussinson, R., Elias, Y., Mentser, S., Bar-Anan, Y., & Gronau, N. (2019). Bidirectional effects of stimulus vertical position and construal level. *Social Psychology, 50*(3), 162–173.

Nussinson, R., Elias, Y., Yosef-Nitsan, E., Mentser, S., Zadka, M., Weinstein, Z., et al. (2021). Somewhere over the rainbow: Vertical position is associated with psychological distance and construal level. *Social Cognition, 39*(5), 632–655.

Nussinson, R., Rozenberg, I., Hatzek, A., Mentser, S., Navon, M., Gilead, M., et al. (2024). The poetry of psychological distance: Bidirectional associations between stimulus speed and its psychological distance and construal level. *Journal of Personality and Social Psychology, 127*(1), 58–83.

Proffitt, D., Stefanucci, J., Banton, T., & Epstein, W. (2003). The role of effort in perceiving distance. *Psychological Science, 14*(2), 106–112.

Rabaglia, C. D., Maglio, S. J., Krehm, M., Seok, J. H., & Trope, Y. (2016). The sound of distance. *Cognition, 152*, 141–149.

Rim, S., Min, K. E., Liu, P. J., Chartrand, T. L., & Trope, Y. (2019). The gift of psychological closeness: How feasible versus desirable gifts reduce psychological distance to the giver. *Personality and Social Psychology Bulletin, 45*(3), 360–371.

Sackett, A. M., Meyvis, T., Nelson, L. D., Converse, B. A., & Sackett, A. L. (2010). You're having fun when time flies: The hedonic consequences of subjective time progression. *Psychological Science, 21*(1), 111–117.

Sharif, M. A., Mogilner, C., & Hershfield, H. E. (2021). Having too little or too much time is linked to lower subjective well-being. *Journal of Personality and Social Psychology, 121*(4), 933.

Slepian, M. L., Masicampo, E., & Ambady, N. (2015). Cognition from on high and down low: Verticality and construal level. *Journal of Personality and Social Psychology, 108*(1), 1.

Stefanucci, J., Proffitt, D., Banton, T., & Epstein, W. (2005). Distances appear different on hills. *Perception & Psychophysics, 67*(6), 1052–1060.

Stephan, E., Liberman, N., & Trope, Y. (2011). The effects of time perspective and level of construal on social distance. *Journal of Experimental Social Psychology, 47*(2), 397–402.

Tonietto, G. N., Malkoc, S. A., & Nowlis, S. M. (2019). When an hour feels shorter: Future boundary tasks alter consumption by contracting time. *Journal of Consumer Research, 45*(5), 1085–1102.

Tonietto, G. N., VanEpps, E. M., Malkoc, S. A., & Maglio, S. J. (2022). Time will fly during future fun (but drag until then). *Journal of Consumer Psychology, 32*(3), 475–483.

Trope, Y., & Liberman, N. (2010). Construal level theory of psychological distance. *Psychological Review, 117*(2), 440–463.

Van Boven, L., & Caruso, E. M. (2015). The tripartite foundations of temporal psychological distance: Metaphors, ecology, and teleology. *Social and Personality Psychology Compass, 9*(11), 593–605.

Van Boven, L., Kane, J., McGraw, A. P., & Dale, J. (2010). Feeling close: Emotional intensity reduces perceived psychological distance. *Journal of Personality and Social Psychology, 98*(6), 872–885.

Wakslak, C. J., & Trope, Y. (2009). The effect of construal level on subjective probability estimates. *Psychological Science, 20*, 52.

Waytz, A., Hershfield, H. E., & Tamir, D. I. (2015). Mental simulation and meaning in life. *Journal of Personality and Social Psychology, 108*(2), 336–355.

Whillans, A. V., Dunn, E. W., Smeets, P., Bekkers, R., & Norton, M. I. (2017). Buying time promotes happiness. *Proceedings of the National Academy of Sciences, 114*(32), 8523–8527.

Witt, J., Proffitt, D., & Epstein, W. (2005). Tool use affects perceived distance, but only when you intend to use it. *Journal of Experimental Psychology: Human Perception and Performance, 31*(5), 880–888.

Zakay, D., & Block, R. A. (1997). Temporal cognition. *Current Directions in Psychological Science, 6*(1), 12–16.

Zauberman, G., Kim, B. K., Malkoc, S. A., & Bettman, J. R. (2009). Discounting time and time discounting: Subjective time perception and intertemporal preferences. *Journal of Marketing Research, 46*(4), 543–556.

Zauberman, G., Levav, J., Diehl, K., & Bhargave, R. (2010). 1995 feels so close yet so far: The effect of event markers on subjective feelings of elapsed time. *Psychological Science, 21*(1), 133–139.

Zhao, M., Lee, L., & Soman, D. (2012). Crossing the virtual boundary: The effect of task-irrelevant environmental cues on task implementation. *Psychological Science, 23*(10), 1200–1207.

CHAPTER 4

From Words to Bonds

The Science of Meaningful Conversations

Sebastian Speer, Laetitia Mwilambwe-Tshilobo, Lily Tsoi,
Shannon Burns, Abigail S. Weber, Emily B. Falk,
and Diana I. Tamir

The human mind is a remarkable thing. It allows us to transcend the boundaries of the here and now, leap across time and space, imagine far-off places and hypothetical worlds, and step into the lives and minds of others. As Trope and colleagues have shown, our ability to mentally travel beyond our immediate experience—to explore the distant past, envision the future, or contemplate abstract realities—gives us a sense of meaning (Trope & Liberman, 2003; Waytz, Hershfield, & Tamir, 2015). By stepping outside of ourselves, we transform our narrow perspectives into something broader and richer. And yet, a life of solitary internal reflection—even in a mind with the capacity for the most elaborate, creative, transcendent mental escapes—would be a lonely journey. Waking each day with no one to talk to, no one to share experiences with, no one to challenge or expand your perspective would be stifling and incomplete. The act of connecting with others—of building bridges across the distances that separate us—creates meaning in ways that individual cognition cannot achieve alone. Conversation is a key tool that makes this connection possible.

Through dialogue, we share our experiences and realities, invite others into our worlds, and step into theirs. Conversations can build bridges—not only across social distance but also across time, space, and abstract realms of thought. When we converse, we have the potential to access information and perspectives unavailable through direct experience (Epley & Schroeder, 2014), escape the confines of our own minds, explore new territories of thought, and construct meaning *together.*

Conversation creates meaning in at least two ways. First, it is a powerful means of connection. Conversations can form and strengthen the social bonds that bolster well-being (Ryff, 1995), self-esteem (Leary & Baumeister, 2000), happiness (Diener & Seligman, 2002), and physical health (Baumeister, Brewer, Tice, & Twenge, 2007) while helping to stave off loneliness and its risks for mortality (Yu, 2023). Second, conversation can itself serve as an act of meaning making. A "good" conversation reshapes how we understand ourselves, others, and the world around us (Heine, Proulx, & Vohs, 2006). It allows people to traverse psychological distance: Close friends reminisce about the distant past, dream about the future, and explore abstract ideas far removed from their immediate surroundings (Speer et al., 2024b). The further a conversation stretches across these distances, the more meaningful it may feel—much like an individual mind finds meaning by transcending the here and now (Waytz, Hershfield, & Tamir, 2015).

In this chapter, we explore how conversation helps people create meaning. We address three central questions: *Why do people have conversations?* We consider the personal, relational, and societal incentives for conversation and the benefits it provides. *How do conversations create social connection?* We identify the features and dynamics that allow conversations to shrink interpersonal distance and expand perspectives. *How can we create more meaningful conversations?* We examine common missteps that prevent people from achieving the full potential of conversation and offer insights into how to converse better.

Through this exploration, we argue that conversation is more than a tool for connection; it is a fundamental act of meaning making, bridging the distances that separate us from each other, our past and future selves, and the larger world. By understanding what makes conversations meaningful, we can better understand the human quest for meaning itself.

WHY DO PEOPLE HAVE CONVERSATIONS?

Conversations permeate human life (Dunbar, Marriott, & Duncan, 1997). From casual coffee shop exchanges to deep discussions with loved ones, people spend a considerable amount of their day in conversation (Mehl, Vazire, Ramírez-Esparza, Slatcher, & Pennebaker, 2007). Why do people spend so many of their waking hours in conversations? There are a multitude of benefits, manifesting at multiple levels, from individuals up to cultural groups (Figure 4.1). Conversations also carry risk, such as miscommunication, hurt feelings, privacy breaches, and cultural misunderstandings that can escalate tensions, damage relationships or

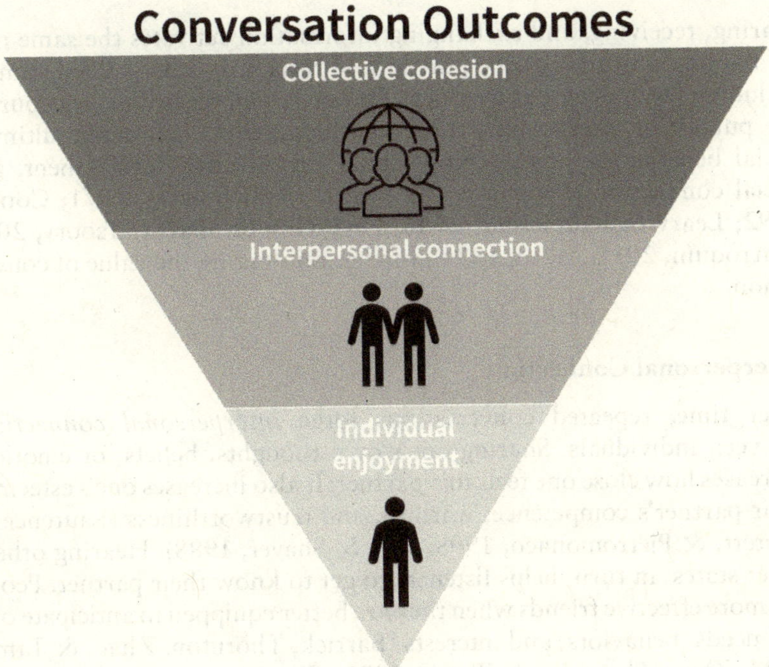

FIGURE 4.1. Why do people have conversations? Conversation benefits outcomes at the individual, dyadic, and collective levels.

reputations, and have legal implications, among others. However, in this chapter, we focus on the benefits of conversations.

Individual Enjoyment

People can derive *individual enjoyment* from conversation. Whether with friends, colleagues, acquaintances, or strangers, people frequently have conversations solely for enjoyment (Epley & Schroeder, 2014). People enjoy even shallow (Epley & Schroeder, 2014; Schroeder, Lyons, & Epley, 2022) and short interactions (Sandstrom & Dunn, 2014), although long and deep conversation with close others can enhance momentary mood (Kardas, Kumar, & Epley, 2022) and offer cognitive benefits such as increased creativity and problem-solving (Ybarra et al., 2008). The short-term enjoyment derived from an interaction provides an immediate reward, observable as reward-related brain activity (Baek, Scholz, O'Donnell, & Falk, 2017; Chan et al., 2023; Scholz et al., 2017; Tamir, Zaki, & Mitchell, 2015; Tamir & Mitchell, 2012). That is, the act of sharing, receiving, and exchanging information activates the same neural regions activated by the pursuit and receipt of other valued stimuli, including food, drugs, and money. This proximal reward may encourage the pursuit of interactions, through which people can derive ultimate social benefits such as emotion regulation, identity development, and social connection (Baumeister & Leary, 1995; Bowlby, 1971; Cooley, 1992; Leary & Baumeister, 2000; Levy-Gigi & Shamay-Tsoory, 2017; Marroquín, 2011; Mead, 1934), further reinforcing the value of conversation.

Interpersonal Connection

Over time, repeated conversations forge *interpersonal connections* between individuals. Sharing one's own thoughts, beliefs, or emotions increases how close one feels to a partner. It also increases one's esteem of their partner's competence, warmth, and trustworthiness (Laurenceau, Barrett, & Pietromonaco, 1998; Reis & Shaver, 1988). Hearing others' inner states, in turn, helps listeners to get to know their partner. People are more effective friends when they are better equipped to anticipate others' needs, behaviors, and interests (Barrick, Thornton, Zhao, & Tamir, 2024; Zhao, Thornton, & Tamir, 2022; Zhao, Sened, & Tamir, 2023). Responding with emotional support is particularly effective in strengthening social bonds between people (Morelli, Lee, Arnn, & Zaki, 2015). This bidirectional exchange of inner states facilitates effective future communication between people, iteratively ratcheting individuals into a shared reality (Garrod & Pickering, 2004)—a mutual understanding of oneself, partner, and perspectives about the external world (Higgins, Rossignac-Milon, & Echterhoff, 2021; Rossignac-Milon, Bolger, Zee, Boothby, & Higgins, 2021; Rossignac-Milon & Higgins, 2018). The more two people experience shared reality, the more they feel connected, close, and "clicked" into each other (Rossignac-Milon et al., 2021).

Collective Cohesion

Beyond building rapport with specific others, conversation fosters collective cohesion by aligning how the group or community views the world (Pizarro et al., 2022; Turner & Reynolds, 2011). Conversation is an effective tool for coordinating opinions, values, and perspectives about the world among a group of individuals (Clark & Brennan, 1991; Higgins et al., 2021). We see clear evidence that conversation aligns perspectives by looking at how it aligns neural activity. In the absence of conversation, each individual shows idiosyncratic responses to an incoming stimulus. The more idiosyncratic, or unaligned, a person's representation is of the world, the lonelier they are (Baek et al., 2023). After having a conversation, however, group members show aligned neural activity while viewing novel movie clips; each idiosyncratic discussion aligns members in an idiosyncratic way, leading to more similar activity between individuals within a group than between groups (Sievers, Welker, Hasson, Kleinbaum, & Wheatley, 2024). Conversation thus offers a powerful tool for aligning perspectives, both within regularly interacting groups and across collective cultures.

Culture may be defined by what people collectively agree is important to talk about (Fast, Heath, & Wu, 2009). This social rehearsal both reflects and elevates the cultural prominence of frequently rehearsed topics within the broader society (Echterhoff, Higgins, & Groll, 2005; Fast et al., 2009; Shteynberg, 2010; Valdesolo & DeSteno, 2011). Although cultures differ in their conversational norms (Floyd, 2021), shared opinions on topics that are frequently rehearsed become institutionalized and widely accepted, and they evolve through ongoing communication, influenced by broader societal contexts, ensuring the continuous construction and reinforcement of culture and collective cohesion (Wan, 2012). For instance, the shared belief in a country's founding myths or national values, such as freedom or democracy, is continuously reinforced through public holidays, education, and political discourse (Coenders & Scheepers, 2003; Fox, 2006). Over time, these shared opinions become deeply institutionalized, shaping the collective identity of a nation. Similar processes also play out in local communities, developing local norms and negotiating shared values.

HOW DO CONVERSATIONS CREATE SOCIAL CONNECTION?

Conversations can have powerful effects on individual well-being, interpersonal connection, and collective cohesion. However, not all conversations are created equal. Some are boring or frustrating, whereas others are calming or energizing; sometimes we wish conversations would keep going for hours, and sometimes we can't wait for them to end (Mastroianni, Gilbert, Cooney, & Wilson, 2021). What makes a conversation succeed? Here, we first consider how *an individual* contributes to a successful conversation by sharing information, making space for others, and bringing positivity (Table 4.1). However, conversation is more than the sum of its individual parts. Next, we highlight how *dyadic interactions* contribute to conversation success as separate individuals dynamically integrate their perspectives and move each other through content at the right moment and the right speed (Table 4.2).

TABLE 4.1. Individual and Dyadic Factors That Can Improve Conversation Outcomes

Conversation Feature	Description	Why It Leads to Success
Individual contributions		
Self-Disclosure	Sharing personal information, feelings, and experiences	Builds trust, fosters intimacy, encourages reciprocal sharing
Providing Space for Others	Making room for partner's input, asking questions, actively listening	Encourages partner disclosure, increases liking, demonstrates genuine interest
Increasing Positivity	Infusing humor, gratitude, and compliments into a conversation	Enhances enjoyment, improves mental and physical health, strengthens social bonds and relationship satisfaction
Dyadic dynamics		
Alignment (Synchrony)	Partners synchronize psychologically, behaviorally, and linguistically	Promotes fluency, reduces cognitive load, fosters similarity and consensus, signals social connection
Misalignment Divergence, Exploration, Complementarity	Partners provide novel ideas, avoid repetition, and adopt distinct roles	Increases engagement, insights, problem-solving, creativity, and emotion regulation
Balancing Alignment and Misalignment	Finding the right mix of alignment and misalignment depending on context and goals	Maximizes interpersonal understanding and deeper connections, creative exploration and problem-solving

What the Individual Contributes to Conversation Success

Sharing One's Perspective

One way of offering one's own perspective in conversation is through self-disclosure. Self-disclosure refers to the act of communicating personal information to another person, such as one's personality, preferences, behaviors, or internal experiences. This is a common activity—up to 40% of everyday speech comprises self-disclosure (Dunbar et al., 1997; Lipinski-Harten & Tafarodi, 2012). People are motivated to share their thoughts, feelings, and experiences with others, in part, because doing so is intrinsically rewarding (Tamir & Mitchell, 2012). Self-disclosure facilitates social bonding and learning, in part because it fosters feelings of liking, caring, and trust with a listener. It allows people to manage their reputation and present their best self to others; it allows people to teach others about their own experience so that others don't have to relearn each lesson on their own (Cozby, 1973; Jourard & Friedman, 1970; Jourard & Rubin, 1968; Tamir et al., 2015). It also allows people to offload intense emotional experiences to others (Nils & Rimé, 2012). Doing so often elicits comfort or advice from a partner, and receiving high-quality support is associated with higher conversation satisfaction and feelings of social connection (Guntzviller, MacGeorge, & Brinker, 2017). Self-disclosure also elicits reciprocal self-disclosure from listeners, feeding a cycle of disclosure that facilitates an intimacy that deepens close relationships (Altman & Taylor, 1973; Cozby, 1973) and staves off loneliness (Leung, 2002; Solano, Batten, & Parish, 1982).

Providing Space for the Other

Establishing social connection is not only about taking space for oneself. One also needs to make space for the other person to share their thoughts, feelings, and opinions. People who actively encourage their partner's disclosure and advice by asking questions are better liked by their partners and are more likely to sustain long-term connections (Brooks, Gino, & Schweitzer, 2015; Miller & Berg, 1983; Yeomans, Brooks, Huang, Minson, & Gino, 2019). For example, daters who ask more questions get more second dates (Huang, Yeomans, Brooks, Minson, & Gino, 2017); physicians who ask more questions to their patients provide more satisfying treatment (Bertakis, Roter, & Putnam, 1991). In contrast, focusing too much on oneself by boasting or dominating the conversation instead of asking questions reduces liking (Berman, Levine, Barasch, & Small, 2015; Vangelisti, Knapp, & Daly, 1990). Open-ended questions are particularly effective at encouraging partners to express their opinions, thoughts, and feelings (Foddy, 1993). After soliciting this disclosure, good conversation partners care to hear the response. Through active listening, listeners more effectively help their partners cope with adverse events (Jones, 2011), are perceived as more liked and attractive (Argyle & Cook, 1976), garner more trust (Mechanic & Meyer, 2000), and perform better at their jobs (Kluger & Itzchakov, 2022), thus fostering the deeper understanding and connection that are fundamental for close relationships (Duncan, Coatsworth, & Greenberg, 2009; Pasupathi, Carstensen, Levenson, & Gottman, 1999).

Increasing Positivity

Satisfaction, connection, and consensus can be built through conversations regarding negative topics, such as venting or seeking emotional support (Nils & Rimé, 2012; Trần, Szabó, Ward, & Jose, 2023). But on average, conversations are most enjoyable when they include positivity, which can come in several forms. First, one effective way of increasing positivity is through humor (Treger, Sprecher, & Erber, 2013). People desire a sense of humor in a conversation partner (Fraley & Aron, 2004) and find humorous partners more sexually attractive (Bressler & Balshine, 2006) and likable (Li et al., 2009). Humor also offers a way of connecting (Curry & Dunbar, 2013) and making shared meaning (Semko & Schulenberg, 2023). Second, people who express positivity through gratitude experience better physical and mental health (Wood, Froh, & Geraghty, 2010), higher life satisfaction (Emmons & McCullough, 2003), and stronger relationship functioning (Algoe, Haidt, & Gabl, 2008; Algoe & Stanton, 2012). Similarly, the simple act of giving a compliment has been shown to increase interpersonal liking and facilitate social connection (Boothby & Bohns, 2021).

How Partners Create Conversation Success

An individual can influence the enjoyment, interpersonal connection, and group consensus that builds from conversation by discussing particular things. However, good conversations are not just about what an *individual* is saying but also how the information flows *between the conversation partners*. Meaningful conversations are not characterized by constant high levels of self-disclosure or joking around, and inflexibility in this respect can lead to awkwardness (Cozby, 1972). Instead, conversation partners have to dynamically and interactively build up to more intimate disclosures and mutually enjoyable topics. To fully understand how social interactions generate connection, we must study the emergent processes between partners and the mutual organization of the interaction. Here we identify two dynamics people use in conversation and their consequences for social connection.

The Social Benefits of Alignment

Alignment is a frequently studied type of integration between partners in which they match each other conceptually and behaviorally. It often occurs spontaneously in natural conversation. People instinctively mimic or synchronize with each other's motor movements, eye movements, language, tone, and physiological responses (Cacioppo et al., 2014;

Prochazkova, Sjak-Shie, Behrens, Lindh, & Kret, 2021; Wynn & Borrie, 2022). Alignment offers a strong predictor of social connection because it reflects and promotes conversation fluency, interpersonal similarity, and shared consensus.

First, alignment in conversation facilitates connection because it reduces the complexity and increases the fluency of the interaction (daSilva & Wood, 2025; Koban, Ramamoorthy, & Konvalinka, 2019). When synchronized, the interaction partners can cognitively "chunk" the many moving parts of their interaction into fewer parts that are less demanding to process, thereby alleviating the cognitive load on the dyad. This simplification through synchronization enables partners to better anticipate and understand each other's actions (Brown-Schmidt, Yoon, & Ryskin, 2015; daSilva & Wood, 2025; Garrod & Pickering, 2009; Templeton, Chang, Reynolds, Cone LeBeaumont, & Wheatley, 2022). For example, linguistic alignment, which happens as dyads converge on matched expressions to refer to objects, as well as shared grammatical structure, facilitates better interpersonal understanding (Branigan, Pickering, & Cleland, 2000; Brennan & Clark, 1996; Garrod & Anderson, 1987; Hawkins, Frank, & Goodman, 2020). Nonverbal synchrony, such as posture, movement, gestures, and vocal tone, promotes better problem-solving in conversations (Shockley, Santana, & Fowler, 2003) and better social outcomes, such as liking (Chartrand & Bargh, 1999; Lakin & Chartrand, 2003; McEllin, Knoblich, & Sebanz, 2020), rapport (Vacharkulksemsuk & Fredrickson, 2012), trust (Cornejo et al., 2018), positivity, and connection (Cacioppo et al., 2014).

Second, alignment offers a cue to interpersonal similarity. People choose social partners to be similar along nearly every attribute, including race, personality, politics, and academic performance (Antonoplis & John, 2022; Huber & Malhotra, 2017; McPherson, Smith-Lovin, & Cook, 2001; Smirnov & Thurner, 2017). Seeing that someone else is similar to you through signals of alignment could serve as a cue for potential social connection. For example, using the same vocabulary, signaling shared traits, and finding common ground are all associated with interpersonal attraction (daSilva & Wood, 2025; Montoya, Horton, & Kirchner, 2008). Alignment of gestures and speech is associated with enhanced rapport, prosocial intentions, and social connection (Chartrand & Bargh, 1999; Cornejo et al., 2018; Lakin & Chartrand, 2003; Vacharkulksemsuk & Fredrickson, 2012). Perceived interpersonal similarity, in turn, further enhances alignment, promoting a positive feedback loop of connection (Cirelli, 2018; daSilva & Wood, 2025).

Finally, alignment arises when two people share similar views of the world (Yeshurun et al., 2017). When people agree on content, this alignment of mental states facilitates shared understanding (Kelsen,

Sumich, Kasabov, Liang, & Wang, 2022). This mental and conceptual alignment is associated with positive conversational outcomes, such as emotional support (Doré & Morris, 2018), interpersonal liking (Ireland et al., 2011; Putman & Street, 1984; Street, Brady, & Putman, 1983), social influence (Ludwig et al., 2013), social cohesion (Konvalinka et al., 2011), intimacy, compliance (Jacob, Guéguen, Martin, & Boulbry, 2011; Ramseyer & Tschacher, 2011), perceptions of similarity (Valdesolo & DeSteno, 2011), and cooperation (Tunçgenç & Cohen, 2018; Valdesolo & DeSteno, 2011; Wiltermuth & Heath, 2009). Neural and physiological synchrony are associated with greater understanding across a range of relationship types, including between strangers (Jiang et al., 2012), between counselors and clients (Zhang, Meng, Hou, Pan, & Hu, 2018), and between managers and employees (Balconi & Fronda, 2020). Conversation thus brings people into alignment (Mwilambwe-Tshilobo et al., 2024; Sievers et al., 2024).

The Social Benefits of Misalignment

However, alignment may not be the full story. If alignment were always a desirable state between people, then most conversations would consist of topics and actions that are easy to align to, like small talk and repetition. But conversations also need to be engaging. Partners need to provide each other with novel ideas, opportunities to learn, and surprising information. This opens up a role for other integrative conversation dynamics, such as divergence, exploration, and complementarity, that allow for individuality while still fostering effective communication.

First, *divergence* allows people to make more interesting, unique contributions to a conversation. People want their conversation partners to make unexpected and unique contributions (See, Roller, Kiela, & Weston, 2019). Surprises and unexpected information tend to capture people's attention, making the conversation more intriguing and less monotonous (Westgate & Wilson, 2018). A recent hyperscanning study showed that friends benefit from sharing common ground with each other from the start of a conversation. This common ground serves as a safe starting point from which they can diverge quickly in neural, linguistic, and topic space and enjoy better conversations as a result. Strangers, on the other hand, frequently start more distant and use the conversation to become mentally aligned over time (Figure 4.2). The more strangers can diverge and explore like friends, however, the more they enjoy the conversation and feel close to the conversation partner (Speer et al., 2024b). Similarly, securely attached children show less autonomic synchrony with their parents than insecurely attached ones (Nguyen, Kungl, Hoehl, White, & Vrtička, 2024). Thus, safely rooted

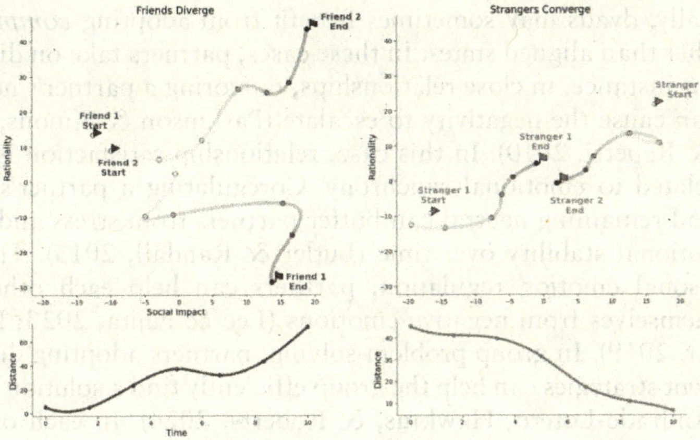

FIGURE 4.2. Friends explore mental space, whereas strangers align mentally. Adapted from Speer et al. (2024b).

relationships may facilitate the kinds of exploratory conversation dynamics that promote more enjoyable, interesting conversations.

Second, *exploration* of a wide range of conceptual space may enable problem-solving. Problem-solving conversations involve less semantic and grammatical repetition than affiliative conversations (Dideriksen, Christiansen, Tylén, Dingemanse, & Fusaroli, 2023). This may be because although synchrony enhances the predictability of social interactions, the increased predictability comes with the trade-off of greater redundancy and less information exchanged (Hoehl, Fairhurst, & Schirmer, 2021; Koban et al., 2019). This is less of an issue when a conversation goal is to signal relatability, but it is a concern when optimal problem-solving depends on partners bringing unique, diverse, and complementary ideas to the table. When partners can notice and react to environmental events independently, the dyad gains the advantage of having multiple perspectives (Gomes & Semin, 2020). For example, a recent hyperscanning study found that dyads discussing solutions to societal problems were more likely to agree on an optimal solution if they explored more ground in conversation and more diverse mental states (Speer et al., 2024a). In contrast, when partners commit too early to a single shared strategy or show too much synchrony, they risk being stuck with a suboptimal solution (Abney, Paxton, Dale, & Kello, 2015; Shirado & Christakis, 2017; Wallot, Mitkidis, McGraw, & Roepstorff, 2016). Thus, escaping similarity by diverging from one's partner in conversation may ultimately aid in agreement and finding new, optimal solutions to tough problems.

Finally, dyads may sometimes benefit from adopting *complementary* rather than aligned states. In these cases, partners take on different roles. For instance, in close relationships, mirroring a partner's negative affect can cause the negativity to escalate (Parkinson & Simons, 2012; Saxbe & Repetti, 2010). In this case, relationship satisfaction is *negatively* related to emotional synchrony. Coregulating a partner's affect by instead remaining neutral can buffer partners from stress and facilitate emotional stability over time (Butler & Randall, 2013). Through interpersonal emotion regulation, partners can help each other distance themselves from negative emotions (Lee & Fujita, 2023; Powers & LaBar, 2019). In group problem-solving, partners adopting different concurrent strategies can help the group efficiently find a solution (Goldstone, Andrade-Lotero, Hawkins, & Roberts, 2024). In each of these cases, adopting distinct, complementary roles can be more beneficial for successful interaction than alignment.

Balancing Alignment and Misalignment

Together, alignment and divergence give minds a virtuosic ability to traverse psychological distance. According to construal-level theory, psychological distance—whether across time, space, social perspectives, or hypothetical possibilities—shapes how people represent experiences. Proximal experiences are construed concretely, with vivid details, whereas distal experiences are construed more abstractly (Trope & Liberman, 2003). Each individual human mind has a fantastic ability to traverse distance at will. This power magnifies in the presence of other minds as conversation partners dynamically draw each other into their own high- or low-level construal. In particular, conversations provide a unique mechanism for modulating this distance by balancing the two core dynamics discussed earlier: alignment and misalignment (Table 4.2).

Conversation spontaneously aligns people—in body, behavior, voice, and mind—and in doing so, it increases interaction fluency, interpersonal similarity, and group consensus (daSilva & Wood, 2025; Kelsen et al., 2022; Prochazkova et al., 2021; Sievers et al., 2024). In this way, alignment is a signal that reflects and generates decreased psychological distance between two people. This affects how people process information about each other and, ultimately, their relationship (Chavez, Guthrie, & Kapustka, 2025). Smaller psychological distance facilitates concrete and detailed representations (Liberman & Trope, 2014; Liviatan, Trope, & Liberman, 2008; Trope, Liberman, & Wakslak, 2007). This makes it easier to take another's perspective and empathize, improving intergroup interactions and conflict resolution (Brewer & Miller, 1983; Ensari &

TABLE 4.2. Proposed Effects of High and Low Construal on Conversation Outcomes

Construal Level	Benefits
High-Level Construal	**Facilitates Creative Problem-Solving:** Enables exploration of diverse ideas and connections, leading to innovative solutions
	Enhances Emotional Support: Focuses on broader emotional states, promoting stability and understanding (Lee & Fujita, 2023)
	Identifies Core Issues: Helps in recognizing essential elements and overarching themes in conversations (Gomes & Semin, 2020)
Low-Level Construal	**Improves Interpersonal Empathy:** Concrete details enhance perspective-taking and emotional connection (Liberman & Trope, 2014).
	Enhances Conversation Fluency: Synchronizing reduces cognitive load and increases interaction fluency (Brown-Schmidt et al., 2015).
	Builds Interpersonal Connection: Shared concrete details foster similarity and rapport among conversation partners (daSilva & Wood, 2024).
	Increases Clarity: Concrete and detailed communication can facilitate mutual understanding (Liberman & Trope, 2014).

Miller, 2002; Firat & Ataca, 2022). Ultimately, the psychological proximity between people and ideas that comes with alignment facilitates bonding and more efficient interpersonal coordination.

At the same time, people also benefit from the psychological distance that comes from conversational polyphony—captured as divergence, exploration, and complementarity. Greater psychological distance leads individuals to think more abstractly, focusing on the broader, essential features rather than specific details (Liberman & Trope, 2014; Trope et al., 2007). In affiliative conversations, abstraction may enable people to see connections between seemingly distant topics, apply ideas across various contexts, and in doing so, generate a conversation that is more informative and engaging because it covers a wider range of topics. In problem-solving conversations, abstraction facilitates the identification of core issues and the generation of creative solutions as associations between initially seemingly unrelated objects become apparent from a greater distance. This can help dyads bridge diverse perspectives and foster more creative and effective collaboration (Gomes & Semin, 2020; Shirado & Christakis, 2017). Thus, the psychological distance afforded by a *lack* of alignment (i.e., wider divergence or exploration) in conversations facilitates more effective and creative problem-solving, emotional support, and more meaningful connections.

Ultimately, conversations need to balance alignment and divergence (Ravreby, Shilat, & Yeshurun, 2022). The optimal strategy may depend on to whom one is talking or what one's conversation goals are. The same dynamics that work for friends may not work for strangers (Templeton, Chang, Reynolds, Cone LeBeaumont, & Wheatley, 2023). At times, alignment and finding common ground may be the sole goal; at other times, divergence, exploration, or complementarity will facilitate positive conversation outcomes more than alignment. Prior work has shown that people's needs for proximity or distance will modulate the kinds of conversation topics, partners, and contexts that they need (Lee & Fujita, 2023). Future work can test the impact of proximity and distance on people's choice for alignment or divergence dynamics and with close or far interlocutors, respectively. Conversation dynamics may also need to change as the conversation unfolds. For example, although strangers might initially look for common ground, once this is established, they will be on stronger footing to explore more novel topics together (Sened, Speer, Cooney, Reece, & Tamir, 2024). In joint tasks, the best approach may be to alternate between alignment and divergence, balancing independent work with collaborative efforts (Paulus, 2000; Pentland et al., 2014; Wiltshire, Butner, & Fiore, 2018). This allows the group to leverage both the unique contributions of individuals and the combined strength of a cohesive team. By alternately shrinking and expanding psychological distance, alignment and misalignment shape the construal of experiences in conversation. This dynamic movement enhances the flexibility and richness of any individual human mind, elevating conversation into a powerful tool for meaning making.

HOW CAN PEOPLE HAVE MORE MEANINGFUL CONVERSATIONS?

People establish social connections and shape each other's perspectives on the world through conversation, but they do not always know what makes for a successful interaction. In many domains of life, people are overly confident in their skills, such as investors in their forecasting ability (Chuang & Lee, 2006; Statman, Thorley, & Vorkink, 2006), students in their academic performance (Dunlosky & Rawson, 2012), or everyone in their ability to detect lies (Bond & DePaulo, 2006; Vrij, Mann, & Fisher, 2006). Conversations are an odd exception in this regard: People commonly underestimate their and their partner's conversational skills and motivation and have overly pessimistic expectations of the value and potential of future conversations, starting before a conversation even begins and continuing until after the conversation ends (Boothby, Cooney, Sandstrom, & Clark, 2018; Mastroianni et al., 2021). As a consequence, people may perceive conversations as more awkward than they are or misjudge the interest of a stranger in having a conversation, both of which can reduce the chance of forming a social connection. Luckily, there are ways people can become better at preparing for and starting a conversation, engaging in deeper conversations, ending conversations, and more accurately evaluating conversations *after* they happen (Figure 4.3).

Preparing for a Conversation

When preparing for a conversation, it is important to be aware of one's conversation goals. In fact, people often fail to clearly identify their own conversational objectives (Yeomans, Schweitzer, & Brooks, 2022). Part of the reason for this failure is that people's goals change over time and sometimes even within a conversation. In addition, people can harbor competing goals in a conversation. For instance, short-term goals such as enjoyment can sometimes be pitted against long-term goals such as maintaining trust in conversations. Failure to identify one's own goal may lead to dissatisfaction in conversation and a potential loss of social connection. One approach to tackling this issue is to prepare by reflecting on one's goals before entering the conversation. Even just half a minute of preplanning can assist individuals in selecting more mutually beneficial and enjoyable conversation topics and aid individuals in effectively pursuing their objectives throughout the conversation (Rogers, Milkman, John, & Norton, 2015).

Congruently, discerning the other partner's conversation goal is an essential aspect of ensuring a successful conversation (Yeomans et al., 2022). People underestimate the extent to which others' goals can diverge from their own. One reason could be that people egocentrically over-rely on their own motives as a guide for the motives of others (Epley, Keysar, Van Boven, & Gilovich, 2004). This overconfidence in inferring others' states may hinder us from seeking more information, exacerbating the issue. In addition, relationships are fluid, and people take on different roles in relationships at different times (Fitzsimons & Finkel, 2018). Therefore, it is crucial to be aware of which role is currently needed and be attentive to the potential for shifts in these needs. Further, conversation partners may not always reveal accurate information about their goals and needs. In some contexts, lack of information, downright deception, or strategic motives for relational concerns may prevent people from gaining access to accurate information (Yeomans et

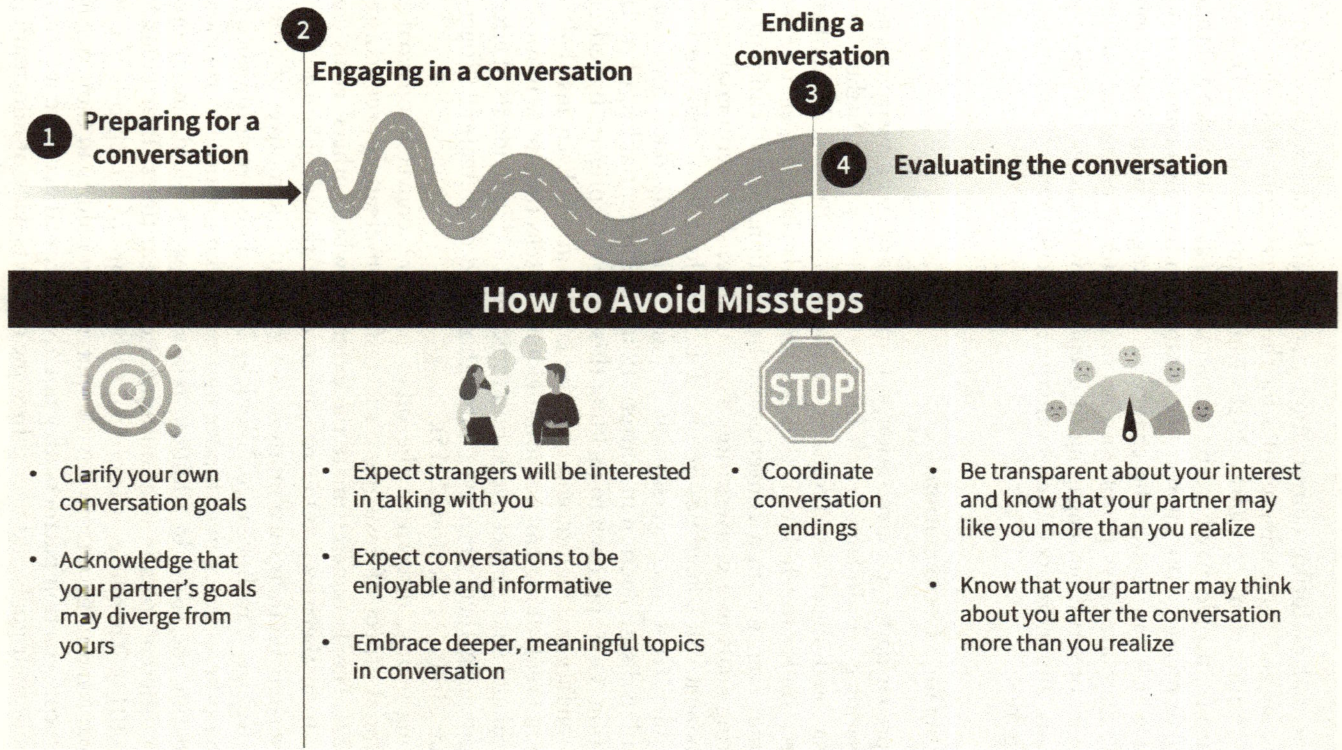

FIGURE 4.3. Steps to creating more meaningful conversation and avoiding common missteps.

al., 2022). Thus, identifying one's own goals and discerning the conversation partner's motives can go a long way in establishing social connection in conversations.

Engaging in Conversation

When people are about to engage in a new conversation, they need to assess whether their partner is interested in interacting. The more interested the partner, the more likely people are to start up a conversation. A common reason to avoid starting a conversation with a stranger might be that people underestimate their interest in connecting. To test this hypothesis, two separate studies (Epley & Schroeder, 2014; Schroeder et al., 2022) instructed commuters on public transport to start a conversation with a stranger near them or to remain disconnected. The authors found that participants reported a more positive experience when they conversed with a stranger than when they remained in solitude. Notably, participants reported anticipating the direct opposite outcome, expecting a more positive experience in solitude. The reason for this inaccurate prediction was that participants underestimated the interest of a stranger in connecting with them through a conversation (Epley & Schroeder, 2014; Schroeder et al., 2022). Relatedly, people underestimate how much they can learn from a conversation (Atir, Wald, & Epley, 2022). This is important because the amount people anticipate to learn predicts their interest in engaging in a conversation. Recalibrating these expectations can help people start conversations that they will ultimately enjoy.

Once people successfully enter a conversation, there are additional obstacles to overcome. People underestimate how much they will enjoy deep conversations with a stranger (Kardas et al., 2022). Conversationalists avoid asking sensitive questions because they overestimate how uncomfortable it will make their conversation partner feel (Hart, VanEpps, & Schweitzer, 2021). People worry that asking sensitive questions will result in negative perceptions. However, people formed similarly favorable impressions of conversational partners who asked more sensitive questions, such as "How much is your salary," as compared with partners who asked nonsensitive questions. In addition, dyads who had deep conversations felt more connected than dyads who remained at a shallow level. Thus, people need not shy away from more sensitive questions. Instead, approaching deeper conversation topics can foster social connection. Together, these studies suggest that interventions targeted at improving the calibration of expectations could help people to engage in more conversations in more meaningful ways to establish new social connections.

Ending a Conversation

When people are nearing the end of a conversation, they are faced with another challenge: When, precisely, should the conversation end? It could be assumed that if people enter the conversation with a clear goal, the conversation ends as soon as the goal is accomplished. However, people might not always be aware of their or their partner's goals, and the goals may differ, which increases the uncertainty about when it is best to end the conversation. Also, because most conversations aim to build or maintain social connections, people usually follow many rules meant to protect each other's feelings (Goffman, 1967). Ending a conversation prematurely or perpetuating a conversation beyond the partner's wishes are both violations of these conventions. Terminating conversations can therefore be thought of as a coordination problem (Friedman, 2012), in which a person's actions are based on what they assume their partner will and wants to do. Empirical evidence shows that conversations almost never conclude when both conversants desire, and they rarely end even when just one participant wants to, with the typical conversation lasting about half as long as desired (Mastroianni et al., 2021). This occurs because conversation partners overestimate the difference between their partners' desires about ending the conversation and their own. This might be due to a failure to correctly identify one's own and the other's motives for the conversation. Clearer communication of one's goals for conversation may facilitate ending the conversation at the right moment.

Evaluating the Conversation

Conversations, especially ones with strangers, rarely feel easy. This (undue) unease persists even after the conversation ends as people evaluate their performance and worry about what conversation partners really think about them. People are often left uncertain about how their partners enjoyed their company and whether they would like to interact again. In fact, Boothby and colleagues (2018) found that people consistently underestimated how much their conversation partners liked them, a miscalibration that has been termed the *liking gap*. This liking gap prevailed over short, medium, and long conversations and even over the course of a year. Why is it so hard for people to gauge their partners' enjoyment and liking? Similar to the uncertainty about ending conversations, politeness conventions in conversation may obscure conversants' true feelings. Relatedly, people may be cautious to convey and signal interest in their partners in case this interest is not reciprocated. This also relates to the problem of ambiguity around the conversation partner's motives. In addition, conversations are cognitively demanding, and conversants may thus fail to pick up on subtle cues their partner is sending because they are too busy planning what to say next and managing the impression they are making. The liking gap may have a functional purpose in that it helps people to focus on conversation mistakes that they can avoid in future conversations.

Another bias that complicates evaluations of past conversations is the *thought gap* (Cooney, Boothby, & Lee, 2022). After a conversation ends, people continue to reflect on their interaction partner. They think about their stories, their advice, and their criticisms. However, conversants systematically underestimate how much their partners think about *them*. Thus, there is an asymmetry in the availability of one's own thoughts compared with the partner's thoughts. With more salient conversations and time to accumulate reflections on a partner's contributions, the thought gap increases (Cooney et al., 2022).

Misconceptions and distorted expectations for conversations prevent people from engaging in conversation with strangers, interfere with people's ability to enjoy conversations and form connections during the interaction, and bias people's evaluations of the conversations. People typically have an overly pessimistic outlook on their own conversation skills, the potential of a conversation, and their partner's interest in them. One way to address these obstacles is by more clearly identifying and communicating one's own goals and more proactively exploring the conversation partner's needs and motives. This may boost people's confidence in their conversation skills and may facilitate engaging in more conversations with strangers to help people grow their social networks.

GENERAL SUMMARY

Conversations are a powerful tool for generating meaning through social connection, offering benefits at individual, dyadic, and collective levels. In this chapter, we have reviewed key insights into how individuals and dyads can contribute to successful conversation outcomes. Effective conversations involve individuals sharing their perspectives, creating space for others, and fostering positivity. Within these interactions, partners can both align their thoughts and explore differing viewpoints—two complementary mechanisms that adjust the psychological distance between people, ideas, and emotions. The success of a conversation hinges on skillfully balancing these dynamics to modulate construal level, tailoring scope to best serve personal and shared goals. Finally, avoiding common misconceptions about conversations can encourage more frequent, effective, and positively evaluated social exchanges.

Together, these insights open new avenues for understanding the psychology of conversation and the processes through which meaningful social connections are formed and maintained.

REFERENCES

Abney, D. H., Paxton, A., Dale, R., & Kello, C. T. (2015). Movement dynamics reflect a functional role for weak coupling and role structure in dyadic problem solving. *Cognitive Processing, 16*(4), 325–332.

Algoe, S. B., Haidt, J., & Gable, S. L. (2008). Beyond reciprocity: Gratitude and relationships in everyday life. *Emotion, 8*(3), 425–429.

Algoe, S. B., & Stanton, A. L. (2012). Gratitude when it is needed most: Social functions of gratitude in women with metastatic breast cancer. *Emotion, 12*(1), 163–168.

Altman, I., & Taylor, D. A. (1973). *Social penetration: The development of interpersonal relationships.* Holt, Rinehart, &Winston.

Antonoplis, S., & John, O. P. (2022). Who has different-race friends, and does it depend on context? Openness (to other), but not agreeableness, predicts lower racial homophily in friendship networks. *Journal of Personality and Social Psychology, 122*(5), 894–919.

Argyle, M., & Cook, M. (1976). *Gaze and mutual gaze.* Cambridge University Press.

Atir, S., Wald, K. A., & Epley, N. (2022). Talking with strangers is surprisingly informative. *Proceedings of the National Academy of Sciences, 119*(34), e2206992119.

Baek, E. C., Hyon, R., López, K., Du, M., Porter, M. A., & Parkinson, C. (2023). Lonely individuals process the world in idiosyncratic ways. *Psychological Science, 34*(6), 683–695.

Baek, E. C., Scholz, C., O'Donnell, M. B., & Falk, E. B. (2017). The value of sharing information: A neural account of information transmission. *Psychological Science, 28*(7), 851–861.

Balconi, M., & Fronda, G. (2020). Morality and management: An oxymoron? fNIRS and neuromanagement perspective explain us why things are not like this.. *Cognitive, Affective, & Behavioral Neuroscience, 20*(6), 1336–1348.

Barrick, E. M., Thornton, M. A., Zhao, Z., & Tamir, D. I. (2024). Individual differences in emotion prediction and implications for social success. *Emotion, 24*(7), 1697–1708.

Baumeister, R. F., Brewer, L. E., Tice, D. M., & Twenge, J. M. (2007). Thwarting the need to belong: Understanding the interpersonal and inner effects of social exclusion. *Social and Personality Psychology Compass, 1*(1), 506–520.

Baumeister, R. F., & Leary, M. R. (1995). The need to belong: Desire for interpersonal attachments as a fundamental human motivation. *Psychological Bulletin, 117*(3), 497.

Berman, J. Z., Levine, E. E., Barasch, A., & Small, D. A. (2015). The braggart's dilemma: On the social rewards and penalties of advertising prosocial behavior. *Journal of Marketing Research, 52*(1), 90–104.

Bertakis, K. D., Roter, D., & Putnam, S. M. (1991). The relationship of physician medical interview style to patient satisfaction. *Journal of Family Practice, 32*(2), 175–181.

Bond, C. F., & DePaulo, B. M. (2006). Accuracy of deception judgments. *Personality and Social Psychology Review, 10*(3), 214–234.

Boothby, E. J., & Bohns, V. K. (2021). Why a simple act of kindness is not as simple as it seems: Underestimating the positive impact of our compliments on others. *Personality and Social Psychology Bulletin, 47*(5), 826–840.

Boothby, E. J., Cooney, G., Sandstrom, G. M., & Clark, M. S. (2018). The liking gap in conversations: Do people like us more than we think? *Psychological Science, 29*(11), 1742–1756.

Bowlby, J. (1971). *Attachment and loss. Vol. 1: Attachment.* Basic Books.

Branigan, H. P., Pickering, M. J., & Cleland, A. A. (2000). Syntactic coordination in dialogue. *Cognition, 75*(2), B13–B25.

Brennan, S. E., & Clark, H. H. (1996). Conceptual pacts and lexical choice in conversation. *Journal of Experimental Psychology: Learning, Memory, and Cognition, 22*(6), 1482–1493.

Bressler, E. R., & Balshine, S. (2006). The influence of humor on desirability. *Evolution and Human Behavior, 27*(1), 29–39.

Brewer, M. B., & Miller, N. (1983). Beyond the contact hypothesis: Theoretical. In N. Miller & M. Brewer (Eds.), *Groups in contact: The psychology of desegregation* (pp. 281–302). Academic Press.

Brooks, A. W., Gino, F., & Schweitzer, M. E. (2015). Smart people ask for (my) advice: Seeking advice boosts perceptions of competence. *Management Science, 61*(6), 1421–1435.

Brown-Schmidt, S., Yoon, S. O., & Ryskin, R. A. (2015). People as contexts in conversation. In *Psychology of Learning and Motivation* (Vol. 62, pp. 59–99). Elsevier.

Butler, E. A., & Randall, A. K. (2013). Emotional coregulation in close relationships. *Emotion Review, 5*(2), 202–210.

Cacioppo, S., Zhou, H., Monteleone, G., Majka, E. A., Quinn, K. A., Ball, A. B., Norman, G. J., Semin, G. R., & Cacioppo, J. T. (2014). You are in sync with me: Neural correlates of interpersonal synchrony with a partner. *Neuroscience, 277*, 842–858.

Chan, Y., Scholz, C., Cosme, D., Martin, R. E., Benitez, C., Resnick, A., Carreras, J., Cooper, N., Paul, A. M., & Falk, E. B. (2023). Neural signals predict information sharing across cultures. *Proceedings of the National Academy of Sciences of the United States of America, 120*(44), 1–3.

Chartrand, T. L., & Bargh, J. A. (1999). The chameleon effect: The perception-behavior link and social interaction. *Journal of Personality and Social Psychology, 76*(6), 893–910.

Chavez, R. S., Guthrie, T. D., & Kapustka, J. M. (2025). Person knowledge is independently encoded by allocentric and egocentric reference frames within separate brain systems. *Psychological Science, 36*(4), 265–277.

Chuang, W.-I., & Lee, B.-S. (2006). An empirical evaluation of the overconfidence hypothesis. *Journal of Banking & Finance, 30*(9), 2489–2515.

Cirelli, L. K. (2018). How interpersonal synchrony facilitates early prosocial behavior. *Current Opinion in Psychology, 20*, 35–39.

Clark, H. H., & Brennan, S. E. (1991). Grounding in communication. In L. B. Resnick, J. M. Levine, & S. D. Teasley (Eds.), *Perspectives on socially shared cognition* (pp. 127–149). American Psychological Association.

Coenders, M., & Scheepers, P. (2003). The effect of education on nationalism and ethnic exclusionism: An international comparison. *Political Psychology, 24*(2), 313–343.

Cooley, C. H. (1992). *Human nature and the social order.* Cornell University Library.

Cooney, G., Boothby, E. J., & Lee, M. (2022). The thought gap after conversation: Underestimating the frequency of others' thoughts about us. *Journal of Experimental Psychology: General, 151*(5), 1069–1088.

Cornejo, C., Hurtado, E., Cuadros, Z., Torres-Araneda, A., Paredes, J., Olivares, H., Carré, D., & Robledo, J. P. (2018). Dynamics of simultaneous and imitative bodily coordination in trust and distrust. *Frontiers in Psychology, 9*, Article 1546.

Cozby, P. C. (1972). Self-disclosure, reciprocity and liking. *Sociometry, 35*(1), 151.

Cozby, P. C. (1973). Self-disclosure: A literature review. *Psychological Bulletin, 79*(2), 73–91.

Curry, O. S., & Dunbar, R. I. M. (2013). Sharing a joke: The effects of a similar sense of humor on affiliation and altruism. *Evolution and Human Behavior, 34*(2), 125–129.

daSilva, E. B., & Wood, A. (2025). How and why people synchronize: An integrated perspective. *Personality and Social Psychology Review, 29*(2), 159–187.

Dideriksen, C., Christiansen, M. H., Tylén, K., Dingemanse, M., & Fusaroli, R. (2023). Quantifying the interplay of conversational devices in building mutual understanding. *Journal of Experimental Psychology: General, 152*(3), 864–889.

Diener, E., & Seligman, M. E. P. (2002). Very happy people. *Psychological Science, 13*(1), 81–84.

Doré, B. P., & Morris, R. R. (2018). Linguistic synchrony predicts the immediate and lasting impact of text-based emotional support. *Psychological Science, 29*(10), 1716–1723.

Dunbar, R. I. M., Marriott, A., & Duncan, N. D. C. (1997). Human conversational behavior. *Human Nature, 8*(3), 231–246.

Duncan, L. G., Coatsworth, J. D., & Greenberg, M. T. (2009). A model of mindful parenting: Implications for parent–child relationships and prevention research. *Clinical Child and Family Psychology Review, 12*(3), 255–270.

Dunlosky, J., & Rawson, K. A. (2012). Overconfidence produces

underachievement: Inaccurate self evaluations undermine students' learning and retention. *Learning and Instruction, 22*(4), 271–280.
Echterhoff, G., Higgins, E. T., & Groll, S. (2005). Audience-tuning effects on memory: The role of shared reality. *Journal of Personality and Social Psychology, 89*(3), 257.
Emmons, R. A., & McCullough, M. E. (2003). Counting blessings versus burdens: An experimental investigation of gratitude and subjective well-being in daily life. *Journal of Personality and Social Psychology, 84*(2), 377–389.
Ensari, N., & Miller, N. (2002). The out-group must not be so bad after all: The effects of disclosure, typicality, and salience on intergroup bias. *Journal of Personality and Social Psychology, 83*(2), 313–329.
Epley, N., Keysar, B., Van Boven, L., & Gilovich, T. (2004). Perspective taking as egocentric anchoring and adjustment. *Journal of Personality and Social Psychology, 87*(3), 327–339.
Epley, N., & Schroeder, J. (2014). Mistakenly seeking solitude. *Journal of Experimental Psychology: General, 143*(5), 1980–1999.
Fast, N. J., Heath, C., & Wu, G. (2009). Common ground and cultural prominence: How conversation reinforces culture. *Psychological Science, 20*(7), 904–911.
Firat, M., & Ataca, B. (2022). Does perceived cultural distance mediate the relationship between intergroup contact and support for refugee rights? A preliminary investigation. *Journal of Community & Applied Social Psychology, 32*(1), 57–72.
Fitzsimons, G. M., & Finkel, E. J. (2018). Transactive-goal-dynamics theory: A discipline-wide perspective. *Current Directions in Psychological Science, 27*(5), 332–338.
Floyd, S. (2021). Conversation and culture. *Annual Review of Anthropology, 50*(1), 219–240.
Foddy, W. (1993). *Constructing questions for interviews and questionnaires: Theory and practice in social research.* Cambridge University Press.
Fox, J. E. (2006). Consuming the nation: Holidays, sports, and the production of collective belonging. *Ethnic and Racial Studies, 29*(2), 217–236.
Fraley, B., & Aron, A. (2004). The effect of a shared humorous experience on closeness in initial encounters. *Personal Relationships, 11*(1), 61–78.
Friedman, J. W. (2012). *Problems of coordination in economic activity* (Vol. 35). Springer Science & Business Media.
Garrod, S., & Anderson, A. (1987). Saying what you mean in dialogue: A study in conceptual and semantic co-ordination. *Cognition, 27*(2), 181–218.
Garrod, S., & Pickering, M. J. (2004). Why is conversation so easy? *Trends in Cognitive Sciences, 8*(1), 8–11.
Garrod, S., & Pickering, M. J. (2009). Joint action, interactive alignment, and dialog. *Topics in Cognitive Science, 1*(2), 292–304.
Goffman, E. (1967). *Interaction ritual: Essays in face-to-face behavior.* Routledge.
Goldstone, R. L., Andrade-Lotero, E. J., Hawkins, R. D., & Roberts, M. E. (2024). The emergence of specialized roles within groups. *Topics in Cognitive Science, 16*(2), 257–281.

Gomes, N., & Semin, G. R. (2020). Mapping human vigilance: The influence of conspecifics. *Evolution and Human Behavior, 41*(1), 69–75.

Guntzviller, L. M., MacGeorge, E. L., & Brinker, D. L. (2017). Dyadic perspectives on advice between friends: Relational influence, advice quality, and conversation satisfaction. *Communication Monographs, 84*(4), 488–509.

Hart, E., VanEpps, E. M., & Schweitzer, M. E. (2021). The (better than expected) consequences of asking sensitive questions. *Organizational Behavior and Human Decision Processes, 162*, 136–154.

Hawkins, R. D., Frank, M. C., & Goodman, N. D. (2020). Characterizing the dynamics of learning in repeated reference games. *Cognitive Science, 44*(6), e12845.

Heine, S. J., Proulx, T., & Vohs, K. D. (2006). The meaning maintenance model: On the coherence of social motivations. *Personality and Social Psychology Review, 10*(2), 88–110.

Higgins, E. T., Rossignac-Milon, M., & Echterhoff, G. (2021). Shared reality: From sharing-is-believing to merging minds. *Current Directions in Psychological Science, 30*(2), 103–110.

Hoehl, S., Fairhurst, M., & Schirmer, A. (2021). Interactional synchrony: Signals, mechanisms and benefits. *Social Cognitive and Affective Neuroscience, 16*(1–2), 5–18.

Huang, K., Yeomans, M., Brooks, A. W., Minson, J., & Gino, F. (2017). It doesn't hurt to ask: Question-asking increases liking. *Journal of Personality and Social Psychology, 113*(3), 430–452.

Huber, G. A., & Malhotra, N. (2017). Political homophily in social relationships: Evidence from online dating behavior. *Journal of Politics, 79*(1), 269–283.

Ireland, M. E., Slatcher, R. B., Eastwick, P. W., Scissors, L. E., Finkel, E. J., & Pennebaker, J. W. (2011). Language style matching predicts relationship initiation and stability. *Psychological Science, 22*(1), 39–44.

Jacob, C., Guéguen, N., Martin, A., & Boulbry, G. (2011). Retail salespeople's mimicry of customers: Effects on consumer behavior. *Journal of Retailing and Consumer Services, 18*(5), 381–388.

Jiang, J., Dai, B., Peng, D., Zhu, C., Liu, L., & Lu, C. (2012). Neural synchronization during face-to-face communication. *Journal of Neuroscience, 32*(45), 16064–16069.

Jones, S. M. (2011). Supportive listening. *International Journal of Listening, 25*(1–2), 85–103.

Jourard, S. M., & Friedman, R. (1970). Experimenter-subject "distance" and self-disclosure. *Journal of Personality and Social Psychology, 15*(3), 278–282.

Jourard, S. M., & Rubin, J. E. (1968). Self-disclosure and touching: A study of two modes of interpersonal encounter and their inter-relation. *Journal of Humanistic Psychology, 8*(1), 39–48.

Kardas, M., Kumar, A., & Epley, N. (2022). Overly shallow?: Miscalibrated expectations create a barrier to deeper conversation. *Journal of Personality and Social Psychology, 122*(3), 367–398.

Kelsen, B. A., Sumich, A., Kasabov, N., Liang, S. H. Y., & Wang, G. Y. (2022).

What has social neuroscience learned from hyperscanning studies of spoken communication? A systematic review. *Neuroscience & Biobehavioral Reviews, 132*, 1249–1262.

Kluger, A. N., & Itzchakov, G. (2022). The power of listening at work. *Annual Review of Organizational Psychology and Organizational Behavior, 9*, 121–146.

Koban, L., Ramamoorthy, A., & Konvalinka, I. (2019). Why do we fall into sync with others? Interpersonal synchronization and the brain's optimization principle. *Social Neuroscience, 14*(1), 1–9.

Konvalinka, I., Xygalatas, D., Bulbulia, J., Schjødt, U., Jegindø, E.-M., Wallot, S., Van Orden, G., & Roepstorff, A. (2011). Synchronized arousal between performers and related spectators in a fire-walking ritual. *Proceedings of the National Academy of Sciences, 108*(20), 8514–8519.

Lakin, J. L., & Chartrand, T. L. (2003). Using nonconscious behavioral mimicry to create affiliation and rapport. *Psychological Science, 14*(4), 334–339.

Laurenceau, J.-P., Barrett, L. F., & Pietromonaco, P. R. (1998). Intimacy as an interpersonal process: The importance of self-disclosure, partner disclosure, and perceived partner responsiveness in interpersonal exchanges. *Journal of Personality and Social Psychology, 74*(5), 1238–1251.

Leary, M. R., & Baumeister, R. F. (2000). The nature and function of self-esteem: Sociometer theory. In M. P. Zanna (Ed.), *Advances in experimental social psychology* (Vol. 32, pp. 1–62). Elsevier.

Lee, D. S., & Fujita, K. (2023). From whom do people seek what type of support? A regulatory scope perspective. *Journal of Personality and Social Psychology, 124*(4), 796–811.

Leung, L. (2002). Loneliness, self-disclosure, and ICQ ("I seek you") use. *CyberPsychology & Behavior, 5*(3), 241–251.

Levy-Gigi, E., & Shamay-Tsoory, S. G. (2017). Help me if you can: Evaluating the effectiveness of interpersonal compared to intrapersonal emotion regulation in reducing distress. *Journal of Behavior Therapy and Experimental Psychiatry, 55*, 33–40.

Li, N. P., Griskevicius, V., Durante, K. M., Jonason, P. K., Pasisz, D. J., & Aumer, K. (2009). An evolutionary perspective on humor: Sexual selection or interest indication? *Personality and Social Psychology Bulletin, 35*(7), 923–936.

Liberman, N., & Trope, Y. (2014). Traversing psychological distance. *Trends in Cognitive Sciences, 18*(7), 364–369.

Lipinski-Harten, M., & Tafarodi, R. W. (2012). A comparison of conversational quality in online and face-to-face first encounters. *Journal of Language and Social Psychology, 31*(3), 331–341.

Liviatan, I., Trope, Y., & Liberman, N. (2008). Interpersonal similarity as a social distance dimension: Implications for perception of others' actions. *Journal of Experimental Social Psychology, 44*(5), 1256–1269.

Ludwig, S., de Ruyter, K., Friedman, M., Brüggen, E. C., Wetzels, M., & Pfann, G. (2013). More than words: The influence of affective content and linguistic style matches in online reviews on conversion rates. *Journal of Marketing, 77*(1), 87–103.

Marroquín, B. (2011). Interpersonal emotion regulation as a mechanism of social support in depression. *Clinical Psychology Review, 31*(8), 1276–1290.

Mastroianni, A. M., Gilbert, D. T., Cooney, G., & Wilson, T. D. (2021). Do conversations end when people want them to? *Proceedings of the National Academy of Sciences, 118*(10), e2011809118.

McEllin, L., Knoblich, G., & Sebanz, N. (2020). Synchronicities that shape the perception of joint action. *Scientific Reports, 10*(1), 15554.

McPherson, M., Smith-Lovin, L., & Cook, J. M. (2001). Birds of a feather: Homophily in social networks. *Annual Review of Sociology, 27*(1), 415–444.

Mead, G. H. (1934). *Mind, self, and society from the standpoint of a social behaviorist.* University Chicago Press.

Mechanic, D., & Meyer, S. (2000). Concepts of trust among patients with serious illness. *Social Science & Medicine, 51*(5), 657–668.

Mehl, M. R., Vazire, S., Ramírez-Esparza, N., Slatcher, R. B., & Pennebaker, J. W. (2007). Are women really more talkative than men? *Science, 317*(5834), 82–82.

Miller, L. C., & Berg, J. H. (1983). Openers: Individuals who elicit intimate self-disclosure. *Journal of Personality and Social Psychology, 44*(6), 1234–1244.

Montoya, R. M., Horton, R. S., & Kirchner, J. (2008). Is actual similarity necessary for attraction? A meta-analysis of actual and perceived similarity. *Journal of Social and Personal Relationships, 25*(6), 889–922.

Morelli, S. A., Lee, I. A., Arnn, M. E., & Zaki, J. (2015). Emotional and instrumental support provision interact to predict well-being. *Emotion, 15*(4), 484–493.

Mwilambwe-Tshilobo, L., Tsoi, L., Speer, S. P. H., Burns, S., Falk, E. B., & Tamir, D. (2024). *Real-time conversation leads to neural alignment in friends and strangers* [Manuscript in preparation].

Nguyen, T., Kungl, M. T., Hoehl, S., White, L. O., & Vrtička, P. (2024). Visualizing the invisible tie: Linking parent–child neural synchrony to parents' and children's attachment representations. *Developmental Science, 27*(6), e13504.

Nils, F., & Rimé, B. (2012). Beyond the myth of venting: Social sharing modes determine the benefits of emotional disclosure. *European Journal of Social Psychology, 42*(6), 672–681.

Parkinson, B., & Simons, G. (2012). Worry spreads: Interpersonal transfer of problem-related anxiety. *Cognition & Emotion, 26*(3), 462–479.

Pasupathi, M., Carstensen, L. L., Levenson, R. W., & Gottman, J. M. (1999). Responsive listening in long-married couples: A psycholinguistic perspective. *Journal of Nonverbal Behavior, 23*(2), 173–193.

Paulus, P. (2000). Groups, teams, and creativity: The creative potential of idea-generating groups. *Applied Psychology, 49*(2), 237–262.

Pentland, D., Forsyth, K., Maciver, D., Walsh, M., Murray, R., & Irvine, L. (2014). Enabling integrated knowledge acquisition and management in health care teams. *Knowledge Management Research & Practice, 12*(4), 362–374.

Pizarro, J. J., Zumeta, L. N., Bouchat, P., Włodarczyk, A., Rimé, B., Basabe, N., Amutio, A., & Páez, D. (2022). Emotional processes, collective behavior, and social movements: A meta-analytic review of collective effervescence outcomes during collective gatherings and demonstrations. *Frontiers in Psychology, 13*, 974683.

Powers, J. P., & LaBar, K. S. (2019). Regulating emotion through distancing: A taxonomy, neurocognitive model, and supporting meta-analysis. *Neuroscience & Biobehavioral Reviews, 96*, 155–173.

Prochazkova, E., Sjak-Shie, E., Behrens, F., Lindh, D., & Kret, M. E. (2021). Physiological synchrony is associated with attraction in a blind date setting. *Nature Human Behaviour, 6*(2), 269–278.

Putman, W. B., & Street, R. L. (1984). The conception and perception of noncontent speech performance: Implications for speech-accommodation theory. *International Journal of the Sociology of Language*, 46, 97–114.

Ramseyer, F., & Tschacher, W. (2011). Nonverbal synchrony in psychotherapy: Coordinated body movement reflects relationship quality and outcome. *Journal of Consulting and Clinical Psychology, 79*(3), 284–295.

Ravreby, I., Shilat, Y., & Yeshurun, Y. (2022). Liking as a balance between synchronization, complexity and novelty. *Scientific Reports, 12*(1), 3181.

Reis, H. T., & Shaver, P. (1988). Intimacy as an interpersonal process. In S. Duck, D. F. Hay, S. E. Hobfoll, W. Ickes, & B. M. Montgomery (Eds.), *Handbook of personal relationships: theory, research and interventions* (pp. 367–389). Wiley.

Rogers, T., Milkman, K. L., John, L. K., & Norton, M. I. (2015). Beyond good intentions: Prompting people to make plans improves follow-through on important tasks. *Behavioral Science & Policy, 1*(2), 33–41.

Rossignac-Milon, M., Bolger, N., Zee, K. S., Boothby, E. J., & Higgins, E. T. (2021). Merged minds: Generalized shared reality in dyadic relationships. *Journal of Personality and Social Psychology, 120*(4), 882–911.

Rossignac-Milon, M., & Higgins, E. T. (2018). Epistemic companions: Shared reality development in close relationships. *Current Opinion in Psychology, 23*, 66–71.

Ryff, C. D. (1995). Psychological well-being in adult life. *Current Directions in Psychological Science, 4*(4), 99–104.

Sandstrom, G. M., & Dunn, E. W. (2014). Social interactions and well-being: The surprising power of weak ties. *Personality and Social Psychology Bulletin, 40*(7), 910–922.

Saxbe, D., & Repetti, R. L. (2010). For better or worse? Coregulation of couples' cortisol levels and mood states. *Journal of Personality and Social Psychology, 98*(1), 92–103.

Scholz, C., Baek, E. C., O'Donnell, M. B., Kim, H. S., Cappella, J. N., & Falk, E. B. (2017). A neural model of valuation and information virality. *Proceedings of the National Academy of Sciences, 114*(11), 2881–2886.

Schroeder, J., Lyons, D., & Epley, N. (2022). Hello, stranger? Pleasant conversations are preceded by concerns about starting one. *Journal of Experimental Psychology: General, 151*(5), 1141–1153.

See, A., Roller, S., Kiela, D., & Weston, J. (2019). *What makes a good conversation? How controllable attributes affect human judgments.* arXiv. *arxiv.org/abs/1902.08654*

Semko, J. H., & Schulenberg, S. E. (2023). Is humor a meaning making process? Investigating the effects of absurd humor and mortality salience on meaning in life, moral identity, belongingness, and belief in a just world. *Psychological Reports, 128*(3), 2000–2020.

Sened, H., Speer, S. P. H., Cooney, G., Reece, A. G., & Tamir, D. I. (2024). *The temporal arc of successful conversations* [Conference presentation]. Society for Personality and Social Psychology 2024 Conference, San Diego, CA, United States.

Shirado, H., & Christakis, N. A. (2017). Locally noisy autonomous agents improve global human coordination in network experiments. *Nature, 545*(7654), 370–374.

Shockley, K., Santana, M.-V., & Fowler, C. A. (2003). Mutual interpersonal postural constraints are involved in cooperative conversation. *Journal of Experimental Psychology: Human Perception and Performance, 29*(2), 326–332.

Shteynberg, G. (2010). A silent emergence of culture: The social tuning effect. *Journal of Personality and Social Psychology, 99*(4), 683.

Sievers, B., Welker, C., Hasson, U., Kleinbaum, A. M., & Wheatley, T. (2024). Consensus-building conversation leads to neural alignment. *Nature Communications, 15*(1), 3936.

Smirnov, I., & Thurner, S. (2017). Formation of homophily in academic performance: Students change their friends rather than performance. *PLOS ONE, 12*(8), e0183473.

Solano, C. H., Batten, P. G., & Parish, E. A. (1982). Loneliness and patterns of self-disclosure. *Journal of Personality and Social Psychology, 43*(3), 524.

Speer, S., Mwilambwe-Tshilobo, L., Tsoi, L., Burns, S. M., Falk, E. B., & Tamir, D. I. (2024a). *Mental state dynamics underlying persuasion and compromise* [Conference presentation]. Social Cognitive and Affective Neuroscience 2024 Conference, Toronto, Ontario, Canada.

Speer, S. P. H., Mwilambwe-Tshilobo, L., Tsoi, L., Burns, S. M., Falk, E. B., & Tamir, D. I. (2024b). Hyperscanning shows friends explore and strangers converge in conversation. *Nature Communications, 15*(1), 7781.

Statman, M., Thorley, S., & Vorkink, K. (2006). Investor overconfidence and trading volume. *Review of Financial Studies, 19*(4), 1531–1565.

Street, R. L., Brady, R. M., & Putman, W. B. (1983). The influence of speech rate stereotypes and rate similarity or listeners' evaluations of speakers. *Journal of Language and Social Psychology, 2*(1), 37–56.

Tamir, D. I., & Mitchell, J. P. (2012). Disclosing information about the self is intrinsically rewarding. *Proceedings of the National Academy of Sciences, 109*(21), 8038–8043.

Tamir, D. I., Zaki, J., & Mitchell, J. P. (2015). Informing others is associated with behavioral and neural signatures of value. *Journal of Experimental Psychology: General, 144*(6), 1114–1123.

Templeton, E. M., Chang, L. J., Reynolds, E. A., Cone LeBeaumont, M. D., & Wheatley, T. (2022). Fast response times signal social connection in conversation. *Proceedings of the National Academy of Sciences, 119*(4), e2116915119.

Templeton, E. M., Chang, L. J., Reynolds, E. A., Cone LeBeaumont, M. D., & Wheatley, T. (2023). Long gaps between turns are awkward for strangers but not for friends. *Philosophical Transactions of the Royal Society B: Biological Sciences, 378*(1875), 20210471.

Trần, V., Szabó, Á., Ward, C., & Jose, P. E. (2023). To vent or not to vent? The impact of venting on psychological symptoms varies by levels of social support. *International Journal of Intercultural Relations, 92*, Article 101750.

Treger, S., Sprecher, S., & Erber, R. (2013). Laughing and liking: Exploring the interpersonal effects of humor use in initial social interactions. *European Journal of Social Psychology, 43*(6), 532–543.

Trope, Y., & Liberman, N. (2003). Temporal construal. *Psychological Review, 110*(3), 403–421.

Trope, Y., Liberman, N., & Wakslak, C. (2007). Construal levels and psychological distance: Effects on representation, prediction, evaluation, and behavior. *Journal of Consumer Psychology, 17*(2), 83–95.

Tunçgenç, B., & Cohen, E. (2018). Interpersonal movement synchrony facilitates pro-social behavior in children's peer-play. *Developmental Science, 21*(1), e12505.

Turner, J. C., & Reynolds, K. J. (2011). Self-categorization theory. In P. A. M. Van Lange, A. W. Kruglanski, & E. T. Higgins (Eds.), *Handbook of theories in social psychology* (Vol. 2, pp. 399–417). Sage.

Vacharkulksemsuk, T., & Fredrickson, B. L. (2012). Strangers in sync: Achieving embodied rapport through shared movements. *Journal of Experimental Social Psychology, 48*(1), 399–402.

Valdesolo, P., & DeSteno, D. (2011). Synchrony and the social tuning of compassion. *Emotion, 11*(2), 262–266.

Vangelisti, A. L., Knapp, M. L., & Daly, J. A. (1990). Conversational narcissism. *Communication Monographs, 57*(4), 251–274.

Vrij, A., Mann, S., & Fisher, R. P. (2006). An empirical test of the behaviour analysis interview. *Law and Human Behavior, 30*(3), 329–345.

Wallot, S., Mitkidis, P., McGraw, J. J., & Roepstorff, A. (2016). Beyond synchrony: Joint action in a complex production task reveals beneficial effects of decreased interpersonal synchrony. *PLOS ONE, 11*(12), e0168306.

Wan, C. (2012). Shared knowledge matters: Culture as intersubjective representations. *Social and Personality Psychology Compass, 6*(2), 109–125.

Waytz, A., Hershfield, H. E., & Tamir, D. I. (2015). Mental simulation and meaning in life. *Journal of Personality and Social Psychology, 108*(2), 336–355.

Westgate, E. C., & Wilson, T. D. (2018). Boring thoughts and bored minds: The MAC model of boredom and cognitive engagement. *Psychological Review, 125*(5), 689–713.

Wiltermuth, S. S., & Heath, C. (2009). Synchrony and cooperation. *Psychological Science, 20*(1), 1–5.

Wiltshire, T. J., Butner, J. E., & Fiore, S. M. (2018). Problem-solving phase transitions during team collaboration. *Cognitive Science, 42*(1), 129–167.

Wood, A. M., Froh, J. J., & Geraghty, A. W. A. (2010). Gratitude and well-being: A review and theoretical integration. *Clinical Psychology Review, 30*(7), 890–905.

Wynn, C. J., & Borrie, S. A. (2022). Classifying conversational entrainment of speech behavior: An expanded framework and review. *Journal of Phonetics, 94*, 101173.

Ybarra, O., Burnstein, E., Winkielman, P., Keller, M. C., Manis, M., Chan, E., & Rodriguez, J. (2008). Mental exercising through simple socializing: Social interaction promotes general cognitive functioning. *Personality and Social Psychology Bulletin, 34*(2), 248–259.

Yeomans, M., Brooks, A. W., Huang, K., Minson, J., & Gino, F. (2019). It helps to ask: The cumulative benefits of asking follow-up questions. *Journal of Personality and Social Psychology, 117*(6), 1139–1144.

Yeomans, M., Schweitzer, M. E., & Brooks, A. W. (2022). The conversational circumplex: Identifying, prioritizing, and pursuing informational and relational motives in conversation. *Current Opinion in Psychology, 44*, 293–302.

Yeshurun, Y., Swanson, S., Simony, E., Chen, J., Lazaridi, C., Honey, C. J., & Hasson, U. (2017). Same story, different story: The neural representation of interpretive frameworks. *Psychological Science, 28*(3), 307–319.

Yu, B. (2023). Social disconnection and mortality: New evidence for old truths. *Trends in Cognitive Sciences, 27*(10), 890–891.

Zhang, Y., Meng, T., Hou, Y., Pan, Y., & Hu, Y. (2018). Interpersonal brain synchronization associated with working alliance during psychological counseling. *Psychiatry Research: Neuroimaging, 282*, 103–109.

Zhao, Z., Sened, H., & Tamir, D. I. (2023). Egocentric projection is a rational strategy for accurate emotion prediction. *Journal of Experimental Social Psychology, 109*, 104521.

Zhao, Z., Thornton, M. A., & Tamir, D. I. (2022). Accurate emotion prediction in dyads and groups and its potential social benefits. *Emotion, 22*(5), 1030–1043.

CHAPTER 5

Constructing Meaning through Communication

On Distance and Gender and Their Impact on Communicative Abstraction

Cheryl Wakslak

Meaning making can take many forms, from the lofty and the spiritual to the everyday and prosaic. In the current chapter, I describe a small attempt to understand meaning making within the context of communication. This research suggests that the way we express ourselves—the meaning we ascribe to experiences as we relate them to others—is sensitive to the expectations of our audience. That is, one's intended audience fundamentally shapes communication and the way that ideas are expressed. We see this as broadly functional: People want to be understood by others, so they adjust the way they describe events to support such interpretability. In doing so, however, people potentially shape the meaning they themselves come to draw about their own experiences because communication comes full circle to shape understanding. Meaning making within communication may furthermore not only be shaped by the static characteristics of the audience but also by the interplay of the speaker and the audience; one manifestation of this is the way that key individual-level characteristics that influence potential ways of relating to an audience can shape this process. Finally, the meaning we ascribe to events as captured in communication may affect how we are seen by others because individuals draw inferences from such meaning making about our characteristics and intentions. In what follows, I describe several projects that have examined these conjectures and point to open questions that continue to fascinate.

THE ROLE OF AUDIENCE DISTANCE IN COMMUNICATION

We have deep experience of our proximal worlds—the time and place that we inhabit, the people we know well and who often share our experiences. Communicating with others who exist within this zone of proximity is thus relatively straightforward; there exists a shared understanding of a concrete, lived experience that another person is likely to understand and be able to relate to. As one's audience becomes more remote, however, a key challenge emerges in that the specific contours of one's own experiences may be less readily understood; our everyday experiences are unlikely to be shared, making them less immediate fodder for common ground.

One way in which we might attempt to solve this problem is by expressing ourselves at a more abstract level. In their seminal work on construal-level theory (CLT), Trope and Liberman (2010) distinguish between high-level construal representations, abstract representations that capture an item's essence and defining characteristics, and low-level construal representations, concrete representations that capture an item's details and specific manifestation; they argue that abstraction or higher-level construal is often recruited to represent distant events because abstract representations are more likely to stay relevant across distance, even as the concrete manifestation of something might change. For example, representing a phone as a "communication device" rather than an "iPhone 16 Pro" makes sense when thinking about a distant context because the concrete form that a phone takes may change across contexts, but the underlying conceptualization of it as a device used for communication is likely to still be relevant across variation in time, space, and social contexts. Although CLT traditionally focused on *intrapersonal* representation—how an individual represents an item or event in their mind as a function of its distance—this logic should extend to the context of interpersonal representation, or how they choose to represent it to other people. To the degree that an audience is more remote from the individual, the concrete manifestation of things might differ in their context; thus, communicating with them in a more abstract fashion might be expected to be more useful.

In a set of related articles, my colleagues and I examined this idea as it applies to both the content and form of communication, arguing that when people's scope of communication is larger (i.e., when their audience is more remote), they will increasingly use abstraction within communication. For example, in one project (Joshi, Wakslak, Raj, & Trope, 2016), we considered how differences in the geographical distance of a message recipient would influence the abstraction of a message, finding that people sent more abstract messages to more distal message recipients. For instance, when asked to describe a day in the life of a student at their university to a prospective student located far away, participants described such a day more abstractly than when instructed to describe this to a prospective student located nearby. We also found similar effects when people communicated with large versus small audiences; large audiences, which were generally judged as more distal, were communicated to more abstractly than small audiences (which were experienced as more proximal; Joshi & Wakslak, 2014). In related research (Amit, Wakslak, & Trope, 2013), we further found that the form of communication was influenced by the distance of the recipient: Specifically, drawing on Amit's prior research linking visual communication with concreteness and verbal communication with abstraction (Amit, Algom, & Trope, 2009), we found in a series of studies that people increasingly used verbal (vs. visual) communication when a message recipient was distal.

The interpersonal context of communication further affords consideration of the functional aspect of adoption of low- versus high-level construals. My colleagues and I tiptoed toward this in a few ways. First, in our research on communicative abstraction and audience size (Joshi & Wakslak, 2014), we showed in two studies that the effects were contingent on people's motivation to do a good job at communicating. For example, in one study, we asked people to try to persuade a 1-person or 20-person audience to recycle using either abstract, high-level arguments (e.g., "Recycling helps sustain the environment for future generations") or concrete, low-level arguments (e.g., "Recycling drop-off centers are conveniently located in most communities"). We found that people increasingly sent high-level rather than low-level arguments to the larger audience, but this was especially the case when they had indicated greater motivation to persuade the audience. Similarly, in another study, we asked people to select arguments to persuade either 1 person or 20 other people to buy a newly launched juice project; we experimentally manipulated motivation to persuade by varying background information about the company producing the product, such that it was described as either being certified or not being certified as having good manufacturing practices. In line with the idea that motivation would moderate the effects of audience size on communicative abstraction, we found that it was only in the high-motivation condition that participants used more abstract descriptions when trying to persuade a large audience than a small audience. Together, these findings provided initial evidence that the effects we observed were not simply about some sort of distance or number priming. Rather, participants seemed to be using a construal-informed communication strategy, particularly when they wanted the communication to be successful. This supports more broadly the idea that people are using such strategies in a functional manner.

A second way in which our research addressed the conceptual issue of functionality was by showing that the effects are contingent on what might make this association more versus less functional. Two different types of studies broadly fit this approach. First, although the vast majority of research has identified "why"-related information as being at a higher level than "how"-related information (cf., Liberman & Trope, 1998), we reasoned that in some interpersonal contexts, that might not be the case (see Eyal, Liberman, and Trope [2014], for a different context in which "why" versus "how" may likewise not map onto high versus low construals). In particular, considering the case of a distributed team that must work together, we reasoned that procedural, "how"-related information might be superordinate to end-related "why"-related information. In line with this, we found that participants who described a new technology to a distal (rather than near) colleague to persuade them to use the technology increasingly described the technology in terms of its "why"-related aspects; however, this effect reversed when they were told that they need to work with the colleague using this tool (Joshi et al., 2016). This finding suggests that people are motivated by the functionality of communication at different levels; when the situational context makes a typically lower-level, subordinate attribute the superordinate defining element, individuals respond by increasingly prioritizing that dimension when communicating across distance.

Our research on audience size also considered the contingency of our effects in a way that speaks to functionality. We speculated in this work that large audiences are presumed to be more distant and that they are also characterized by greater heterogeneity. Variability has been argued to be core to the functional relationship between abstraction and distance (Gilead, Trope, & Liberman, 2020); across distance, one presumes more variability, and therefore representations shift toward what is most defining and thus likely to manifest across distance. Drawing on these ideas, we manipulated the relative presence of heterogeneity within an audience (Joshi & Wakslak, 2014); to the degree that variability across individuals is responsible for higher-level communication with a large audience, describing a sizeable audience as low in heterogeneity should minimize this effect. Findings were in line with this prediction, suggesting that heterogeneity plays an important role in driving this specific effect of audience size and, more generally, supporting a functional approach to the relationship between scope and communicative abstraction.

In recent work, my colleagues and I have also begun to explore people's intuitions surrounding such functionality more directly.

For example, inspired by recent research considering metacognitive beliefs about the functionality of construal in self-control contexts (e.g., Nguyen et al., 2019; see also Carnevale & Fujita, this volume), we recently examined the lay theories that people may have regarding the utility of high-level construal for interacting with groups high in diversity (Ferragamo, Yin, & Wakslak, 2025). According to the general argument that abstraction is useful for addressing anticipated variability, people should appreciate abstraction as a tool that might help them connect with a diverse range of others (i.e., to connect with others across difference). We find evidence for this across a number of different manifestations. For example, people believe that an exercise that will help them attain a high-level construal orientation will be more useful preparation for working in a diverse (but not nondiverse) group compared with an exercise that will help them attain a low-level construal orientation; they are also more likely to assign an employee who self-describes as high in abstraction (rather than concretization) to work in a diverse group, believing this employee will more strongly prefer to work in such a group and be more effective at doing so. We also find a similar effect at the level of communication choices; for example, people indicate that they will turn to more abstract communication topics when interacting across more versus less difference. Intriguingly, similar to the aforementioned work suggesting boundary conditions that support a functional perspective on such effects, we identified here, once again, important boundary conditions that suggest people are more likely to turn to abstraction where it is most functional. For example, although the presence of difference might generally suggest that abstract communication is more effective than concrete communication, this may not be the case in situations where people—despite their differences—have a shared concrete experience. Indeed, we found that respondents were sensitive to this distinction when considering their communication choices. In one study, for instance, participants considered attending a conference with people from many different schools/majors at their university; although they were interested in talking about more abstract topics when they considered interacting across difference (having a conversation with students attending other schools rather than their own school), this was no longer the case when they were asked to consider a potential conversation about the shared experience itself (i.e., the event they were concurrently attending).

In addition to considering how the scope of one's communication (i.e., whether one is communicating with a more distal or broad audience) affects abstraction within communication, we also considered the opposite relationship: whether framing a communication more abstractly would lead people to want to communicate the message to more distal others. We found that this indeed was the case; people were increasingly inclined to prefer distal (versus near) recipients when communication was more (versus less) abstract, was communication was verbal (rather than visual), and when they had been placed into a more abstract (rather than concrete) general orientation. These findings support the idea that the link between communicative scope and abstraction is bidirectional: Communicative abstraction supports an expansion of scope, in addition to scope evoking greater communicative abstraction.

We also proceeded to take a different perspective on this bidirectional relationship by considering the presence of communicative abstraction as a cue that signals a speaker's distance. In this fashion, we extended from thinking about how the scope of communication shapes meaning making within the context of communication to thinking about how observers make sense of a communicator's tendency to speak abstractly or concretely. We did this in a number of ways. For instance, we considered whether people would use concretization in the form of picture-based communication to try to signal proximity with a message recipient (Torrez, Wakslak, & Amit, 2019). In this study, we asked people to imagine wanting to signal closeness (vs. distance) from a message recipient and to then indicate how they would respond to a text message. We found that participants asked to adopt a proximity rather than distance motivation were more likely to indicate they would send a message containing an emoji. Similarly, when asked to imagine themselves as managers wanting to establish closeness with (vs. distance from) employees, participants increasingly opted to use a visual (rather than text-based) biography when meeting a new hire. Similar effects emerged in an online interactive context; when told that it is useful for online workers who are far from each other to compensate for their distance and try to create a sense of proximity, versus it being important for them to respect their distance, participants increasingly chose to introduce themselves to another online worker using visual rather than text-based information. These findings suggest that people seek to establish proximity by using more visual-based forms of communication.

We also looked at the general idea of linguistic abstraction as a potential cue for distance versus proximity within the specific context of power assessments. Work by Smith and Trope (2006) had previously established that power is associated with construal level, such that people with greater power represent information more abstractly, potentially because power acts as a distance dimension. In follow-up research, we considered how communicative abstraction may influence power assessments (Wakslak, Smith, & Han, 2014). Across a range of operationalizations, we found that people ascribed more power to individuals who communicated abstractly rather than concretely. For example, people read about an ostensibly earlier participant who described an activity using a more ends-related, abstract identification or a more means-related, concrete identification and were asked to judge that person's characteristics. Those who had used the more abstract, end-related descriptions were perceived as more powerful. We saw similar effects when the descriptions were depicted as being made by politicians and the topics related to politics: Again, those who used more abstract, big-picture language were seen as more powerful. We further considered underlying reasons for why this might be and found support for the idea that communicative abstraction signaled that the speaker is likely a big-picture thinker, and this mediated the impact of communicative abstraction on power judgments. Additionally, we found some support for the idea that communicative abstraction portrayed a willingness to make judgments (given that abstract language is often more decisive about the meaning of a behavior or an event) and that this, too, played a role in informing power judgments.

GENDER AND COMMUNICATIVE ABSTRACTION

As the previously described research linking distance, communication, and power perceptions accumulated, I found myself, on a personal level, reflecting on my own tendency to communicate concretely and what this might inadvertently be signaling about my power-related potential. As someone who has been long interested in gender but never made it a focus of my research, I began to especially notice how my own tendencies contrasted with those of my male colleagues. One area where this especially stood out was over email, where I noticed that my responses were often more detail oriented than those of my male colleagues, who seemed less hesitant than I was to answer in a more high-level fashion.

Wondering if this might be a more general pattern that extended beyond anecdotal personal experience, my colleagues and I considered whether there might be a general tendency for men to speak more abstractly than women. As we mulled over this question, we began to appreciate that, conceptually, several different lines of existing research would support such an association, especially considering our earlier work on audience distance and size as precursors to communicative abstraction. For example, prior research argues for differences in how men and women use language, with men focusing more on content and control and women having more relational intentions (e.g., Rubin, Perse, & Barbato, 1988; Tannen, 1991, 1994). This, to us, broadly fit an argument that women might be more proximally oriented in communicative contexts. Other research has suggested that women often operate in tighter, more close-knit networks compared with men, and even as young children, they socialize in a more relational, tight-knit fashion in contrast to the more "pack-driven" tendencies of boys (Marsden, 1987; Maccoby, 2002; McPherson & Smith-Lovin, 1982, 1986). Thus, to the degree that women often socialize in more intimate, tight-knit contexts, this might be another reason for them to have developed a more concrete style of speech. Additionally, historically, men and women have differed in their social roles and ascribed power (Carli, 1999; Eagly & Wood, 1999; Ridgeway, 2001); to the degree that power is associated with more abstract communication, this would also point to a similar effect of women speaking more concretely than men. Conversations with women highlighted even more mechanisms that might further support such an effect. For example, some women described concerns about either showing their competence or not wanting to make judgments for others. Such women expressed an interest in "sticking to the facts," to the concrete details of what had occurred, rather than trying to interpret an event for others, a tendency that could be influenced by a desire to show competence *vis-à-vis* mastery of details, concerns that any judgments they made might be questioned, or simply a desire to act more humbly by laying out information for others to process without presuming to impose their own higher-level meaning.

Having appreciated that there were strong conceptual reasons to expect this effect, above and beyond anecdotal personal experience, we started to explore this idea by meta-analyzing our prior data on communicative abstraction across audience distance and size. Across these data, we found that women tended to speak more concretely than men, in particular when the audience was proximal. This suggested to us that it was not that women couldn't speak more abstractly if they so desired, such as when an audience's distance or size was made especially salient, as in our prior experimental contexts. But without this particular salience of audience distance, women and men seemed to use different levels of communicative abstraction when speaking with others. Building on these findings, we proceeded to explore this effect across a range of contexts, including both lab-based and archival datasets (Joshi, Wakslak, Appel, & Huang, 2020). For example, in one study, we asked participants to persuade another student from their university to recycle by selecting arguments from a list that we provided; we found that men chose more abstract, ends-related arguments (and correspondingly, fewer concrete, means-related arguments) compared with women. We also found that the effects persisted across contexts that varied in power. For example, we found similar effects with online panel participants, in an analysis of everyday bloggers' writings, and in the speech of congresspeople on the floor of the U.S. Congress. We also experimentally manipulated sense of power and did not find this to moderate the effects. Although we strongly suspect that these effects are multidetermined, at reviewers' request, we conducted a measurement-based mediation study to see if support emerged for some or all of the processes we had outlined. Our findings offered the strongest support for an effect of current social network size; however, this finding should be taken with caution because these findings are only as reliable as our measures, and we are not convinced that it is readily plausible to model how deeply seated, culturally supported tendencies influence communication with this sort of current-snapshot design.

In describing these findings to audiences, I note anecdotally and completely nonscientifically that the women in the audience often nod their heads along as they hear of these findings (while the men mostly look at me blankly). This is fascinating to me because it suggests that women are aware of their tendency to be more concrete—or at least recognize it immediately when they learn of it. I recall one especially interesting conversation, which went something like this[1]: A female executive in the audience excitedly came up to me after I had mentioned these findings during a session, explaining that she had recently presented to a board meeting and had an eye-opening experience. She said that normally, she would have presented all the relevant details related to the topic she was addressing, but in this case, she actually didn't have all of the detailed information. So, she instead let someone else present the details, whereas she herself presented a higher-level view of the issue. At the end of the meeting, the response she got was: "We needed to hear more of what you were saying and less of what the other person was saying." She explained that this was shocking to her—she only went to the bigger-picture, high level because in that situation, she had no choice; she didn't have command of the details. And yet, the audience's reaction helped her to understand that the higher level was more compelling for her audience, more of what they wanted to hear from her as a leader.

Indeed, given our earlier research on the social impression implications of speaking abstractly and our findings that it is men who tend to speak more abstractly, we believe that speaking style may be an especially important consideration for women striving to be seen as leaders. In one unpublished study, we saw some intriguing initial evidence for this. We had one group of online participants write a paragraph, then coded these for linguistic abstraction; in line with the general finding that women speak more concretely than men, we found the communications written

[1]I sadly don't know the executive's name and also did not write down the story immediately after the fact; details may thus be incorrect—and yes, I note the irony of my comment on the details.

by women to be more concrete than those written by men. We then had a separate group of participants, each yoked to two respondents in the first set, read these individuals' communication and evaluate them for managerial and administrative assistant positions. Critically, we didn't mention anything about the initial writer's gender. Despite gender not being explicitly communicated, we found a gender effect on assessments for the positions, such that participants doing the evaluating increasingly favored men over women for the managerial (vs. administrative assistant) position. Moreover, the effects of gender on perceived fitness for the managerial position were mediated by linguistic abstraction; that is, we found evidence of a preference for men over women in a leadership position—without telling people the gender of the writer—and this was driven by the writer's tendency to communicate abstractly.

Findings from other research teams also dovetail with the idea that gender differences in abstraction could have important downstream consequences. In particular, Kolev, Fuentes-Medel, and Murray (2019) conducted an intriguing study of the grant review process at the Gates Foundation. They first noted that despite the blinded review process, a gender gap had emerged at the foundation, in which applications submitted by men were more successful than those submitted by women. This gender gap was not explained by the proposal topics or *ex ante* measures of applicant quality, raising the perplexing question of what was leading to these differences. In a bottom-up analysis, Kolev and colleagues sought to understand what factors might drive these effects, observing that they were explained by the tendency of male applicants to use broad language and female applicants to use narrow language. Critically, variation in applicants' linguistic style predicted reviewer scores, but they did not predict innovative performance after an accepted proposal, suggesting that this signal might be harming qualified women. What is especially intriguing to me is that the researchers here approached this issue in a completely atheoretical fashion; that is, they were puzzled by a gender difference that emerged in a context where the blinding of the applications suggests it was unlikely to be driven by explicit or implicit gender biases per se. They thus sought to understand whether there might be content or quality differences in the applications (or applicants) and to understand, if not, what stylistic differences could explain the divergence in success. That they ultimately landed on a pattern highly consistent with our findings was quite exciting!

Intrigued by the potential implications of linguistic gender differences, in related work, we considered how the tendency of women to speak more concretely than men might play out in the context of entrepreneurial pitching (Huang, Joshi, Wakslak, & Wu, 2021). As a key mechanism by which start-ups are able to access critical investment resources, entrepreneurial pitching is inherently important, and findings suggest women tend to receive many fewer venture capital dollars than men (Silano, 2023; Teare, 2024). Moreover, from a social psychological perspective, entrepreneurial pitching is also an amazingly intriguing setting within which to consider basic phenomena, especially around impression formation. It is a high-stakes context where the impressions that are formed can have critical consequences; despite the due diligence that venture capitalists (VCs) perform on the companies that they invest in, decisions are often based on impressions of the "jockey" (i.e., the entrepreneur) as much as the "horse" (i.e., the idea; Vaynerchuk, 2014) and may be surprisingly based on gut intuition (Huang, 2018). Thus, small differences in social perceptions are not just a few tenths of a point on a scale in a crowd-sourced study; they truly have the potential to shape critical outcomes.

Considering our prior findings suggesting that women speak more concretely than men, we sought to demonstrate whether (1) this occurs within the entrepreneurial pitching context and (2) what downstream consequences this may have. We found that, much as in other contexts, women tended to pitch their companies more concretely compared with men. Moreover, we found that this seemed to affect how they were seen; for example, in a study looking at one VC firm's deal flow for 2018, we considered the companies that got past the initial screening phase, which was done through an online platform. The firm focused on early-stage companies and was especially interested in the long-term growth and scalability of companies; investors from the firm thus rated potential deals on growth potential. We found that female-led firms were less likely to make it through this initial phase. Female founders presented their ventures less abstractly, abstract speech was positively associated with being perceived as growth oriented, and growth orientation predicted the likelihood of making it through to the next stage, with evidence of the serial mediation of the overall gender effect.

Intriguingly, at some point in the research process on this project, we learned of a session at South by Southwest featuring female VCs, where a VC named Susan Lyne made the following observation: "I see men pitch unicorns, and women pitch businesses" (Bellstrom, 2017). We used this as an epigraph in our eventual article because it so perfectly captured our basic effect and its implications. Men seem to be explaining the big-picture vision of how their idea will turn into a billion-dollar company; women, in contrast, are focusing on the more concrete details, the mechanics of the business, rather than the broader vision of where this will evolve.

One question that follows from these prior findings, however, is whether advising women to use abstract language could create any potential backlash. That is, to the degree that this is a relatively masculine style of communication, would big-picture speech from women be associated with negative consequences as a result of this style not fitting what we expect from women or seeming more masculine, or would it have positive consequences? In preliminary research on this question, our findings suggest that speaking abstractly has similar implications for men and women, specifically *vis-à-vis* power and leadership judgments. For example, in one study, we presented participants with résumés from men and women in which candidates described their prior work experience using more high-level or low-level descriptions (e.g., managing business correspondence in order to maintain good client relationships vs. managing business correspondence by emailing clients). We found that participants were more likely to favor candidates with high-level (rather than low-level) descriptions for a management position, an effect that was similar in magnitude for male and female candidates. (When assessing candidates for an administrative assistant position, in contrast, abstraction did not predict perceived suitability.) Although such findings do not rule out that there may be cases where a fit effect or backlash emerges, they suggest that in many situations, women may reap potential benefits for assessments of their power by speaking more abstractly.

At the same time, the previously described findings, as a whole, do not preclude the idea that there are times when speaking more concretely may be beneficial, even in a leadership context. Indeed, in line with this, Palmeira (2015) found that abstract communication did signal power, that concrete communication signaled a greater action orientation, and that both of these assessments could be important for overall perceptions related to leadership. Research also suggests that concrete communication can increase trustworthiness (Larrimore, Jiang, Larrimore, Markowitz, & Gorski, 2011; Toma & Hancock, 2012). For example, Pan, McNamara, Lee, Haleblian, and Devers (2018) demonstrated that the chief executive officer's concrete communication on earning calls was associated with positive investor reactions for firms with high-financial-risk profiles (whereas for those with low-financial-risk profiles, the opposite pattern emerged). Intriguingly, a real-world example where female leadership seemed to emerge positively was during the COVID-19 pandemic, when many of the world leaders who received strong reviews were women, a pattern striking enough to receive commentary from several mainstream media outlets (Bear & Agner, 2021; Orme, 2021). An intriguing possibility to consider in future research is whether some forms of crisis might evoke a desire for the concrete style of communication that women often favor and whether that may explain women's success in situations such as this historic event. More broadly, it seems plausible that in favorable environments, leadership assessments may be more highly linked to judgments of power, and abstract speech may be favored; in contrast, in environments where uncertainty is salient and/or trustworthiness is a focal issue, assessments may be linked to judgments of veracity and action orientation, and concrete communication may be favored (see Wakslak & Joshi [2020] for a similar argument).

As a whole, this work on gender and communicative abstraction highlights several important points. First, it brings home the degree to which meaning making performed during communication is not a static function of the qualities of the audience; rather, a communicator's general tendencies and specific communication goals may play a critical role in whether they describe things more concretely or more abstractly. Second, observers are often not aware of the communicator's reasons for turning to greater concretization or abstraction, and they may therefore be willing to draw broad conclusions—even in fairly high-stakes contexts—about a person's motivations and/or enduring characteristics from their choice of abstract or concrete speech. Thus, a multiperson, complex meaning-making process can co-occur, with communicators creating meaning in a way that they think will resonate with their audience and observers drawing meaning from such communicator choices.

FROM COMMUNICATIVE ABSTRACTION TO GENDERED EXPECTATIONS

To the degree that women speak more concretely than men, another intriguing possibility emerges: that people may be sensitive to this association and come to expect women to be more concrete than men. Intriguingly, this may extend not only to expectations of verbal concreteness but also to greater expectations more generally of women to adopt a lower-level construal orientation. A series of studies (Dodson, Goodwin, Wakslak, Diekmann, & Graham, et al., in press) recently explored this possibility. For example, in studies directly considering the possibility that women are associated with concreteness and men with abstraction, findings supported such an association at both an implicit level (i.e., using an Implicit Association Test [IAT] measure) and an explicit level. Such patterns also emerged when participants were asked to consider the typical man and woman within a range of occupations (e.g., the typical male/female accountant, the typical male/female realtor, etc.) and rate the likelihood of them possessing high-level versus low-level tendencies (using items adapted from Nguyen and Fujita [2020]). Strikingly, although overall expectations of individuals having abstract versus concrete tendencies varied across occupations, as one might expect, within occupations, people generally expected the typical woman in that occupation to have increasingly lower-level, concrete tendencies than the typical man within that occupation; indeed, at a descriptive level, this was the case in 45 of the 48 occupations examined. Effects also emerged within real-world contexts. For example, a large study of recommendations on LinkedIn found that recommendations for women increasingly highlighted aspects of their performance related to concreteness rather than abstractness when compared with men. We also found that this difference in how people consider men and women *vis-à-vis* construal influences their assignment of men and women to tasks (i.e., increased assignment to women of detailed tasks, even when such tasks are identified as undesirable for the task assignee). This phenomenon may help us understand why women often get assigned office housework and other low-level tasks not associated with promotability (e.g., Babcock, Recalde, Vesterlund, & Weingart, 2017; Jang, Allen, & Regina, 2020; Kaplan, 2022). In this way, women's presumed detail orientation may be something of a double-edged sword; on the one hand, this is a way for women to demonstrate competence, while on the other hand, it may lead them to get pigeonholed into the sorts of tasks that don't lead to being seen as a leader or visionary in the long term. Thus, while it may be a neutral or even positive thing for women in the short term, there may be long-term negative consequences of this association. Future research will hopefully continue to explore these implications.

Interestingly, however, in another related project (Dodson, Goodwin, Tideman, et al., 2025), we found that once women were established as leaders, they might be seen in a particularly abstract fashion. We suggest that this may occur because, as exceptions to the norm, female leaders may be seen as more atypical and thus viewed at a distance. We see evidence for this pattern across varied contexts. For example, *New York Times* profiles written about female leaders use more abstract language than those written about male leaders. A large corpus of quarterly earnings conference calls shows a related pattern, with analysts asking female leaders more abstract questions compared with male leaders, especially when their firm's performance exceeds analysts' expectations. These findings are intriguing in that they suggest that although the typical woman may be seen as being more concrete than the typical man, once a woman is seen as a leader, they may be approached with a relatively abstract mindset.

The association people hold between gender and concreteness may also have additional interesting implications. For example, in recent research, we considered the relationship between gender and stimulus complexity (Amit, Rubinstein, Appel, & Wakslak, 2025). Complex objects are more disorganized and less predictable than simple objects (Casti, 1995; Cilliers, 1998; Shannon, 1948). If men are seen as more abstract and women as more concrete, then men may be more likely to be associated with simpler stimuli—because these fit more with schematic and gist-like abstract representation—and women with more complex stimuli. A number of studies that operationalized complexity in different ways found support for this relationship. For example, participants expected that a medication with a simpler rather than more complex name was increasingly likely to be one that targets men (rather than women). Likewise, an employee was judged as more increasingly likely to be male (rather than female) when they had selected a T-shirt with a more simple rather than complex company logo (a grid in which columns alternated between two colors vs. a grid in which the two colors alternated in a checkerboard pattern). We also found that the association between gender and complexity had a number of downstream implications. First, we found evidence for a congruency effect between complexity and gender when it came to predicting others' preferences. More specifically, participants who thought about purchasing a gift for a female rather than male friend expected the friend to have a relatively greater preference for a gift with complex packaging (a visually complex lotion bottle) rather than simple packaging (a visually simple lotion bottle). Second, we also found that people's communications with men and women were in line with a gender/complexity association. For example, product listings on Amazon were more likely to be complex (more characters, longer words) when the product was targeted to women versus those targeted to men. We found similar results when we considered people's everyday communications; for instance, in a study of transactions on the payment platform Venmo, we found that messages sent to women (whether from men or women) were more likely to be characterized by complexity than messages sent to men.

In addition to our findings linking gender with expectations of construal, current complementary research (Ferragamo & Wakslak, 2025) finds that people associate gender and distance. For example, across four different IATs considering temporal distance, spatial distance, social distance, and hypotheticality, people are more likely to associate women with proximity. Interestingly, this effect is consistently moderated across all four distances by participant gender. Women tend to show a very strong linkage between the concepts of female and proximity (and male and distance); men, in contrast, show a reverse pattern that is weaker in size (linking men with proximity, but to a considerably smaller degree). Further research explicitly asking people about each of these associations has yielded broadly consistent findings, suggesting this is not an artifact of the IAT procedure but something more enduring. Interestingly, although the pattern is not as strong, in our research on the gender/construal association (Dodson, et al., in press), we similarly find in a meta-analysis that these effects are stronger for female participants. This suggests, interestingly, that it is women rather than men who may have stronger associations between their own gender and both proximity and detail-oriented thinking.

ABSTRACT SPEECH, SCOPE, AND GENDER

I argued earlier that people turn to abstract speech to connect across distance because abstract speech is more likely to transcend one's own direct concrete experience and allow a person to connect with a broader group of individuals. In recent research (Yin, Wakslak, & Joshi, 2022), my colleagues and I considered the implications that this might have for the types of pronouns people use in communication, particularly differentiating between whether people would use singular or plural first-person pronouns (*I* language vs. *we* language). To the degree that *I* language signals that one is presenting one's individuated thoughts and experiences, this should fit well with concrete language that is more specific to direct experience. On the flip side, to the degree that *we* language suggests an attempt to go beyond the self and adopt a broader scope, this should fit well with abstract language that extends beyond the specific context. Intriguingly, prior literature on pronoun usage has found that women tend to use more first-person singular pronouns than men (*I*'s rather than *we*'s; Newman, Groom, Handelman, & Pennebaker, 2008). This has been a bit puzzling, given that many people might assume that women—who are presumed to be more relational (Gabriel & Gardner, 1999; Wood & Eagly, 2012)—might be more inclined to use *we* language. In addition, another group shown in prior research to use more first-person singulars is those low in power (Kacewicz, Pennebaker, Davis, Jeon, & Graesser, 2014), which again might be surprising because low-power individuals are generally presumed to be less self-oriented than high-power individuals (Galinsky, Magee, Inesi, & Gruenfeld, 2006; Van Kleef et al., 2008). Intriguingly, a perspective on first-person pronouns that sees such speech as adopting a narrower rather than broader scope may provide a useful perspective on these prior effects, given our prior work linking both gender (Joshi et al., 2020) and power (Wakslak et al., 2014) with linguistic abstraction. That is, women and those low in power may be more inclined to describe their own idiosyncratic experience and less inclined to speak for others in a broad and general way; such a tendency may be associated, on the one hand, with an increase in concrete speech and, on the other hand, with a tendency to use more first-person singular pronouns rather than plural pronouns (i.e., to use *I* rather than *we*).

We first set out to consider the pronoun/abstraction link by considering whether messages that contain more concrete language would tend to have greater relative usage of *I* versus *we* pronouns. We found this was indeed the case across several archival datasets, including a dataset of Airbnb listings, a dataset of Twitter posts about COVID-19, and a dataset of congressional speech. We also followed up these correlational findings by running experiments showing that (a) prompting people to write about more abstract versus concrete topics was associated with greater relative use of *we* (compared with *I*) pronouns, and (b) people were more concrete when prompted to write using *I* rather than *we* pronouns (specifically, when asked to write about "What I do at work" rather than "What we do at work").

Having established the relationship between pronoun usage and linguistic abstraction, we next sought to consider one implication of this association: whether communications would benefit from a fit between pronoun usage and linguistic abstraction. For example, in a dataset of tweets that included how many people favorited each tweet, we first replicated the basic effect that greater concreteness was associated with greater use of *I* relative to *we* pronouns. We then examined how relative pronoun usage and linguistic concreteness might interact to predict the odds of being favorited. We found that concrete language was positively associated with a tweet's likeability at average levels of *I* versus *we* pronoun usage; this positive association increased as tweets used more *I* (vs. *we*) pronouns. We also explored the same idea using a laboratory paradigm. Participants read abstract or concrete messages about recycling that used either *we* or *I* pronouns. They then rated the message on a variety of dimensions, including their liking for the message, the message's persuasiveness, perceptions of the writer, and the degree to which the message felt natural or right (i.e., message "fit"). We found that abstraction and pronoun usage interacted to predict how natural and compelling the message was perceived to be. Concrete messages were more compelling than abstract messages, but only in the *I* condition; when messages used *we* pronouns, this difference did not emerge. (Or, looking at the alternative simple effects, *we* messages were found more compelling than *I* messages, but only when the message was abstract and not when it was concrete.) Intriguingly, although we find that in general, these two linguistic aspects tend to go together in natural language use, a notable example of not following this norm confronted me when I returned to campus after COVID-19. Signs and posters had been placed across campus with various messages. One flyer posted in the stairwell of my parking garage caught my eye. The text read: "Here we take the stairs if able, otherwise. . . . we don't crowd others and we wait for others to exit; we cover our faces; we sanitize hands before and after touching buttons." The "nonfit" exemplified in the copy—a mixing of *we* pronouns and very concrete language regarding what it is "we" do—immediately jumped out. Presumably, the goal of using *we* in this context was to activate a shared identity and signal that we were all bound together in the fight against COVID-19; although the messaging was undoubtedly well intentioned, the pairing of *we* use with very concrete language made it awkward.

OPEN QUESTIONS AND CONCLUDING THOUGHTS

As noted at the start of this chapter, meaning making can take many forms. In this review, I have mostly focused on two perspectives and two accompanying types of meaning making: that of the communicator, who attempts to meaning make within the communicative context in order to communicate effectively with an audience, and of an observer, who draws inferences about a communicator from what they say. A key missing perspective is, of course, that of the audience itself, the conceptual center of much of our argument, which has nonetheless been largely missing in our empirical investigations to date. Indeed, while we argue that people see abstraction as functional when communicating across distance, we have done less to examine directly whether it *is* functional. On the one hand, audience members may, in some contexts, be sensitive to the dynamics I describe here; on the other hand, it is also possible that they are more influenced by the message itself and relatively insensitive to the distance of its source and other related variations. Future studies focused on the audience's experience will dramatically expand our understanding of this key perspective.

Another important opportunity is to consider how effects related to communication, such as those summarized here, may come to affect understanding. That is, I focused here on exploring meaning making as it is informed by communication, noting that the goals that people bring to communication—the desire to be understood, but also potentially to create a sense of proximity and connection—can shape the way we ascribe meaning to experiences as we describe them to others. What we have not yet done is take this work to the next critical step: to understand how communicative meaning making may shape the very way that one comes to understand the thing oneself. That is, to the degree that I turn to either abstraction or concretization to support communication, does this shape my own understanding of what has happened? Consider, for example, our research on gender and communicative abstraction. That women and men communicate differently does not inherently mean they have different capabilities, or even preferences, for abstract and concrete thought. However, if I develop my thinking as I seek to communicate with others, my communicative tendencies toward abstraction or concretization may affect how I come to think of things, above and beyond my communication per se. Indeed, it is plausible that even the mere anticipation of communication—knowing that I will communicate this information to someone else—might shape my cognitive approach as I seek to process information and understand something that has occurred (see Grinfeld, Usher, and Liberman [2024] for a similar argument applied to the way that knowing one will receive communicated information from others may affect how people process experienced self-relevant information). Drawing a more direct line from the meaning making that occurs within the context of communication to how this may shape one's fundamental understanding would dramatically extend the implications of this work and is an exciting area for continued investigation.

Related to the previous argument, at an even broader level, it is fascinating to consider how the meaning of concepts and ideas—through the way that they may at least be partially constructed via acts of communication—may be influenced by regularities within a cultural context of proximal versus distal communication. That is, if the meaning of an idea or concept to at least some degree emerges from what people say when they talk about that concept, this suggests that persistent patterns of proximal and distal communication may fundamentally shape a concept's emergent meaning. Consider, for example, the meaning of a concept like "patriotism." To the degree that people in a culture may tend to primarily communicate with close others—and thus be concrete in their communication—the emergent meaning of "patriotism" in that culture is likely to be more concrete than the same concept would be within a culture in which people communicate more with distal others. Thus, regularities associated with the scope of communication—the degree to which people in a context tend to communicate with others who are close versus distant—may fundamentally come to influence the meaning that ideas within that context take on. This suggests a number of important implications about how patterns of communication shape our basic cognition; for example, information bubbles, which lead us to spend more time talking to others like us (and less time talking to those unlike us), may not only affect persuasion and other outcomes of communication but also shape the very fabric of meaning itself. Future research should continue to explore these and other ideas, unearthing how communicative scope may drive not only what is said at a given moment but also what comes to be fundamentally understood.

REFERENCES

Amit, E., Algom, D., & Trope, Y. (2009). Distance-dependent processing of pictures and words. *Journal of Experimental Psychology: General, 138*(3), 400.

Amit, E. Rubinstein, T., Appel, G. & Wakslak, C. (2025). *Unveiling the social dimension of complexity: Complexity as a gender cue in consumer behavior* [Working paper]. Tel Aviv University.

Amit, E., Wakslak, C., & Trope, Y. (2013). The use of visual and verbal means of communication across psychological distance. *Personality and Social Psychology Bulletin, 39*(1), 43–56.

Babcock, L., Recalde, M. P., Vesterlund, L., & Weingart, L. (2017). Gender differences in accepting and receiving requests for tasks with low promotability. *American Economic Review, 107*(3), 714–747.

Bear, A., & Agner, R. (2021, March 8). Why more countries need female leaders. *US News and World Report. www.usnews.com/news/best-countries/articles/2021-03-08/why-countries-with-female-leaders-have-responded-well-to-the-pandemic*

Bellstrom, K. (2017, March 15). Investors explain why "men pitch unicorns and women pitch businesses." *Fortune. fortune.com/2017/03/15/sxsw-2017-funding-tips-women-entreprenuers*

Carli, L. L. (1999). Gender, interpersonal power, social influence. *Journal of Social Issues, 55*(1), 81–99.

Casti, J. L. (1995). *Complexification: Explaining a paradoxical world through the science of surprise.* HarperCollins.

Cilliers, P. (1998). *Complexity and postmodernism: Understanding complex systems.* Routledge.

Dodson, S., Goodwin, R., Tideman, S., Graham, J., Diekmann, K., & Wakslak, C. (2025). *Extraordinary executive women: leader gender, atypicality, and elicited abstraction* [Working paper]. University of Calgary.

Dodson, S., Goodwin, R., Wakslak, C., Diekmann, K, & Graham, J. (in press). She sees the trees, he sees the forest: Descriptive gender stereotypes of concreteness and abstractness. *Journal of Personality and Social Psychology.*

Eagly, A. H., & Wood, W. (1999). The origins of sex differences in human behavior: Evolved dispositions versus social roles. *American Psychologist, 54*(6), 408–423.

Eyal, T., Liberman, N., & Trope, Y. (2014). Thinking of why a transgression occurred may draw attention to extenuating circumstances: A comment on Žeželj & Jokić replication. *Social Psychology, 45*(4), 329–331.

Ferragamo, A., & Wakslak, C. (2025). *On the association between gender and distance* [Working paper]. University of Southern California.

Ferragamo, A., Yin, Y., & Wakslak, C. J. (2025). *Abstraction in service of connection: On people's recruitment of abstraction to facilitate interaction across difference* [Working paper]. University of Southern California.

Gabriel, S., & Gardner, W. L. (1999). Are there "his" and "hers" types of interdependence? The implications of gender differences in collective versus relational interdependence for affect, behavior, and cognition. *Journal of Personality and Social Psychology, 77*(3), 642–655.

Galinsky, A. D., Magee, J. C., Inesi, M. E., & Gruenfeld, D. H. (2006). Power and perspectives not taken. *Psychological Science, 17*(12), 1068–1074.

Gilead, M., Trope, Y., & Liberman, N. (2020). Above and beyond the concrete: The diverse representational substrates of the predictive brain. *Behavioral and Brain Sciences, 43*, Article e121.

Grinfeld, G., Usher, M., & Liberman, N. (2024). Expecting to integrate additional information improves averaging of experience. *Scientific Reports, 14*(1), 16627.

Huang, L. 2018. The role of investor gut feel in managing complexity and extreme risk. *Academy of Management Journal, 61*(5), 1821–1847.

Huang, L., Joshi, P., Wakslak, C., & Wu, A. (2021). Sizing up entrepreneurial potential: Gender differences in communication and investor perceptions of long-term growth and scalability. *Academy of Management Journal, 64*(3), 716–740.

Jang, S., Allen, T., & Regina, J. (2020). Office housework, burnout, and promotion: Does gender matter? *Journal of Business and Psychology, 36*(5), 793–805.

Joshi, P., & Wakslak, C. J. (2014). Communicating with the crowd: Speakers use abstract messages when addressing larger audiences. *Journal of Experimental Psychology: General, 143*(1), 351–362.

Joshi, P., Wakslak, C., Appel, G., & Huang, L. (2020). Gender differences in communicative abstraction. *Journal of Personality and Social Psychology, 118*(3), 417–435.

Joshi, P., Wakslak, C. J., Raj, M., & Trope, Y. (2016). Communicating with distant others: The functional use of abstraction. *Social Psychological and Personality Science, 7*(1), 37–44.

Kacewicz, E., Pennebaker, J. W., Davis, M., Jeon, M., & Graesser, A. C. (2014). Pronoun use reflects standings in social hierarchies. *Journal of Language and Social Psychology, 33*(2), 125–143.

Kaplan, A. (2022). Just let it pass by and it will fall on some woman: Invisible work in the labor market. *Gender & Society, 36*(6), 838–868.

Kolev, J., Fuentes-Medel, Y., & Murray, F. (2019). *Is blinded review enough? How gendered outcomes arise even under anonymous evaluation* (NBER Working Paper #25759). National Bureau of Economic Research. *www.nber.org/papers/w25759*

Larrimore, L., Jiang, L., Larrimore, J., Markowitz, D., & Gorski, S. (2011). Peer to peer lending: The relationship between language features, trustworthiness, and persuasion success. *Journal of Applied Communication Research, 39*(1), 19–37.

Liberman, N., & Trope, Y. (1998). The role of feasibility and desirability considerations in near and distant future decisions: A test of temporal construal theory. *Journal of Personality and Social Psychology, 75*(1), 5–18.

Maccoby, E. E. (2002). Gender and group process: A developmental perspective. *Current Directions in Psychological Science, 11*(2), 54–58.

Marsden, P. V. (1987). Core discussion networks of Americans. *American Sociological Review, 52*(1), 122–131.

McPherson, J. M., & Smith-Lovin, L. (1982). Women and weak ties: Differences by sex in the size of voluntary organizations. *American Journal of Sociology, 87*(4), 883–904.

McPherson, J. M., & Smith-Lovin, L. (1986). Sex segregation in voluntary associations. *American Sociological Review, 51*(1), 61–79.

Newman, M. L., Groom, C. J., Handelman, L. D., & Pennebaker, J. W. (2008). Gender differences in language use: An analysis of 14,000 text samples. *Discourse Processes, 45*(3), 211–236.

Nguyen, T., Carnevale, J. J., Scholer, A. A., Miele, D. B., & Fujita, K. (2019). Metamotivational knowledge of the role of high-level and low-level construal in goal-relevant task performance. *Journal of Personality and Social Psychology*, 117(5), 876–899. *https://doi.org/10.1037/pspa0000166*

Nguyen, T., & Fujita, K. (2020). *Subjective construal level measure* [Unpublished manuscript]. Ohio State University.

Orme, G. (2021). Women leaders have shone during the pandemic: Men, take note. *Forbes. www.forbes.com/sites/gregorme/2021/08/04/women-leaders-have-shone-during-the-pandemicambitious-men-should-take-note/*

Palmeira, M. (2015). Abstract language signals power, but also lack of action orientation. *Journal of Experimental Social Psychology, 61*, 59–63.

Pan, L., McNamara, G., Lee, J. J., Haleblian, J., & Devers, C. E. (2018). Give it to us straight (most of the time): Top managers' use of concrete language and its effect on investor reactions. *Strategic Management Journal, 39*(8), 2204–2225.

Ridgeway, C. L. (2001). Gender, status, and leadership. *Journal of Social Issues, 57*(4), 637–655.

Rubin, R. B., Perse, E. M., & Barbato, C. A. (1988). Conceptualization and measurement of interpersonal communication motives. *Human Communication Research, 14*(4), 602–628.

Shannon, C. E. (1948). A mathematical theory of communication. *Bell System Technical Journal*, 27(3), 379–423.

Silano, S. (2023, March 6). *Women founders get 2% of venture capital funding in U.S.* Morningstar. *www.morningstar.com/alternative-investments/women-founders-get-2-venture-capital-funding-us*

Smith, P. K., & Trope, Y. (2006). You focus on the forest when you're in charge of the trees: Power priming and abstract information processing. *Journal of Personality and Social Psychology, 90*(4), 578–596.

Tannen, D. (1991). *You just don't understand: Women and men in conversation*. William Morrow.

Tannen, D. (1994). *Talking from 9 to 5: How women's and men's conversational styles affect who gets heard, who gets credit, and what gets done at work*. William Morrow.

Teare, G. (2024, June 6). *The portion of US VC funding that went to female founders hit a new peak in 2023, thanks to massive AI deals.*

Crunchbase News. *news.crunchbase.com/diversity/us-vc-funding-female-founders-peaked-2023-ai-openai-anthropic/*

Toma, C. L., & Hancock, J. T. (2012). What lies beneath: The linguistic traces of deception in online dating profiles. *Journal of Communication, 62*(1), 78–97.

Torrez, B., Wakslak, C. J., & Amit, E. (2019). Dynamic distance: Use of visual and verbal means of communication as social signals. *Journal of Experimental Social Psychology, 85,* 103849.

Trope, Y., & Liberman, N. (2010). Construal-level theory of psychological distance. *Psychological Review, 117*(2), 440–463.

van Kleef, G. A., Oveis, C., van der Löwe, I., LuoKogan, A., Goetz, J., & Keltner, D. (2008). Power, distress, and compassion: Turning a blind eye to the suffering of others. *Psychological Science, 19*(12), 1315–1322.

Vaynerchuk, G. (2014, October 29). *Betting on the jockey, not the horse.* Medium. *medium.com/the-entrepreneurs-journey/the-way-i-evaluate-startups-and-their-founders-7b0770cc0f22*

Wakslak, C., & Joshi, P. (2020). Expansive and contractive communication scope: A construal level perspective on the relationship between interpersonal distance and communicative abstraction. *Social and Personality Psychology Compass, 14*(5), 271–284.

Wakslak, C. J., Smith, P. K., & Han, A. (2014). Using abstract language signals power. *Journal of Personality and Social Psychology, 107*(1), 41–55.

Wood, W., & Eagly, A. H. (2012). Biosocial construction of sex differences and similarities in behavior. In J. M. Olson & M. P. Zanna (Eds.), *Advances in experimental social psychology* (Vol. 46, pp. 55–123). Academic Press.

Yin, Y., & Wakslak, C. J., & Joshi, P. (2022). "I" am more concrete than "we": Linguistic abstraction and first-person pronoun usage. *Journal of Personality and Social Psychology, 122*(6), 1004–1021.

PART II

CREATING MEANING TO FIND DIRECTION IN PERSONAL STRIVING

CHAPTER 6

Making Meaning through Motivated Perception

The Role of Construal

Jenna P. Landy, Jordan S. Daley, and Emily Balcetis

Nearly 900 years ago, in India's southernmost state of Tamil Nadu, King Rajaraja Chola II constructed a site that is famous for kindling visual disagreement. This site, the Airavatesvara Temple, pays homage to the Hindu deity Shiva. The temple's original architecture included a complex system of seven roads and seven courts. In these courts, thick stone walls are covered in inscriptions and carvings of bulls, acrobats, chariots, sundials, nymphs, and yalis—mythological beasts with the combined features of a lion and an elephant. Over the years, many of the temple's wonders have been lost, perhaps to the ravages of time or war. But preserved inside remains what is considered to be the world's oldest optical illusion: a bas-relief carving depicting an enigmatic creature. For hundreds of years, countless visitors to the temple have, at first glance, seen that carving as a muscular bull. But at the same time, many others have looked upon the same stone relief and perceived a trumpeting elephant. How can it be that any two people can look at the same depiction and see something so entirely different?

This illusion is, of course, not the only famous example of divergence in visual interpretation of the same focal object. Nearly a century later and half a world over, in Manchester, England, Cecilia Bleasdale went shopping for a dress. In a changing room, she snapped photos of a few options, then sent the pictures to her daughter (Jinks, 2024). The conversation that followed was the beginning of a worldwide debate:

"What do you think?"
"The third one, but I thought you said it was blue."
"It's blue and black."
"The photo you sent is white and gold."

With this conversation, a controversy exploded. In just 24 hours, #TheDress was the subject of nearly 5 million tweets (Warzel, 2016). A BuzzFeed poll (Holderness, 2015) tallying results from 4 million respondents found that about two-thirds of people saw the dress as white and gold, and one-third saw it as blue and black. Casual viewers and neuroscientists alike found themselves perplexed. The dress even drove vision scientist Jay Neitz to make an audacious commitment: "Now, I'm going to spend the rest of my life working on this. I thought I was going to cure blindness, but now I guess I'll do this" (Pardes & Pearl, 2015).

Although these visual illusions may amuse a lone viewer, they become so much more powerful when viewed by a group. After all, humans are innately social beings; they regularly call on others around them to confirm that they are perceiving the world in the same way. When there is a mismatch—when a person sees something different from someone beside them—the experience calls into question the reliability of the human eyes and mind and the way in which people make meaning of the world. This may be confusing or even troubling because people tend to believe that their sensory experiences accurately and completely correspond to the world as it really is (Granot & Igliozzi, 2023; Lehar, 2003; L. Ross & Ward, 1995, 1996) and that their sensory-based conclusions should and will correspond with others' experiences (L. Ross & Ward, 1995, 1996).

Indeed, among individuals' sensory experiences, vision takes precedence. People value their sense of sight over their other senses, and many even report that they would prefer to live 5 years with perfect sight over 10 years with complete loss of sight (Enoch, McDonald, Jones, Jones, & Crabb, 2019). From an early age, we make sense of the world foremost in terms of what we see, evidenced by the fact that vision verbs, like *see* and *look*, emerge in child language before verbs pertaining to other senses, like *hear* and *touch* (San Roque, Norcliffe, & Majid, 2024). Because people place such primacy on vision, they hope that they are seeing the world just as anyone else would see it. Consensus brings people assurance that their eyes have not deceived them. But what should one believe when there is no consensus—when they disagree with others on a visual experience?

In this chapter, we explore how people make meaning of what they see around them. We probe the source of disagreements regarding the visual world, given that consensus in visual experience can sometimes be hard to reach. Strong evidence across cultures shows that people interpret what they see based on what they want to be true. People's visual experiences vary as a function of what they value (e.g., Bruner & Goodman, 1947), what they need (e.g., Bhalla & Proffitt, 1999; Hancock & McNaughton, 1986), what they expect (e.g., Howansky, Albuja, & Cole, 2020), what they are hoping for (e.g., Balcetis & Dunning, 2006, 2007), and what they like (e.g., Balcetis, Dunning, & Granot, 2012). Although a spirited debate surrounds the question of whether idiosyncrasies in visual experience are the result of perception, attention, or judgment (Firestone, 2013; Firestone & Scholl, 2016; Teufel & Nanay, 2017; but see the 34 commentaries following Firestone and Scholl [2016], including Balcetis and Cole [2016] and Qu-Lee and Balcetis [2022]), evidence points to the conclusion that people see the world not for what it really is but instead for what they want it to be. In other words, people make meaning of the visual world through motivated perception.

THE PUZZLE OF MOTIVATED PERCEPTION

People use visual experience as a tool in the regulation of their thoughts, intentions, and behaviors directed at pursuing their active goals. For example, dieters see unhealthy foods as being farther away (Cole, Dominick, & Balcetis, 2021), as if out of arm's reach. Similarly, people in relationships see potential alternative partners as less attractive (Cole, Trope, & Balcetis, 2016), reducing any temptation or threat they may pose to the monogamy they promised their partner. In addition, individuals selectively search for information that facilitates positive self-concepts (Rajsic, Wilson, & Pratt, 2015, 2018; Wilson, Young, Rule, & Hugenberg, 2018), supports original beliefs and expectations (e.g., Granot, Balcetis, Schneider, & Tyler, 2014; Granot, Jones, & Balcetis, 2022; Kassin, Dror, & Kukucka, 2013; Kukucka & Kassin, 2014; Qu-Lee, Seidel, Harel, Granot, & Balcetis, 2022), or aligns with their social identities (e.g., Granot et al., 2014). In other words, visual experiences are in service of self-regulation (Cole & Balcetis, 2021). However, in serving the self, visual experiences are likely to diverge from the visual experiences others have.

The assumption of and desire for consensus in visual experience is so strong that in fact, it is stressful for people when they realize that their visual experiences do not align with others' experiences. In this way, motivated perception may leave people feeling that they lack shared reality with others (Echterhoff, 2012; Echterhoff, Higgins, & Levine, 2009; Hardin & Higgins, 1996; Higgins & Echterhoff, 2019). In the landmark Asch conformity experiments (Asch, 1951), participants were led to believe that they lacked shared reality with their peers as they reported their visual experience of the length of a drawn line. Their peers, all actors, claimed to see the line as being notably longer or shorter than the participants saw it. This lack of visual shared reality heightened participants' discomfort and made them feel undue pressure to conform to the status quo, vocalizing agreement with their peers' obviously incorrect assessments of the line length. In other studies, a lack of shared reality with close social others has been associated with reduced self-concept clarity, impaired well-being and physical health, and increased stress (Campbell et al., 1996; Light & Goldberg, 2020).

Our preference for consensus in visual experience can in fact be so extreme that differing interpretations of visual experiences fuel social conflict. People often think that those who disagree with them are biased or objectively wrong (Kennedy & Pronin, 2008), even if the topic of their disagreement is subjective (Cheek, Blackman, & Pronin, 2021). As people perceive more bias in others, conflict escalates, and cooperation declines (Kennedy & Pronin, 2008). In addition, disparate visual experiences can drive miscarriages of justice (Granot et al., 2022) and personal and societal health complications (Balcetis, Cole, & Duncan, 2020; Balcetis, Riccio, Duncan, & Cole, 2020). Having visual experiences that contradict others' experiences can interfere with healthy social functioning.

The Biology of Visual Experience

The idea that people make meaning of their visual world through a motivated lens also conflicts with some biological arguments about how sight *should* work. Some might argue that the human eyes and brain are designed to provide a consistent and reliable account of the world. Humans, much like their anatomically similar *Hominidae* family members, including chimpanzees and gorillas, rely on the same basic biology and neurological processes in order to see (Kaas, 2020), suggesting that these systems have been evolutionarily optimized. Indeed, species with different environmental constraints have evolved to support quite different anatomical visual structures; similarities within a species are high, and differences across species that live under vastly different environmental constraints are substantial. Most fish, for instance, have eyes on either side of a flat face, and flounder even have migrating eyes that move during their lives to be on the same side of the face (Zimmer, 2024); this is so that fish can see predators from any angle and camouflage themselves on the ocean floor. Owls have classic front-facing eyes, but they are set in a head that rotates nearly all the way around so that they can detect potential prey on all sides (Bloudoff-Indelicato, 2013).

Dragonflies have compound eyes made up of hundreds of lenses so that they can rapidly detect motion (Ruck, 1965). Lobsters have compound eyes, too, but in this case so that they can see through the murkiest of waters (Cronin & Porter, 2008), a feat so aspirational that humans have copied the design of lobster eyes when building x-ray equipment to identify contraband through walls and to spot cosmic events happening galaxies away (Bugos, 2021; U.S. Department of Homeland Security, 2007). Evolution optimizes biological structures for species to see what is most important in ways that best fit their specific environmental conditions.

Although we are not evolutionary theorists, we believe that evolutionary pressures in fact pushed for humans to have perceptual experiences that would help them to work through objective environmental constraints while simultaneously engaging in subjective goal pursuit. To understand how differences in perceptual experience may have come to be, researchers must study more than just what people are seeing and instead shift focus to the cognitive processes that underlie differences in what people see. It is important to consider not only the objects of perception but also the manner of cognitive processing itself. Ultimately, the way that people make meaning of the world is informed by the world itself *and* by the mindsets that people bring to the perceptual table.

Differences in representation among perceivers are not mistakes in interpreting the world. Rather, these differences serve as evidence that the visual system has been designed to accommodate both the objective demands of the external environment and each individual's idiosyncratic psychological demands. Individuals' different styles of representing the world—their construals—are fundamentally connected to the way that they make meaning of the world. By examining the levels of construal that underlie perceivers' interpretative efforts, researchers can understand how individuals may come to perceive the world's contents in fundamentally different ways. Adding construal level to the study of motivated perception may provide more traction on when, how, and why individuals see the world not as it is but, instead, as how they wish it to be.

ADDING CONSTRUAL LEVEL TO MOTIVATED PERCEPTION

To understand how perceivers can gaze upon the same object yet fail to reach consensus on what they are seeing, we argue that we must attend to an individual's mindset or style of cognitive processing. As illustrated by construal-level theory (Liberman & Trope, 2008; Trope & Liberman,

2010), people make meaning of what they perceive in concrete terms at lower levels of construal, focusing on the specifics, including immediate actions, contextual details, and relevant practicalities (Trope, Liberman, & Wakslak, 2007). When people mentally represent a cocktail at a lower level of construal, for example, they may represent it as "a clear bubbly liquid supporting a floating lime." They focus on details relevant to how the object could be engaged with, the specific properties that describe it, and the distinctive elements that are unique to this specific instantiation of a cocktail. They see the shine of the ice, the clarity of the substance, and the specific hue of the skin of the citrus.

In contrast, at higher levels of construal, people make meaning of what they perceive in abstract terms. The focus is on the big picture—this includes goals, values, and key takeaways (Liberman & Trope, 2008). When people mentally represent the cocktail at a higher level of construal, they may represent it as "a celebratory beverage." They focus on central features relevant to the object's significance and how it could be defined. They think about its thirst-quenching capabilities or its use as a tool for socialization. Importantly, many different drinks match these high-level capabilities, from a gin and tonic to a Kool-Aid pouch for kids. When represented in terms of their low-level details, these two drinks are quite different—no experienced adult would ever confuse the two. But when represented in terms of their high-level functions, perceivers will find that they check many of the same boxes. Indeed, in experimental paradigms, when perceivers were cognitively engaged at higher levels of construal, they grouped objects into fewer, more general categories (Liberman, Sagristano, & Trope, 2002, Study 1). They saw similarities, connections, and homogeneity where they might not otherwise.

That said, consensus on visual experiences is not more likely to occur at any particular level of construal. High-level construals can give rise to discordant perceptual experiences when the process of abstraction for any one perceiver omits details that other perceivers continue to rely on or consider central to interpretation. Similarly, perceivers assuming low-level mindsets might attend to different visual details, producing disagreements in visual experience. For instance, individuals assuming a low-level mindset may all be attending to the lines, edges, and contours of the Necker cube shape shown in Figure 6.1. However, those honing their focus on the thick black line may see a box as if viewing it from above, whereas those honing their focus on the dashed line may see a box as if viewing it from below (e.g., Balcetis & Dale, 2007). Low-level construals could reduce consensus among perceivers who are oriented toward different features that are diagnostic of distinct interpretations.

Rather than using construal level as an indicator of likelihood of perceiver consensus, we encourage the consideration of construal level in

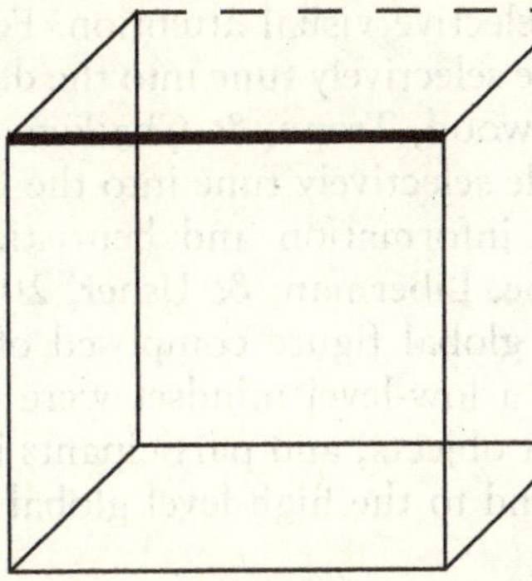

FIGURE 6.1. Necker cube that can be interpreted as a box viewed from above or from below.

probing the process of motivated perception. Even when construal level is held constant, individuals may attend to unique feature sets that still produce divergence in perceptual conclusions. However, considering the mindsets that individuals engage may offer diagnostic capabilities for the processes that underlie motivated perception.

THE ROLE OF CONSTRUAL LEVELS IN SELECTIVE ATTENTION AND AMBIGUITY RESOLUTION

Cognitive construal can guide perceivers through the unique challenges of the messy visual world as they try to make meaning of it. Such challenges include the necessity to engage selective attention and resolve ambiguity.

Selective Attention. Like the packed pictures in a child's I Spy game book, the world is crammed with relevant and irrelevant objects, only some of which require urgent observation. There is a limit to how much low-level information people can attend to. People cannot give equal weight to all of the contents of their environment at once (Carrasco, 2011); they could not afford the cost of the neurological computations if they did (Lennie, 2003). In the midst of a cluttered environment, people may struggle to recognize familiar objects, a phenomenon known as *visual crowding* (Whitney & Levi, 2011). Further complicating things, people can keep track of only a few moving visual elements at once (Alvarez & Franconeri, 2007). Ultimately, people must selectively attend to only a subset of the visual world around them.

Construal level serves as one primary psychological factor that directs the process of selective visual attention. For example, at a low level of construal, people selectively tune into the details of a scene (Ledgerwood, 2014; Ledgerwood, Trope, & Chaiken, 2010), but at a high level of construal, people selectively tune into the Gestalt and are more sensitive to aggregated information and heuristics (Anderson, 1971; Hadar, Glickman, Trope, Liberman, & Usher, 2022; M. Ross, 1989). Indeed, when shown a global figure composed of smaller constituent objects, participants in a low-level mindset were quicker to attend to the low-level constituent objects, and participants in a high-level mindset were quicker to attend to the high-level global figure (Liberman & Förster, 2009).

Construal level shifts individuals' attention as they make judgments about the self and others around them. People are readily able to think about themselves in concrete, low-level terms and about distal others in high-level, abstract terms. So, in our lab's work, when we presented participants with high-level aggregated statistics—or base rates—about cybercrime risk in the general population, we expected participants to differentially incorporate these base rates into their self- versus social judgments (Cox, Zhu, & Balcetis, 2020). Specifically, we expected that when predicting others' risk of succumbing to a cyberattack, participants would be operating at a higher level of construal; this is because the target of consideration (other people) is more psychologically distant (Liberman & Förster, 2009; Trope & Liberman, 2010) than the comparison (the participants themselves). As such, the participants would find utility in attending to the aggregate base rates, relying on them while forming their predictions. On the other hand, when predicting their own risk of succumbing to a cyberattack, participants would be operating at a lower level of construal. As such, they would find little utility in attending to the aggregate base rates, disregarding them while forming their predictions and instead overweighting incidental beliefs about their own skill level or infallibility (Dunning, 2011; Greening & Chandler, 1997; Kruger & Dunning, 1999).

Indeed, using covert eye tracking, we found that participants selectively oriented their visual attention, looking less often at the base rates when predicting their own risk and more often when predicting others' risk. As a result, participants' predictions of others' risk statistically tracked the base rates we provided, whereas participants' predictions of their own risk did not (Cox et al., 2020). This bore consequences for the accuracy of their judgments: Participants woefully underestimated their own risk, which might get them into cyber-trouble down the line.

Handling Ambiguity. At times, visual input can be too ambiguous for fast and reliable resolution. For example, visual input can be degraded or blurry, perhaps because it is blocked by a window screen, viewed on a low-resolution device, shrouded by darkness, or being perceived by someone with poor eyesight. People tend to grow confused and irritated when visual information is ambiguous to the point of being undecipherable—as evidenced by a viral image from 2019, posted to Twitter (now X) with a caption challenging viewers to "name one thing in this photo" (Weisberger, 2019). The image, likely generated by artificial intelligence, depicts . . . some things. Perhaps clothing, jewelry racks, or food items? Maybe piles of shopping bags? Possibly a stuffed teddy bear? These things, whatever they may be, are arranged like a still life, clustered together. But viewers struggle to recognize and name any single one of the items depicted—the resolution of any particular bit of the image into a single identifiable object is impossible. Many have called the image "creepy" or even "cursed" and written off the whole viewing experience as "uncomfortable" or "disturbing" (Cliff, 2019). People want to make sense of what they are seeing and grow ill at ease when they cannot.

The anatomical structure of the eye does little to remedy concerns that people are getting an incomplete look at the world around them. A dip at the back of the retina, called the *fovea*, holds the highest concentration of light-receptive cells (known as *photoreceptors*); as a result, light hitting the fovea produces the sharpest images. But most of the world is seen through peripheral vision, which is strong at detecting motion but weak at picking up fine-grained details about objects and their exact positions (Knotts, Odegaard, Lau, & Rosenthal, 2019; Stewart, Valsecchi, & Schütz, 2020; Strasburger, Rentschler, & Jüttner, 2011). Light is blocked from reception in some parts of the eye altogether, creating blind spots; blood vessels cast shadows over some photoreceptors, and there are areas, including the optic disc, that do not contain photoreceptors at all (Smith & Czyz, 2024).

When presented with unclear or ambiguous visual input, people attempt to hone in on low-level features that are central to an interpretation—particularly, an interpretation that aligns with and advances their active goals (Balcetis & Dunning, 2006). By handling ambiguity in this way, people lose access to any low-level details deemed irrelevant to the interpretation they are forming—their abstraction. But this loss of detail comes with a newfound ability to see the bigger picture, which is why Trope and Liberman (2010, p. 441) wrote that "higher level construals are not simply more impoverished or vague than lower level construals. They often convey additional information about the value of the stimulus and its relations to other stimuli . . . [there is] ascription of new meaning." In the end, by attempting to make meaning out of an ambiguous visual stimulus, two perceivers driven by different active goals may encode information in entirely distinct ways, each losing access to alternate interpretations in the process.

Our lab group demonstrated this point in a study involving an ambiguous image of an animal (Balcetis & Dunning, 2006). We used a line drawing that could be interpreted as either a horse or a seal, and we motivated participants to have particular visual experiences by informing them about the rewards and costs of these visual experiences. Specifically, they knew that if they saw a farm animal, they would go on to complete a taste test of fresh-squeezed orange juice, but if they saw a sea animal, they would go on to complete a taste test of a gelatinous, chunky, pickle-scented, green beverage. Suffice it to say, these participants were hoping to see a farm animal. We then showed them the line drawing for 1,000 milliseconds—just long enough for them to reach one perceptual conclusion but not so long that they were able to recognize that there were multiple interpretative possibilities. In those 1,000 milliseconds, participants formed a high-level representation of the line drawing, dropping low-level details (e.g., the particular pattern of spots on the horse's nose) that bore no critical relevance to their chosen abstraction. At this stage, if we had asked them what animal they were shown, we would have expected participants' interpretations to agree with the most rewarding outcome. On the whole, they would have seen horses.

However, instead of assessing perceptual interpretations at this stage, we engaged in a bit of experimental trickery. We simulated a computer crash. As a result of the crash, we claimed that we had to reassign the categories. Seeing the once-disfavored sea animal would now yield fresh-squeezed orange juice, and seeing the once-favored farm animal would now yield an unfortunate assault on participants' tastebuds. Only then did we ask participants what animal they were shown. With the ultimate reward structure flipped, these participants, who would have initially seen a horse, likely wanted nothing more in this moment than to have seen an ocean-dwelling creature. But the low-level features that defined the seal's face were incidental to the original horse interpretation, and these details had been lost during the process of abstraction. As a result, we expected that participants would not simply be able to think back to the image, retrieve these now-crucial low-level features, and formulate an alternate perceptual abstraction. Instead, we expected that most participants would dejectedly confess that they had been shown a horse and brace themselves for a noxious drink (that, thankfully, would never come). Indeed, 70% of these participants reported that they had seen something other than a seal. This majority had leveled and sharpened the low-level details they originally encoded to such a degree that they could not form a different high-level abstraction. That is, they could not simply decide to see the seal after the fact. As Trope and Liberman (2010) argue, when details are lost to abstraction, they are unlikely to be made available again.

CONCLUSION

By several logical and biological accounts, people should see the world as it is. Species develop visual hardware that is optimized for the physical and social environments they live in and that is conserved across members of the species. Visual discrepancies can fuel irresolvable conflict, miscarriages of justice, and a stressful lack of shared reality. With all of this in mind, it seems like people should see the world just as everyone else does all of the time.

But they don't. How do idiosyncratic visual experiences come to be? We argue that idiosyncrasies in visual perception are not a vestigial tail of development; they are an adaptation. These differences are the result of a process that helps people satisfy their motivations while overcoming visual overload and resolving visual ambiguity. Sometimes, perceivers shift from lower to higher levels of construal—for instance, when goals become active and impinge on perceptual processes. These perceivers are bound to omit details that seem superfluous to whatever abstraction they are forming; as they sharpen the features that remain accessible, omitted details can be lost for good. At other times, perceivers shift from higher to lower levels of construal—for instance, when deliberating precisely how to pursue a goal. These perceivers are bound to focus on a small subset of details; these details may be different from those perceived by their neighbor, facilitating different conclusions. Ultimately, construal levels, as do motivations, guide attention, placing a metaphorical spotlight on specific portions of the visual world.

Appreciating a perceiver's level of mental construal adds an additional predictive factor in modeling idiosyncrasies in visual experience. We can understand differences in visual interpretation as artifacts of an adaptive cognitive tool that helps perceivers navigate the challenges of a rich and complex visual world while prioritizing their various goals, needs, and desires. Ultimately, looking at motivated perception through the lens of construal has provided even more support for the claim that perception is not just in the eye of the beholder.

REFERENCES

Alvarez, G. A., & Franconeri, S. L. (2007). How many objects can you track?: Evidence for a resource-limited attentive tracking mechanism. *Journal of Vision, 7*(13), 14.

Anderson, N. H. (1971). Integration theory and attitude change. *Psychological Review, 78*(3), 171–206.

Asch, S. E. (1951). Effects of group pressure upon the modification and distortion of judgments. In H. Guetzkow (Ed.), *Groups, leadership and men; research in human relations* (pp. 177–190). Carnegie Press.

Balcetis, E., & Cole, S. (2016). Task demand not so damning: Improved techniques that mitigate demand in studies that support top-down effects. *Behavioral and Brain Sciences, 39*, e230.

Balcetis, E., Cole, S., & Duncan, D. T. (2020). How walkable neighborhoods promote physical activity: Policy implications for development and renewal. *Policy Insights from the Behavioral and Brain Sciences, 7*(2), 173–180.

Balcetis, E., & Dale, R. (2007). Conceptual set as a top-down constraint on visual object identification. *Perception, 36*(4), 581–595.

Balcetis, E., & Dunning, D. (2006). See what you want to see: Motivational influences on visual perception. *Journal of Personality and Social Psychology, 91*(4), 612–625.

Balcetis, E., & Dunning, D. (2007). Cognitive dissonance and the perception of natural environments. *Psychological Science, 18*(10), 917–921.

Balcetis, E., Dunning, D., & Granot, Y. (2012). Subjective value determines initial dominance in binocular rivalry. *Journal of Experimental Social Psychology, 48*(1), 122–129.

Balcetis, E., Riccio, M. T., Duncan, D. T., & Cole, S. (2020). Keeping the goal in sight: Testing the influence of narrowed visual attention on physical activity. *Personality and Social Psychology Bulletin, 46*(3), 485–496.

Bhalla, M., & Proffitt, D. R. (1999). Visual-motor recalibration in geographical slant perception. *Journal of Experimental Psychology: Human Perception and Performance, 25*(4), 1076–1096.

Bloudoff-Indelicato, M. (2013). How owls twist their heads almost 360 degrees. *National Geographic. www.nationalgeographic.com/animals/article/how-owls-twist-heads-almost-360-degrees*

Bruner, J. S., & Goodman, C. C. (1947). Value and need as organizing factors in perception. *Journal of Abnormal and Social Psychology, 42*(1), 33–44.

Bugos, C. (2021, June 23). How lobster eyes can help astronomers get a wider view of the cosmos. *Astronomy Magazine. www.astronomy.com/space-exploration/how-lobster-eyes-can-help-astronomers-get-a-wider-view-of-the-cosmos/*

Campbell, J. D., Trapnell, P. D., Heine, S. J., Katz, I. M., Lavallee, L. F., & Lehman, D. R. (1996). Self-concept clarity: Measurement, personality correlates, and cultural boundaries. *Journal of Personality and Social Psychology, 70*(1), 141–156.

Carrasco, M. (2011). Visual attention: The past 25 years. *Vision Research, 51*(13), 1484–1525.

Cheek, N. N., Blackman, S. F., & Pronin, E. (2021). Seeing the subjective as objective: People perceive the taste of those they disagree with as biased and wrong. *Journal of Behavioral Decision Making, 34*(2), 167–182.

Cliff, M. (2019, April 24). Viral tweet asking people to "name one thing in the photo" leaves the internet stumped—but can you identify anything? *The Sun. www.thesun.co.uk/fabulous/8930936/viral-tweet-asking-people-to-name-one-thing-in-the-photo-leaves-the-internet-stumped-but-can-you-identify-anything/*

Cole, S., & Balcetis, E. (2021). Motivated perception for self-regulation: How visual experience serves and is served by goals. In B. Gawronski (Ed.), *Advances in experimental social psychology* (Vol. 64, pp. 129–186). Elsevier.

Cole, S., Dominick, J. K., & Balcetis, E. (2021). Out of reach and under control: Distancing as a self-control strategy. *Personality and Social Psychology Bulletin, 47*(6), 939–952.

Cole, S., Trope, Y., & Balcetis, E. (2016). In the eye of the betrothed: Perceptual downgrading of attractive alternative romantic partners. *Personality and Social Psychology Bulletin, 42*(7), 879–892.

Cox, E. B., Zhu, Q., & Balcetis, E. (2020). Stuck on a phishing lure: Differential use of base rates in self and social judgments of susceptibility to cyber risk. *Comprehensive Results in Social Psychology, 4*(1), 25–52.

Cronin, T. W., & Porter, M. L. (2008). Exceptional variation on a common theme: The evolution of crustacean compound eyes. *Evolution: Education and Outreach, 1*(4), Article 4.

Dunning, D. (2011). The Dunning-Kruger effect: On being ignorant of one's own ignorance. In J. M. Olson & M. P. Zanna (Eds.), *Advances in experimental social psychology* (Vol. 44, pp. 247–296). Academic Press.

Echterhoff, G. (2012). Shared-reality theory. In P. A. M. Van Lange, A. W. Kruglanski, & E. T. Higgins (Eds.), *Handbook of theories of social psychology* (pp. 180–199). Sage.

Echterhoff, G., Higgins, E. T., & Levine, J. M. (2009). Shared reality: Experiencing commonality with others' inner states about the world. *Perspectives on Psychological Science, 4*(5), 496–521.

Enoch, J., McDonald, L., Jones, L., Jones, P. R., & Crabb, D. P. (2019). Evaluating whether sight is the most valued sense. *JAMA Ophthalmology, 137*(11), 1317–1320.

Firestone, C. (2013). How "paternalistic" is spatial perception? Why wearing a heavy backpack doesn't—and couldn't—make hills look steeper. *Perspectives on Psychological Science, 8*(4), 455–473.

Firestone, C., & Scholl, B. J. (2016). Cognition does not affect perception: Evaluating the evidence for "top-down" effects. *Behavioral and Brain Sciences, 39*, e229.

Granot, Y., Balcetis, E., Schneider, K. E., & Tyler, T. R. (2014). Justice is not blind: Visual attention exaggerates effects of group identification on legal punishment. *Journal of Experimental Psychology: General, 143*(6), 2196–2208.

Granot, Y., & Igliozzi, D. (2023). Psychological perspectives on the presentation of video evidence: How perceivers weight what is seen and unseen. *First Monday, 28*(7).

Granot, Y., Jones, K. A., & Balcetis, E. (2022). Sight unseen, justice unobserved: How naïve realism in visual attention affects legal decision-making. In N. Ballantyne & D. Dunning (Eds.), *Reason, bias, and inquiry: The crossroads of epistemology and psychology* (pp. 129–149). Oxford University Press.

Greening, L., & Chandler, C. C. (1997). Why it can't happen to me: The base rate matters, but overestimating skill leads to underestimating risk. *Journal of Applied Social Psychology, 27*(9), 760–780.

Hadar, B., Glickman, M., Trope, Y., Liberman, N., & Usher, M. (2022). Abstract thinking facilitates aggregation of information. *Journal of Experimental Psychology: General, 151*(7), 1733–1743.

Hancock, S., & McNaughton, L. (1986). Effects of fatigue on ability to process visual information by experienced orienteers. *Perceptual and Motor Skills, 62*(2), 491–498.

Hardin, C. D., & Higgins, E. T. (1996). Shared reality: How social verification makes the subjective objective. In *Handbook of motivation and cognition, Vol. 3: The interpersonal context* (pp. 28–84). Guilford.

Higgins, E. T., & Echterhoff, G. (2019). Shared reality: Motivated connection and motivated cognition. In P. A. M. Van Lange, E. T. Higgins, & A. W. Kruglanski (Eds.), *Social psychology: Handbook of basic principles* (3rd ed., pp. 181–201). Guilford.

Holderness, C. (2015, February 26). *What colors are this dress?* BuzzFeed. *www.buzzfeed.com/catesish/help-am-i-going-insane-its-definitely-blue*

Howansky, K., Albuja, A., & Cole, S. (2020). Seeing gender: Perceptual representations of transgender individuals. *Social Psychological and Personality Science, 11*(4), 474–482.

Jinks, P. (2024). *Behind the dress.* The Dress Illusionist. *www.tumblr.com/meatybeefy*

Kaas, J. H. (2020). Evolution of visual cortex in primates. In J. Kremers (Ed.), *Evolutionary neuroscience* (2nd ed., pp. 547–564). Academic Press.

Kassin, S. M., Dror, I. E., & Kukucka, J. (2013). The forensic confirmation bias: Problems, perspectives, and proposed solutions. *Journal of Applied Research in Memory and Cognition, 2*(1), 42–52.

Kennedy, K. A., & Pronin, E. (2008). When disagreement gets ugly: Perceptions of bias and the escalation of conflict. *Personality and Social Psychology Bulletin, 34*(6), 833–848.

Knotts, J. D., Odegaard, B., Lau, H., & Rosenthal, D. (2019). Subjective inflation: Phenomenology's get-rich-quick scheme. *Current Opinion in Psychology, 29*, 49–55.

Kruger, J., & Dunning, D. (1999). Unskilled and unaware of it: How difficulties in recognizing one's own incompetence lead to inflated self-assessments. *Journal of Personality and Social Psychology, 77*(6), 1121–1134.

Kukucka, J., & Kassin, S. M. (2014). Do confessions taint perceptions of handwriting evidence? An empirical test of the forensic confirmation bias. *Law and Human Behavior, 38*(3), 256–270.

Ledgerwood, A. (2014). Evaluations in their social context: Distance regulates consistency and context dependence. *Social and Personality Psychology Compass, 8*(8), 436–447.

Ledgerwood, A., Trope, Y., & Chaiken, S. (2010). Flexibility now, consistency later: Psychological distance and construal shape evaluative responding. *Journal of Personality and Social Psychology, 99*(1), 32–51.

Lehar, S. (2003). Gestalt isomorphism and the primacy of subjective conscious experience: A Gestalt Bubble model. *Behavioral and Brain Sciences, 26*(4), 375–408; discussion 408–443.

Lennie, P. (2003). The cost of cortical computation. *Current Biology: CB, 13*(6), 493–497.

Liberman, N., & Förster, J. (2009). The effect of psychological distance on perceptual level of construal. *Cognitive Science, 33*(7), 1330–1341.

Liberman, N., Sagristano, M. D., & Trope, Y. (2002). The effect of temporal distance on level of mental construal. *Journal of Experimental Social Psychology, 38*(6), 523–534.

Liberman, N., & Trope, Y. (2008). The psychology of transcending the here and now. *Science, 322*(5905), 1201–1205.

Light, A. E., & Goldberg, M. H. (2020). Failure to share reality and its consequences for self-concept clarity. *Social Cognition, 38*(1), 62–96.

Pardes, A., & Pearl, M. (2015, February 27). *We asked a color vision expert about the color of that dress.* Vice. *www.vice.com/en/article/mv58kx/heres-whats-happening-with-that-dress-with-the-confusing-colors-882*

Qu-Lee, J., & Balcetis, E. (2022). The call for ecological validity is right but missing perceptual idiosyncrasies is wrong. *Behavioral and Brain Sciences, 45*, e88.

Qu-Lee, J., Seidel, B., Harel, D., Granot, Y., & Balcetis, E. (2022). The relationship between visual confirmation bias, belief consistency, and belief polarization. *Comprehensive Results in Social Psychology, 6*(1–3), 1–38.

Rajsic, J., Wilson, D. E., & Pratt, J. (2015). Confirmation bias in visual search. *Journal of Experimental Psychology: Human Perception and Performance, 41*(5), 1353–1364.

Rajsic, J., Wilson, D. E., & Pratt, J. (2018). The price of information: Increased inspection costs reduce the confirmation bias in visual search. *Quarterly Journal of Experimental Psychology, 71*(4), 832–849.

Ross, L., & Ward, A. (1995). Psychological barriers to dispute resolution. In M. P. Zanna (Ed.), *Advances in experimental social psychology* (Vol. 27, pp. 255–304). Academic Press.

Ross, L., & Ward, A. (1996). Naive realism in everyday life: Implications for social conflict and misunderstanding. In E. S. Reed, E. Turiel, & T. Brown (Eds.), *Values and knowledge* (pp. 103–135). Erlbaum.

Ross, M. (1989). Relation of implicit theories to the construction of personal histories. *Psychological Review, 96*(2), 341–357.

Ruck, P. (1965). The components of the visual system of a dragonfly. *Journal of General Physiology, 49*(2), 289–307.

San Roque, L., Norcliffe, E., & Majid, A. (2024). Vision verbs emerge first in English acquisition but touch, not audition, follows second. *Cognitive Science, 48*(6), e13469.

Smith, A. M., & Czyz, C. N. (2024). Neuroanatomy, cranial nerve 2 (optic). In *StatPearls*. StatPearls Publishing. *www.ncbi.nlm.nih.gov/books/NBK507907/*

Stewart, E. E. M., Valsecchi, M., & Schütz, A. C. (2020). A review of interactions between peripheral and foveal vision. *Journal of Vision, 20*(12), 2.

Strasburger, H., Rentschler, I., & Jüttner, M. (2011). Peripheral vision and pattern recognition: A review. *Journal of Vision, 11*(5), 13.

Teufel, C., & Nanay, B. (2017). How to (and how not to) think about top-down influences on visual perception. *Consciousness and Cognition, 47*, 17–25.

Trope, Y., & Liberman, N. (2010). Construal-level theory of psychological distance. *Psychological Review, 117*(2), 440–463.

Trope, Y., Liberman, N., & Wakslak, C. (2007). Construal levels and psychological distance: Effects on representation, prediction, evaluation, and behavior. *Journal of Consumer Psychology, 17*(2), 83–95.

U.S. Department of Homeland Security. (2007). *Eye of the lobster. www.dhs.gov/science-and-technology/eye-lobster*

Warzel, C. (2016). *2/26: How two llamas and a dress gave us the internet's greatest day.* BuzzFeed. *www.buzzfeednews.com/article/charliewarzel/226-how-two-runaway-llamas-and-a-dress-gave-us-the-internets*

Weisberger, M. (2019, April 25). *Why is this viral image of unrecognizable objects so creepy?* LiveScience. *www.livescience.com/65317-unidentifiable-objects-viral-photo.html*

Whitney, D., & Levi, D. M. (2011). Visual crowding: A fundamental limit on conscious perception and object recognition. *Trends in Cognitive Sciences, 15*(4), 160–168.

Wilson, J. P., Young, S. G., Rule, N. O., & Hugenberg, K. (2018). Configural processing and social judgments: Face inversion particularly disrupts inferences of human-relevant traits. *Journal of Experimental Social Psychology, 74*, 1–7.

Zimmer, C. (2024, June 21). How flounder wound up with an epic side-eye. *New York Times. www.nytimes.com/2024/06/21/science/flounder-flatfish-evolution.html*

CHAPTER 7

The Meaning of Multitasking

Why Activity Identification Matters When Engaging in Multiple Activities

Emily Nakkawita and E. Tory Higgins

Modern life seems to involve constantly being pulled in different directions by activities that compete for one's time and attention. Beyond perennial demands to engage in the behaviors needed to sustain a successful professional, personal, and family life, the advent of digital technology has enabled new systems that continually notify individuals about a wide range of items to which they could attend (Mark, 2022). It is no surprise, then, that these ever-present distractions might lead individuals to frequently choose to shift from one activity to another within a short period of time—a behavior commonly described as *multitasking* (Oswald, Hambrick, & Jones, 2007).

Research on the prevalence of media multitasking bears out this notion: 23% of the time U.S. adults spend using media involves engaging in more than one activity at the same time (Papper, Holmes, & Popovich, 2004), and this rate is even higher among children (Uncapher et al., 2017). Multitasking trends appear similar even beyond the confines of the media ecosystem. Among participants asked to report their behavior at four time points throughout a 24-hour period, 45% of responses indicated multitasking (Sastre Gomez, Defina, Garrett, Zacks, & Dennis, 2023). Furthermore, a casual scan of employment opportunities posted online reveals that multitasking is frequently highlighted as a desired skill in job requisitions: "Excellent organizational and multitasking abilities"; "A gift for multitasking in a way that leverages problem solving, being solution oriented and flexible"; "Ability to multitask, prioritize and manage multiple projects" (LinkedIn, n.d.). In one recent study that polled a representative U.S. sample, more than 84% of participants responded that the ability to multitask is an important trait to have (Srna, Schrift, & Zauberman, 2018). Overall, multitasking is both prevalent and considered to be desirable.

Despite its ubiquity and common reputation, research indicates that multitasking has numerous drawbacks. For instance, dividing one's focus between activities is challenging because cognitive activity related to one task persists after switching to another—a phenomenon termed *attention residue* (Leroy, 2009). As such, it is no surprise that multitasking has been shown to lead to inattentional blindness, whereby the individual neglects even unusual, potentially important aspects of their experience (Hyman, Boss, Wise, McKenzie, & Caggiano, 2010). Additionally, multitasking tends to be relatively inefficient because of the cognitive demands and time involved in switching between activities (Rogers & Monsell, 1995; see also Rubinstein, Meyer, & Evans, 2001). (For a thorough review of multitasking research encompassing both dual-task and task-switching paradigms, see Koch, Poljac, Müller, & Kiesel [2018].) As a result, productivity experts often encourage individuals to forsake multitasking for longer stretches of "deep work" focused on a single activity at a time (e.g., Crenshaw, 2021; Newport, 2016). But is such a solution really feasible?

Some multitasking is optional, driven by motives of information seeking (e.g., searching the internet for more information on an actor while watching a film in which they are featured), social connection (e.g., popping onto Facebook to feel a sense of belonging while toiling alone in the office), or enjoyment (e.g., minimizing boredom by bouncing between activities; Hwang, Kim, & Jeong, 2014). In these cases, it seems that a shift toward "single-tasking" would be a possibility for individuals who decide that the benefits for attention and productivity outweigh these other concerns. However, in other situations, multitasking may be unavoidable, such as when activity switching is required to successfully perform one's job duties. In such a case, individuals might find that there are emails to be scrutinized, task lists to be maintained, articles to be explored, and projects to be launched—all at once. In cases like these, avoidance of multitasking may not be an option. For instance, communications from supervisors and clients cannot be left to linger without negative consequences, even if at the expense of one's focus on other activities. As a result, individuals might ask: *If multitasking is a necessity, how can one minimize its costs?*

ACTIVITY ENGAGEMENT THEORY

The present chapter addresses this question through the lens of Higgins and Trope's (1990) activity engagement theory and its extensions (Higgins, Lee, Kwon, & Trope, 1995; Higgins, Trope, & Kwon, 1999), which build on a range of classic theories that propose that any referent can vary in its identification (e.g., Brown, 1958; Bruner, 1957; Rosch, 1978), including actions taken by oneself or others (e.g., Kruglanski, 1975; Newtson, 1976; Trope, 1986; Wegner & Vallacher, 1986). It is grounded in the proposition that although people can identify their engagement in a particular activity in many distinct ways, only one of these identifications will be primary for the individual at any given point in time. For instance, an account manager at a technology firm could conceptualize a particular instance of checking their email at distinct hierarchical levels, from as abstract as "accomplishing my job duties" to as concrete as "reading words on my computer screen." Furthermore, this same account manager could identify the email-checking activity in a variety of alternative ways on the same level, such as "preserving important client relationships," "reviewing 'to-do' items for today," "discovering unexpected product promotions in my inbox," or "taking a break from drafting a contract." With this said, only one of these potential identifications will be treated by the individual as primary while engaging in the activity, whereas one or more other identifications may be treated as secondary.

What is it that determines which of the possible activity identifications will be primary during a particular engagement instance? According to Higgins and Trope (1990), in addition to well-established factors that influence the identification of any input, such as usefulness (Brown, 1958), the maximization of cue validity (Rosch, 1978), or a general preference for categorization at the most general level possible (Wegner & Vallacher, 1986), activity identification is influenced by both chronic individual differences and situational demands that affect the availability and accessibility of different constructs (e.g., Higgins, 1989, 1996; Kruglanski, 1990; Wyer & Srull, 1986). Notably, some of these differences may relate to the individual's motivational orientation—for instance, a focus on attaining gains versus maintaining non-losses (Higgins, 1997)—a point we will return to after first completing this introduction to the theory.

Higgins and Trope (1990) further posit that the activity's primary identification will determine the properties of the activity or related stimuli that are most motivationally relevant. Although properties related to the primary identification will likely capture most of the individual's attention, properties related to the secondary identification are also expected to compete for this attention—and because of this distraction, both sets of properties might be experienced by the individual more negatively than they would otherwise. To again consider the example of the account manager checking their email, the property of "delivers immediate push notifications from priority senders" would likely be highly relevant when the activity's primary identification is "preserving important client relationships" but not necessarily when it is "taking a break from drafting a contract." Additionally, a property more relevant to the latter identification, such as "collects interesting newsletter subscriptions into an easily accessible folder," may be seen as diverting rather than useful when the email-checking activity is primarily identified as "carefully sustaining relationships with important clients." The theory posits that over time, individuals form associative networks that connect each activity identification to its relevant properties and related affective responses, and the strongest and most positive responses will be to those properties related to the primary activity identification.

Finally, activity engagement theory specifies that people use the information contained within these associative networks to make inferences about their orientation toward the activity (Higgins & Trope, 1990). Importantly, because these networks differ for each potential identification, the inferences that individuals draw about how they feel about an activity will differ depending on how it is identified. These inferences then affect the individual's motivation to engage in the activity again in the future, assuming that they are experienced as relevant to the activity based on its identification at that point. To exemplify the consequences of this inferential process, Higgins and Trope (1990) described how activity engagement theory might serve as an alternative explanation for classic research in which an expected "extrinsic" reward for assisting an adult in coloring pictures apparently undermined children's "intrinsic" interest in the coloring activity (Lepper, Greene, & Nisbett, 1973). They argued that children in the expected-reward condition would have primarily identified the coloring activity during the initial experimental session as the extrinsically motivated activity of "winning an award from a stranger," whereas the intrinsically motivated identification of "playing" would have been identified as secondary. Because the "playing" identification would have competed with the "winning an award" identification, "playing" would likely have been associated with more negative affective responses among children in this condition. As a result, during a subsequent open engagement session when no stranger was present (and thus the "winning an award from a stranger" identification could no longer be applied), these children would likely have identified the activity as "playing"—and because of the associations learned in the initial session, their desire to engage in the intrinsically motivated coloring activity would decrease, consistent with the pattern of results found in the study (Lepper et al., 1973).

IMPLICATIONS OF ACTIVITY SWITCHING

Beyond scenarios involving a combination of extrinsically and intrinsically motivated activity identifications, activity engagement theory also generates important, and perhaps counterintuitive, predictions in scenarios involving simultaneous activity identifications that are *both intrinsically motivated.* In such cases, Higgins and Trope (1990) argue that the competition and distraction that the positive properties of the secondary identification can pose to the primary identification will decrease the positivity of the individual's responses to the properties of the primary identification. Higgins et al. (1995) expand on this line of argument, proposing that the inherent emphasis that the primary activity identification receives will prompt the individual to make the inference that the secondary activity identification is, by contrast, less attractive. For this reason, when people switch from an interesting or enjoyable primary identified activity to a secondary identified activity, they assume that the switch is meaningful and informative, and they thus infer that the primary activity must not be quite as interesting as they would have thought otherwise. In line with classic work on attribution (e.g., Jones & Davis, 1965), such inferences will be particularly likely when the secondary activity identification isn't especially attractive (because a highly attractive secondary identified activity would be experienced as a strong situational force, which may lead to weaker inferences about the attractiveness of the primary activity).

To test this proposal that people make inferences about their attitudes toward activities based on the supposed meaning of their having *switched* from one identification to another, Higgins et al. (1995) conducted a series of experiments in which grade school children simultaneously engaged in two intrinsically motivated tasks: *reading* and *coloring* within an activity booklet. In the first of these studies, the researchers manipulated children's primary and secondary activity identifications within the instructions that were provided prior to working on a booklet in a preliminary session, telling the children: "I have here two fun stories (pictures) for you to read (color) [. . .] By the way, along with the stories there are also pictures (stories) you can color (read)" (Higgins et al., 1995, p. 752). To serve as a control condition, a third group of children did not complete this first session. Additionally, among the children who participated in the first session, the attractiveness of the coloring activity was manipulated: Half of the children received six marker pens, a condition in which coloring was an especially attractive activity, whereas the other half only received two marker pens. Then, approximately 1 week later, all children participated in a session in which they received a similarly structured booklet with new stories and pictures. In this second session, the researchers again manipulated activity identification; as a result, among participants from the preliminary session, some children received the same primary versus secondary activity identification instructions in both sessions, and for other children, the activity identification changed between the two sessions. (The number of coloring pens was held constant across both sessions for participants outside the control condition.)

Results revealed an interaction between the assigned activity identifications in the first and second sessions: As predicted, changing primary versus secondary activity identifications between sessions led to less time spent on the primary activity in the second session compared with children in the control condition. (See Figures 7.1 and 7.2 for visualizations of the effects of activity identification in each session on time spent reading and coloring, respectively, in the second session.) Furthermore, the undermining effect of changing primary versus secondary activity identifications on time spent reading was reduced in the six-pen condition in which reading was primary but coloring was especially attractive.

Importantly, these undermining effects only emerged in conditions that might be considered multitasking—that is, when both identified activities were considered simultaneously rather than successively. In the first session of a follow-up study, one group of children received booklets with both coloring and reading on alternating pages of the same booklet and instructions simultaneously identifying coloring as primary and reading as secondary, as in the first experiment. Other groups of children were presented with reading booklets containing only stories separately from coloring booklets containing only pictures; although the order of these activities was counterbalanced, in both groups, each booklet was identified only as comprising a single, primary activity in

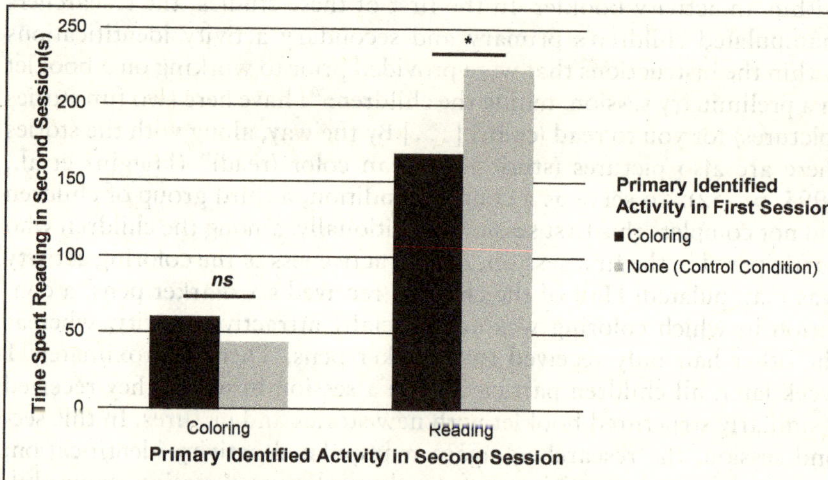

FIGURE 7.1. Time spent reading in second session.

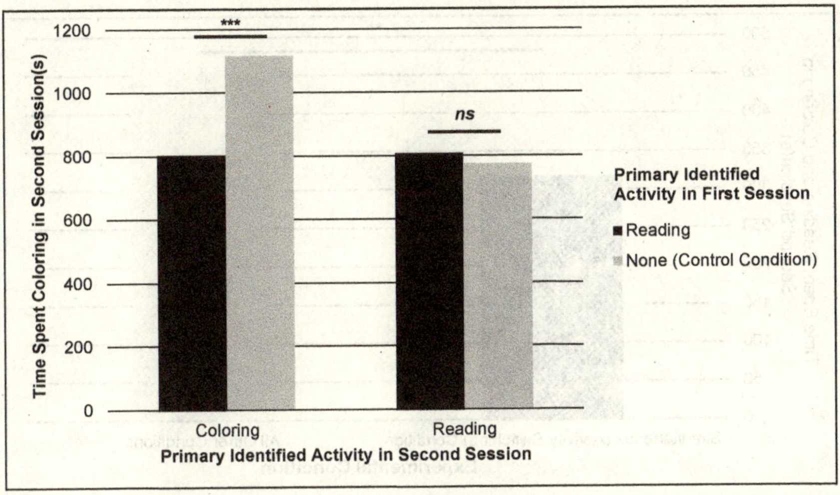

FIGURE 7.2. Time spent coloring in second session.

the instructions ("I have four fun stories [pictures] for you to read [color] [. . .] I hope you will enjoy reading [coloring] them"; Higgins et al., 1995, p. 757). To ensure that the activities in these latter conditions were experienced as successive rather than simultaneous, participants played a counting game during a brief 2-minute break between them. Additionally, two more groups of children only completed one of the activities—either reading or coloring—with the same single-activity identification instructions in the first session.

Results revealed that children in the simultaneous condition involving activity switching (i.e., multitasking) spent less time both reading and coloring in a second session 1 week later compared with children in all other conditions (see Figure 7.3). Additionally, these children in the simultaneous activity-switching condition spent more time in the second session engaging in an unenjoyable penmanship activity. Collectively, the results of this study suggest that the attractiveness of both the coloring and the reading alternatives in the simultaneous condition were undermined by the inferences the children drew about the meaning of their having *switched* from one activity to another: "If I have switched away from reading (coloring), it must not have been that interesting or enjoyable."

The results of these first two studies by Higgins et al. (1995) provide converging evidence that multitasking—that is, shifting between multiple attractive activities within a short period of time—could lead people to infer that the switch is meaningful. That is, they must not have

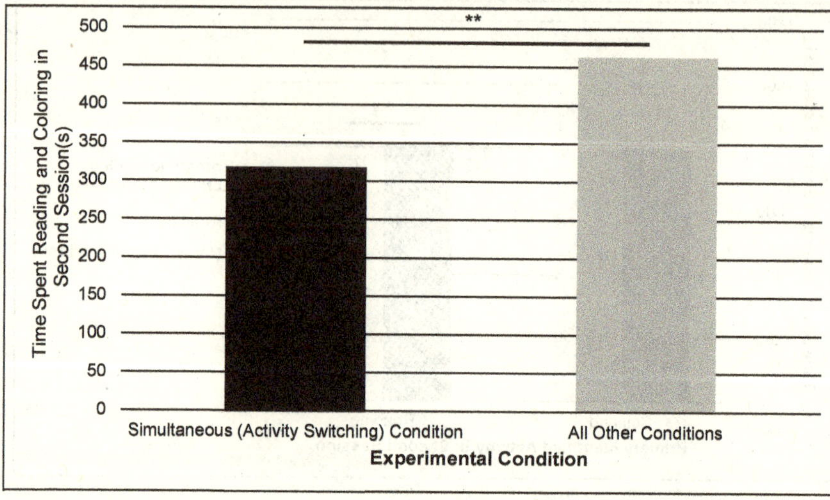

FIGURE 7.3. Time spent reading and coloring in second session.

completely enjoyed the activity from which they switched away; why else would they have decided to stop and engage in a different activity? Notably, this inference emerges even when the switching behavior does not originate from the individual's own decision making, such as when it is solely prompted by the instructions one is given. These findings raise an important question for multitaskers (as well as those who direct their activities, such as their employers and teachers): How might the undermining effects of activity switching be mitigated?

Based on the second study described previously, one option could be to segment one's work or learning into discrete successive activity blocks that clearly delineate one primary identification at a time, without simultaneously presented alternatives. For instance, the busy account manager might reserve the first 10 minutes of every hour for the sole activity of email checking and schedule other activities (e.g., drafting contract revisions, meeting with collaborators) in separate blocks that take place before and after their email-focused work.

Additionally, a third experiment by Higgins and colleagues (1995) provides an alternative solution: to identify the multitasking behavior as a *superordinate activity* that subsumes each of the component tasks. In this third and final study, children whose instructions identified engagement with the coloring storybook as a single, higher-level playbook activity ("There are pictures in this playbook, and there are stories in this playbook. So, you can play with this book by reading the stories and by coloring the pictures"; Higgins et al., 1995, p. 761) did not demonstrate any undermining, despite having engaged in and switched between reading and coloring simultaneously. These results suggest that by representing their engagement in the alternating tasks of reading and coloring as a *singular higher-level activity*, children avoid the deleterious undermining effect that arises from the inferred meaning of having chosen to switch activities. Applied to the prior example of the multitasking account manager at a technology firm, this person might avoid developing more negative attitudes toward their work tasks by identifying all of these behaviors as an overarching activity, such as "successfully overseeing my clients' accounts."

And that is not the end of the story. Importantly, subsequent theorizing and research by Higgins, Trope, and Kwon (1999) reveal that activity switching produces the opposite effect when the valence of individuals' attitudes about the activities is reversed. That is, rather than undermining, switching between two *unattractive* activities actually *augments* people's attitudes about the activities. In one study that validated this proposal, children were presented with activity booklets similarly structured to those in Higgins et al.'s (1995) studies, with both simultaneous and successive activity conditions, but only negatively valenced activities were included (i.e., "finding misspelled words" and "sentence copying"). As predicted, children in the simultaneous conditions who switched between the two disliked activities in the first session spent *more* time engaging in these same activities during a free play period a week later compared with children in the successive conditions (see Figure 7.4).

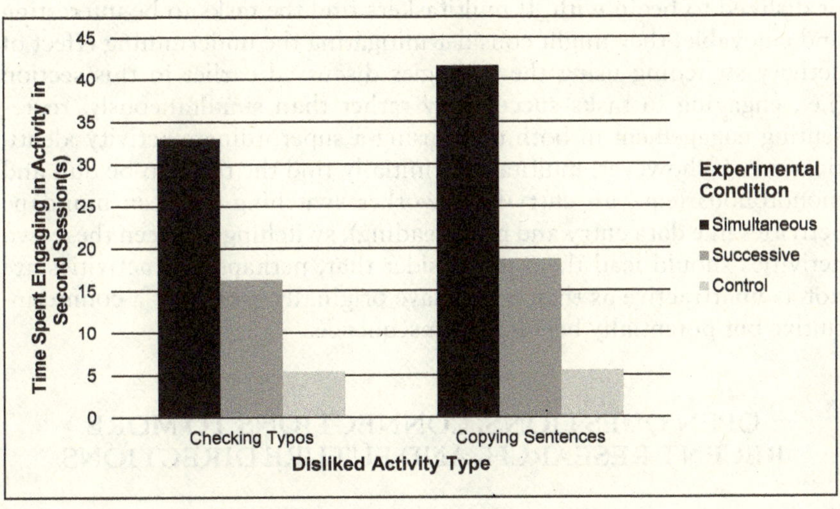

FIGURE 7.4. Time spent engaging in activities in second session.

The authors argued that this effect arises in the meaning-making process and depends on the source of information gain. As posited by information theorists (e.g., Cherry, 1957; Shannon & Weaver, 1949), a signal is informative to the extent that it resolves uncertainty or adds something new or surprising beyond what is already known. Higgins et al. (1999) proposed that activity engagement decisions serve as such a signal. More specifically, the extent to which decisions to shift activities are informative depends on the motivational concerns associated with the activities in question. When activities are attractive, because the activities will already be associated with an approach orientation, decisions *not to approach* these liked activities will be more informative than decisions to approach the same liked activities. Thus, switching between liked activities leads individuals to infer that the activities must not be as attractive as they would have thought otherwise. In contrast, when activities are unattractive, because the activities are already associated with an avoidance orientation, decisions *not to avoid* these disliked activities are more informative than decisions to avoid the same disliked activities. Thus, switching between two disliked activities leads individuals to infer that each activity they switch to must be more attractive than they would have thought otherwise.

Collectively, the results of this research have important implications for multitaskers who, by necessity, must engage in more than one activity within a relatively brief span of time. They suggest that the effects of such multitasking on individuals' attitudes about the activities between which they are shifting will depend on whether those activities are liked or disliked to begin with. If multitaskers find the tasks to be interesting and enjoyable, they might consider mitigating the undermining effect of activity switching using the strategies discussed earlier in this section (i.e., engaging in tasks successively rather than simultaneously, representing engagement in both tasks using a superordinate activity identification). If, however, multitaskers initially find the tasks to be dull and monotonous (e.g., an entry-level worker switching between mundane activities like data entry and proofreading), switching between these two activities should lead them to consider that, perhaps, the activities are not as unattractive as they might have originally thought—a counterintuitive but potentially beneficial consequence.

OPEN QUESTIONS, CONNECTIONS TO MORE RECENT RESEARCH, AND FUTURE DIRECTIONS

Activity engagement theory makes valuable contributions to our understanding of how people derive meaning from multitasking behavior, as well as how they make inferences about their enjoyment of the component activities as a result. Despite these strengths, research on the topic has been limited, and a number of important questions remain. Additionally, more recent theorizing and research on task switching and its consequences for motivation and goal pursuit provide important insight into potential moderators of the meaning-making process posited within activity engagement theory.

Further Validating the Mechanism

First, although the results of existing research testing activity engagement theory are consistent with predictions derived from the theory (Higgins et al., 1995, 1999), more work is needed to more completely validate the theory's postulates. One limitation is that the inferences that participants drew based on their having shifted between two activities were not explicitly assessed in these studies. Instead, the researchers relied on behavioral measures alone, such as the time spent on each activity in a subsequent session and the decision to take home a similar activity. Future work should examine participants' inferences *directly* to provide stronger support for the theory.

Along similar lines, based on the postulates of activity engagement theory (Higgins & Trope, 1990) and its extensions (Higgins et al., 1995, 1999), there is no reason to assume that the inferences drawn from activity switching would be limited to the first switching instance. Instead, it seems to follow that each time an individual shifts between activities, another inference could be drawn. As such, it would seem to follow that the strength of the undermining and augmentation effects (for attractive and unattractive activities, respectively) should be intensified each time another switch is made. To put it another way, the more that a multitasker switches between two distinctly identified activities, the more their attitudes toward those activities should be affected. Researchers could test this proposal by measuring the number of activity switches that take place during the first experimental session. Should an association between the number of activity switches and the strength of attitudinal inferences be detected, this relation could have important consequences for individuals in real-world scenarios involving everyday multitasking, such as those whose job duties require it. Given that 77% of global employees report that they are either not engaged or are actively disengaged in their work, a number that has continued to grow steadily (Gallup, 2024), it raises the question of whether these increasing negative attitudes toward work might be influenced by increases in multitasking expectations that are afforded by ever-advancing technology. Further research is needed to investigate this proposal.

Investigating Moderators of the Effect of Switching on Activity Attitudes

Since the inception of activity engagement theory, a range of additional literature has emerged that offers additional insight into the interplay between activity switching, motivation, and goal pursuit. We propose that these newer lines of work offer intriguing clues into potential moderators of the inferential process posited within activity engagement theory.

Whether Switching Is a Choice

One such line of research derives from Kurzban, Duckworth, Kable, and Myers (2013) theorizing on the relations among the calculation of opportunity costs while engaging in a given task, the subjective experience of mental effort during such task engagement, task performance, and the choice to switch to a different activity. These authors propose that when people engage in mental activities ranging from the basic (e.g., completing Stroop tasks) to the complex (e.g., making difficult decisions), they monitor the benefit-to-cost ratio of continuing to engage in the current activity on an ongoing basis. Additionally, they compare this benefit-to-cost ratio for the current activity to the same ratio for the next-best alternative activity, which functions as a calculation of the opportunity cost of continued engagement in the current activity. Furthermore, this process of monitoring and calculating opportunity costs is posited to produce the phenomenological experience of subjective effort, which can manifest as subjective feelings like boredom, frustration, or mental fatigue with the current activity. These feelings, in turn, motivate people to reallocate their mental resources to activities that are relatively more valuable—thus leading to decrements in their performance of the current activity and, ultimately, the choice to shift to the next-best alternative activity.

We propose that Kurzban et al.'s (2013) opportunity cost theory is broadly consistent with Higgins and Trope's (1990) activity engagement theory because both posit that people's evaluations of activities relate not only to the activities themselves but also to their consideration of alternatives to which they could switch, as well as their actual choices to make such a shift. With this said, the two theories consider these evaluations and switching choices from different directions: The opportunity cost model proposes that ongoing evaluations of activities affect decisions to shift to a next-best alternative, whereas activity engagement theory proposes that switching to a next-best alternative will affect people's evaluations of the activity from which they have switched away.

However, it is important to note that the applicability of Kurzban et al.'s (2013) model appears to be constrained to situations in which it is possible for the individual to make a decision between activity alternatives. In cases such as these, when considered in conjunction with activity engagement theory, we would predict that the inferences the person draws about their having switched between activities would have an especially strong effect on their attitudes about the activities because these inferences would be based on the knowledge that they had chosen to make the switch (i.e., because the opportunity costs of the alternative were too high). However, in cases that involve an activity switch that was not personally driven, such as a switch driven by another person (e.g., when a teacher instructs students to stop their work on a given activity and begin a new one), the effect of activity switching may be attenuated.

When Switching Takes Place Within the Context of the Goal-Pursuit Process

Beyond the simple role of choice in activity switching, we propose that the point within the goal-pursuit process when activity shifts take place may have important consequences for the inferential effect posited within activity engagement theory. This proposal is grounded in theorizing and research on the "goal-gradient" or "goal-looms-larger" effect, which indicate that individuals' motivation to attain a focal goal, and thus their effort and persistence, increase as they approach their desired end state (Förster, Higgins, & Idson, 1998; Heath, Larrick, & Wu, 1999; Hull, 1932; Touré-Tillery & Fishbach, 2011). Similarly, recent research by Emmanuel, Katzir, & Liberman (2022) indicates that individuals tend to engage in tasks more effortfully as they approach task deadlines and that the presence of an alternative task strengthens this gradient effect.

When considered together, we propose that this work suggests that the inferences that people draw about their decisions to switch activities may be affected by where they are within the goal-pursuit process when they make such a choice. More specifically, the decision to shift to an alternative activity near the end of a goal-pursuit process or very close to a deadline should lead to very strong inferences about their interest in the original activity because it would be especially surprising to make a switch at that point in the process when they are most strongly motivated to complete their goal pursuit. By contrast, earlier switching decisions that are further away from goal completion or the deadline should lead to relatively weaker inferences. Future research is needed to test these proposals.

Considering Additional Motivational Factors

Beyond additional work validating the postulates of the theory and examining potential moderators, we also suggest that there are opportunities to extend the theory. One such opportunity relates to the motivational orientations that individuals consider when drawing inferences based on their activity-switching decisions. When introducing activity engagement theory, Higgins et al. (1999) posit that a person's approach versus avoidance motivational orientation with regard to an activity serves as a reference point when making these inferences. We propose that although this approach or avoidance orientation *toward* the activity plays an important role in the meaning-making process, there is no reason to assume that these are the only motivational dimensions that might matter in this process. Indeed, the motivational underpinnings of the activities *themselves* might also play an important role.

How do we know which types of motivation support engagement in different kinds of activities? Regulatory fit theory (Higgins, 2000) proposes that when people pursue their goals using strategic means that align with and sustain their motivational orientation, they experience a sense of regulatory fit that has numerous consequences for engagement, as well as their feelings about the "rightness" of the process. As a result, regulatory fit research, which frequently manipulates both individuals' motivational orientations and the activities in which they engage, provides some insight into this question.

Two of the motivational orientations most commonly studied within regulatory fit research are the promotion regulatory focus and the prevention regulatory focus (Higgins, 1997). According to regulatory focus theory, promotion motivation is grounded in basic needs for growth and nurturance, and as a result, it drives the individual to pursue gains ("+1" or more) as opposed to non-gains ("0" or less). By contrast, prevention motivation is grounded in basic needs for safety and security, and as a result, it drives the individual to ensure non-losses ("0" or more) as opposed to losses ("–1" or less). A promotion (versus prevention) focus involves a strategic preference for eager (versus vigilant) means (Crowe & Higgins, 1997), and research reveals that the activities that fit each regulatory focus align with these broad strategic preferences. For instance, when pursuing academic goals, promotion-focused students prefer activities that embody eagerness, such as "attending all classes" and "completing schoolwork promptly," whereas prevention focused students prefer activities that embody vigilance, such as "spending less time at social gatherings/parties" and "avoiding being unprepared for tests" (Freitas & Higgins, 2002). Similarly, promotion-focused consumers are more persuaded by products that claim to help them engage in the activity of "enjoying life," whereas prevention-focused consumers are more persuaded by products that claim to help them engage in the activity of "being safe" (Lee & Aaker, 2004).

Beyond the realm of regulatory focus, additional regulatory fit research provides insight into the kinds of activities that fit other motivational orientations. For example, consider the assessment and locomotion orientations posited within regulatory mode theory (Kruglanski et al., 2000). Research on regulatory fit reveals that a truth-oriented assessment motivation prompts activities involving careful evaluation (e.g., fully appraising each and every option in one's consideration set before making a decision), whereas a control-oriented locomotion motivation prompts activities involving the enactment of change (e.g., progressively eliminating options throughout the process of making a decision; Avnet & Higgins, 2003). Even less formally studied motivational orientations have been shown to fit distinct activities, such as concerns with fun versus importance (e.g., Higgins, Cesario, Hagiwara, Spiegel, & Pittman, 2010).

Additionally, more recent research of our own provides new insight into how these different motives collectively underlie types of goal-pursuit activities (Nakkawita & Higgins, 2021). This work is grounded in the theory of motivational effectiveness (Higgins, 2012), which argues that fundamental needs to feel effective in three domains—value, truth, and control—work in concert to drive motivated activity. Based on this starting point, we identified and validated a 2 (promotion-value vs. prevention-value) × 2 (truth vs. control) framework of goal-pursuit activities. This research reveals that people oriented toward the combination of promotion and truth are motivated to engage in activities involving knowledge growth and generation (e.g., exploring, wondering, imagining). People oriented toward the combination of prevention and truth are motivated to engage in activities involving scrutiny and verification (e.g., examine, assess, judge). People oriented toward the combination of promotion and control are motivated to engage in activities involving the management of movement and change progress (e.g., leading, accelerating, progressing). Finally, people oriented toward the combination of prevention and control are motivated to engage in activities involving *status quo* preservation (e.g., maintaining, protecting, preserving).

Considered in light of activity engagement theory, we suggest that this 2 × 2 framework provides a new opportunity to further investigate Higgins et al.'s (1999) proposal that motivation-related information gain affects individuals' inferences about their attitudes toward activities. When considering how the activity framework might be applied to do so, it is first important to note that it comprises only positive, approach-oriented activities in its current form. More specifically, it features the kinds of activities that people with the four combinations of motivational orientations want to perform in order to experience effectiveness, and it is silent on the kinds of activities that these same combinations of motives want to avoid. As such, in contrast to Higgins et al.'s (1999) research (but in line with Higgins et al.'s [1995] work), given that people expect to want to approach these activities, it is only informative when they choose *not to approach* them.

Because the activities in the 2 × 2 framework are multiply motivated (e.g., by promotion *and* control, or prevention *and* truth, etc.), it offers clarity into the extent to which a shift in activities should be considered surprising and thus informative—that is, by examining whether the switch involves a change in two, one, or zero motivational dimensions. For instance, if an attorney in a small law firm tends to be most strongly motivated toward promotion and truth, switching away from the promotion-truth activity of "*exploring* solutions to a client's legal challenge" to the prevention-control activity of "*maintaining* the accounts payable/receivable" during a multitasking experience should be especially surprising because it involves deciding not to approach an activity that fits two typically preferred motivational dimensions. As a result, activity engagement theory might predict that the attorney will strongly infer that they must not find "exploring" that interesting and thus will engage in this activity far less in the future. In contrast, shifting from the same promotion-truth activity to the promotion-control activity of "*launching* a new business development plan" or the prevention-truth activity of "*scrutinizing* records for a case review" while multitasking should be less surprising because both choices would involve deciding not to approach only one typically preferred motivational dimension while switching to an activity that still fits the other typically preferred motivational dimension. As a result, the theory might predict that the attorney in this case might make only a moderately strong inference about how uninteresting "exploring" must be, with reduced effects of switching on future activity engagement decisions. Finally, a shift from one promotion-truth activity to another promotion-truth activity should produce the weakest inference of all. Future research should test this predictive logic by directly manipulating the number of motivational dimensions involved in participants' activity shifts.

With this said, as we have noted elsewhere (Nakkawita & Higgins, 2024), we provide a cautionary suggestion that the consequences of engaging multiple cells from this 2 × 2 framework may depend on whether or not the motivational orientations underlying the activities are experienced as competitive. For instance, because the promotion and prevention systems experience the same reference points differently (e.g., a "0" *status quo* is an undesirable non-gain value state for promotion, whereas it is a desirable non-loss value state for prevention; Higgins, 2018) and motivate distinct strategic responses (e.g., the strategic preferences for eagerness vs. vigilance described in greater detail earlier; Crowe & Higgins, 1997), the activities that they motivate are likely to be experienced as conflicting. As a result, undermining effects may be especially likely when an individual chooses to forego an activity that fits their regulatory focus for one that competes with it. By contrast, because truth and control functions work together harmoniously to facilitate the process of goal pursuit, as noted in many theories of self-regulation (e.g., Carver & Scheier, 1998; Gollwitzer, 1990; Kruglanski et al., 2000; Miller, Galanter, & Pribram, 1960), it is possible that truth- and control-oriented activities may be relatively more amenable to superordinate identification, at least as long as they are working toward the same valued end state (i.e., promotion gain or prevention non-loss). As a result, shifting between activities in each domain may not produce undermining effects as reliably as promotion–prevention switches. Further research is needed to test this proposal.

Investigating Consequences for Performance

Finally, activity engagement theory is somewhat restricted in its scope; although it makes predictions about people's attitudes toward activities and their consequent behavioral proclivities to reengage in those activities, it is silent on how effectively they perform the activities in question. For instance, consider the example of exercising while listening to a podcast, with the assumption that the individual finds both activities at least somewhat attractive. If a person simultaneously identifies this activity as "running" (primary) and "podcast listening" (secondary) but switches in their focus again and again throughout the run (e.g., sometimes they are more focused on the exercise and thus identify "running" as the primary activity and "podcast listening" as secondary; sometimes they are more focused on the podcast content and thus identify "podcast listening" as primary and "running" as secondary), activity engagement theory would predict that over time, the individual will infer that they like both activities less than they originally thought.

However, based on Higgins et al.'s (1995) Study 3, if they instead identify the same running and podcast-listening tasks as a superordinate activity, such as "enjoying well-deserved 'me' time," this multitasking behavior should not affect their attitudes about the activities because no switching is occurring. However, it leaves open the question of whether performance (e.g., running speed, comprehension of and memory for the podcast content) would also be affected by the adoption of this kind of superordinate activity identification. Although the research briefly reviewed at the very beginning of this chapter indicates that multitasking hurts performance (Hyman et al., 2010; Koch et al., 2018; Leroy, 2009; Rogers & Monsell, 1995; Rubinstein et al., 2001), might changing one's activity identification mitigate some of these negative consequences?

One recent study suggests that the answer might be yes. More specifically, research by Srna et al. (2018) indicates that when the actual activity is held constant (as it was in Higgins et al.'s [1995] "playbook" study), the mere perception of multitasking improves performance. For instance, in one of these studies, participants in a "perceived multitasking" condition were told that they would work on two tasks simultaneously: a learning task that involved watching an educational video and a transcribing task that involved typing exactly what was said in the same video (i.e., coordinate identification alternatives). In the "perceived single-tasking" condition, participants performed the same activities, but they were collectively described as a learning task that involved watching and transcribing an educational video (i.e., a superordinate identification). Participants then received a small monetary reward for the number of words that they correctly transcribed and answered questions about the video's content. Results revealed that participants in the "perceived multitasking" condition performed better on both measures than participants who were given a superordinate activity identification in the "perceived single-tasking" condition.

Additional studies in this line of research suggest that this performance effect derives from increased task engagement among participants in the "perceived multitasking" condition. Srna et al. (2018) propose that this increase in engagement may result from the fact that people tend to expect multitasking to be challenging, and as a result, they become more motivated and attentive. In addition to this potential mechanism of expected difficulty, activity engagement theory might be extended to predict that individuals' inferences about the meaning of activity switches will affect engagement strength. More specifically, because these tasks were likely not particularly enjoyable (particularly the transcribing aspect), as per Higgins et al. (1999), decisions not to avoid the tasks would be more informative than decisions to avoid them. As such, each decision to shift between learning and transcribing would lead participants to infer that perhaps these tasks aren't quite as unattractive as they originally thought. This decrease in the unattractiveness of the task might then lead participants to be more committed and engaged in the process of performing it. Of course, additional research would be needed to test this proposal.

CONCLUSION

Multitasking is an unavoidable part of modern life for many people (Mark, 2022), and despite its deleterious consequences for cognitive processing (e.g., Koch et al., 2018), it is a common practice that is valued by individuals and employers alike (e.g., Sastre Gomez et al., 2023; Srna et al., 2018). For these reasons, it is important to understand how to help people make the most of multitasking, as well as reduce its potential costs when it cannot be avoided. We propose that activity engagement theory (Higgins et al., 1995, 1999; Higgins & Trope, 1990) offers unique and valuable insights into how the *meaning* of multitasking—that is, the inferences that people draw based on their activity switches—plays an important role in people's attitudes toward and interest in the activities themselves. Despite this promise, research testing this theory has been limited, and far more work is needed to validate more fully the inferential mechanism underlying the theory, test a range of hypothesized moderators, investigate how combinations of distinct motivational forces influence these inferences, and examine the implications of these inferences for performance. We hope that this chapter reignites excitement about the promise of this understudied theory in order to spur new lines of research.

REFERENCES

Avnet, T., & Higgins, E. T. (2003). Locomotion, assessment, and regulatory fit: Value transfer from "how" to "what." *Journal of Experimental Social Psychology, 39*(5), 525–530.

Brown, R. (1958). How shall a thing be called? *Psychological Review, 65*(1), 14–21.

Bruner, J. S. (1957). On perceptual readiness. *Psychological Review, 64*(2), 123–152.

Carver, C. S., & Scheier, M. F. (1998). *On the self-regulation of behavior.* Cambridge University Press.

Cherry, C. (1957). *On human communication: A review, a survey, and a criticism.* Technology Press of Massachusetts Institute of Technology.

Crenshaw, D. (2021). *The myth of multitasking: How "doing it all" gets nothing done.* Mango.

Crowe, E., & Higgins, E. T. (1997). Regulatory focus and strategic inclinations: Promotion and prevention in decision-making. *Organizational Behavior and Human Decision Processes, 69*(2), 117–132.

Emanuel, A., Katzir, M., & Liberman, N. (2022). Why do people increase effort near a deadline? An opportunity-cost model of goal gradients. *Journal of Experimental Psychology: General, 151*(11), 2910–2926.

Förster, J., Higgins, E. T., & Idson, L. C. (1998). Approach and avoidance strength during goal attainment: Regulatory focus and the "goal looms larger" effect. *Journal of Personality and Social Psychology, 75*(5), 1115–1131.

Freitas, A. L., & Higgins, E. T. (2002). Enjoying goal-directed action: The role of regulatory fit. *Psychological Science, 13*(1), 1–6.

Gallup. (2024). State of the global workplace: The voice of the world's employees. *www.gallup.com/workplace/349484/state-of-the-global-workplace.aspx*

Gollwitzer, P. M. (1990). Action phases and mind-sets. In E. T. Higgins & R. M. Sorrentino (Eds.), *Handbook of motivation and cognition: Foundations of social behavior* (Vol. 2, pp. 53–92). Guilford Press.

Heath, C., Larrick, R. P., & Wu, G. (1999). Goals as reference points. *Cognitive Psychology, 38*(1), 79–109.

Higgins, E. T. (1989). Knowledge accessibility and activation: Subjectivity and suffering from unconscious sources. In J. S. Uleman & J. A. Bargh (Eds.), *Unintended thought* (pp. 75–123). Guilford Press.

Higgins, E. T. (1996). Knowledge activation: Accessibility, applicability, and salience. In E. T. Higgins & A. W. Kruglanski (Eds.), *Social psychology: Handbook of basic principles* (pp. 133–168). Guilford Press.

Higgins, E. T. (1997). Beyond pleasure and pain. *American Psychologist, 52*(12), 1280–1300.

Higgins, E. T. (2000). Making a good decision: Value from fit. *American Psychologist, 55*(11), 1217–1230.

Higgins, E. T. (2012). *Beyond pleasure and pain: How motivation works.* Oxford University Press.

Higgins, E. T. (2018). What distinguishes promotion and prevention? Attaining "+1" from "0" as non-gain versus maintaining "0" as non-loss. *Polish Psychological Bulletin, 49*(1), 40–49.

Higgins, E. T., Cesario, J., Hagiwara, N., Spiegel, S., & Pittman, T. (2010). Increasing or decreasing interest in activities: The role of regulatory fit. *Journal of Personality and Social Psychology, 98*(4), 559–572.

Higgins, E. T., Lee, J., Kwon, J., & Trope, Y. (1995). When combining intrinsic motivations undermines interest: A test of activity engagement theory. *Journal of Personality and Social Psychology, 68*(5), 749–767.

Higgins, E. T., & Trope, Y. (1990). Activity engagement theory: Implications of multiply identifiable input for intrinsic motivation. In E. T. Higgins & R. M. Sorrentino (Eds.), *Handbook of motivation and cognition: Foundations of social behavior* (Vol. 2, pp. 229–264). Guilford Press.

Higgins, E. T., Trope, Y., & Kwon, J. (1999). Augmentation and undermining from combining activities: The role of choice in activity engagement theory. *Journal of Experimental Social Psychology, 35*(3), 285–307.

Hull, C. L. (1932). The goal-gradient hypothesis and maze learning. *Psychological Review, 39*(1), 25–43.

Hwang, Y., Kim, H., & Jeong, S.-H. (2014). Why do media users multitask?: Motives for general, medium-specific, and content-specific types of multitasking. *Computers in Human Behavior, 36*, 542–548.

Hyman, I. E., Jr., Boss, S. M., Wise, B. M., McKenzie, K. E., & Caggiano, J. M. (2010). Did you see the unicycling clown? Inattentional blindness while walking and talking on a cell phone. *Applied Cognitive Psychology, 24*(5), 597–607.

Jones, E. E., & Davis, K. E. (1965). From acts to dispositions: The attribution process in person perception. In L. Berkowitz (Ed.), *Advances in experimental social psychology* (Vol. 2, pp. 219–266). Academic Press.

Koch, I., Poljac, E., Müller, H., & Kiesel, A. (2018). Cognitive structure, flexibility, and plasticity in human multitasking—An integrative review of dual-task and task-switching research. *Psychological Bulletin, 144*(6), 557–583.

Kruglanski, A. W. (1975). The endogenous-exogenous partition in attribution theory. *Psychological Review, 82*(6), 387–406.

Kruglanski, A. W. (1990). Motivations for judging and knowing: Implications for causal attribution. In E. T. Higgins & R. M. Sorrentino (Eds.), *Handbook of motivation and cognition: Foundations of social behavior* (Vol. 2, pp. 333–368). Guilford Press.

Kruglanski, A. W., Thompson, E. P., Higgins, E. T., Atash, M. N., Pierro, A., Shah, J. Y., & Spiegel, S. (2000). To "do the right thing" or to "just do it": Locomotion and assessment as distinct self-regulatory imperatives. *Journal of Personality and Social Psychology, 79*(5), 793–815.

Kurzban, R., Duckworth, A., Kable, J. W., & Myers, J. (2013). An opportunity cost model of subjective effort and task performance. *Behavioral and Brain Sciences, 36*(6), 661–679.

Lee, A. Y., & Aaker, J. L. (2004). Bringing the frame into focus: The influence of regulatory fit on processing fluency and persuasion. *Journal of Personality and Social Psychology, 86*(2), 205–218.

Lepper, M. R., Greene, D., & Nisbett, R. E. (1973). Undermining children's intrinsic interest with extrinsic reward: A test of the "overjustification" hypothesis. *Journal of Personality and Social Psychology, 28*(1), 129–137.

Leroy, S. (2009). Why is it so hard to do my work? The challenge of attention residue when switching between work tasks. *Organizational Behavior and Human Decision Processes, 109*(2), 168–181.

LinkedIn. (n.d.). Jobs. LinkedIn. Retrieved June 18, 2024, from *www.linkedin.com/jobs/*

Mark, G. (2022). *Multitasking in the digital age.* Springer.

Miller, G. A., Galanter, E., & Pribram, K. H. (1960). *Plans and the structure of behavior.* Henry Holt and Co.

Nakkawita, E., & Higgins, E. T. (2021). Motivating the journey: An integrative framework of prevention versus promotion goal pursuit activities. *PsyArXiv. doi.org/10.31234/osf.io/eut2k*

Nakkawita, E., & Higgins, E. T. (2024). Marketplace solutions to motivational threats: Helping consumers with four distinct types of vulnerability. In A. Y. Lee (Ed.), *The vulnerable consumer* (Vol. 21, pp. 97–112). Emerald.

Newport, C. (2016). *Deep work: Rules for focused success in a distracted world.* Grand Central.

Newtson, D. (1976). Foundations of attribution: The unit of perception of ongoing behavior. In J. H. Harvey, W. J. Ickes, & R. F. Kidd (Eds.), *New directions in attribution research* (Vol. 1, pp. 223–247). Erlbaum.

Oswald, F. L., Hambrick, D. Z., & Jones, L. A. (2007). Keeping all the plates spinning: Understanding and predicting multitasking performance. In D. H. Jonassen (Ed.), *Learning to solve complex scientific problems* (pp. 77–96). Routledge.

Papper, R. A., Holmes, M., & Popovich, M. (2004). Middletown media studies: Media multitasking . . . and how much people really use the media. *International Digital Media & Arts Association Journal, 1*(1), 5–56.

Rogers, R. D., & Monsell, S. (1995). Costs of a predictable switch between simple cognitive tasks. *Journal of Experimental Psychology: General, 124*(2), 207–231.

Rosch, E. (1978). Principles of categorization. In E. Rosch & B. B. Lloyd (Eds.), *Cognition and categorization* (pp. 27–48). Erlbaum.

Rubinstein, J. S., Meyer, D. E., & Evans, J. E. (2001). Executive control of cognitive processes in task switching. *Journal of Experimental Psychology: Human Perception and Performance, 27*(4), 763–797.

Sastre Gomez, V., Defina, R., Garrett, P. M., Zacks, J. M., & Dennis, S. (2023). The prevalence of multitasking presents challenges for theories of event segmentation. *Proceedings of the Annual Meeting of the Cognitive Science Society, 45*, 2050–2056.

Shannon, C. E., & Weaver, W. (1949). *The mathematical theory of communication*. University of Illinois Press.

Srna, S., Schrift, R. Y., & Zauberman, G. (2018). The illusion of multitasking and its positive effect on performance. *Psychological Science, 29*(12), 1942–1955.

Touré-Tillery, M., & Fishbach, A. (2011). The course of motivation. *Journal of Consumer Psychology, 21*(4), 414–423.

Trope, Y. (1986). Identification and inferential processes in dispositional attribution. *Psychological Review, 93*(3), 239–257.

Uncapher, M. R., Lin, L., Rosen, L. D., Kirkorian, H. L., Baron, N. S., Bailey, K., Cantor, J., Strayer, D. L., Parsons, T. D., & Wagner, A. D. (2017). Media multitasking and cognitive, psychological, neural, and learning differences. *Pediatrics, 140*(Suppl. 2), S62–S66.

Wegner, D. M., & Vallacher, R. R. (1986). Action identification. In R. M. Sorrentino & E. T. Higgins (Eds.), *Handbook of motivation and cognition: Foundations of social behavior* (pp. 550–582). Guilford Press.

Wyer, R. S., & Srull, T. K. (1986). Human cognition in its social context. *Psychological Review, 93*(3), 322–359.

CHAPTER 8

Goals Shape Meaning

Ayelet Fishbach and Jiabi Wang

When evaluating a tropical vacation, one considers not just the anticipated pleasure of reading a book on a sunny beach but also the potential pain that is associated with a shrinking savings account. When evaluating a decadent dessert, one considers not only the texture of melting chocolate but also the potential guilt of failing to adhere to a healthy eating resolution. These various goals shape the meaning of the vacation or the dessert. The same activity may be evaluated and experienced positively in relation to a goal it supports and negatively in relation to a goal it hinders. When goals disagree, the meaning of related stimuli becomes unstable. People may experience attitude ambivalence (Cacioppo, Gardner, & Berntson, 1997) and mixed emotions (Berrios, Totterdell, & Kellett, 2015; Mejía & Hooker, 2017), and they will change their evaluations across contexts and over time (Ferguson & Bargh, 2004).

This chapter examines how the coexistence of and relationships between goals shape the meaning of stimuli. It begins by exploring the cognitive organization of goals and the means by which they are pursued. We then propose that goals can exist in states of harmony or conflict, with their perceived relationships influencing the meaning of associated objects, actions, ideas, and people.

Next, we explore the cognitive representation of a specific type of goal conflict—the self-control dilemma—and its impact on the meaning attached to goal-related stimuli. In a self-control dilemma, a high-priority, long-term goal conflicts with a low-priority and immediate desire. The individual strives to adhere to the high-priority goal while simultaneously wanting to pursue the immediate desire. The perception of conflict between these two goals is a prerequisite for exercising self-control.

However, these high- and low-priority goals may sometimes appear to be in harmony. For example, although saving money and going on a tropical vacation may pose a self-control conflict, these goals can also be perceived as complementary if the purpose of saving is to afford a desired lifestyle. Similarly, eating healthily and enjoying food may seem conflicting but can align harmoniously if the individual enjoys healthy food.

Crucially, perceiving goal conflict—which triggers self-control and reshapes the meaning of goal-related stimuli—is not always the optimal route for pursuing long-term interests. At times, perceiving conflict may even undermine these interests, whereas perceiving harmony can be more motivating. We examine and provide examples of both scenarios: when perceptions of harmony versus conflict enhance motivation to adhere to long-term interests. As a test case, we demonstrate that healthy eating is more likely when individuals perceive health and taste as in harmony, whereas patience in intertemporal choices is more likely when individuals perceive smaller-sooner and larger-later rewards as conflicting, prompting the exercise of self-control.

PART I: THE RELATIONSHIP BETWEEN GOALS

Our big and small goals are cognitively organized in goal systems (Kruglanski, Chernikova, Babush, Dugas, & Schumpe, 2002). In a goal system, each goal is connected to a set of subordinate means (subgoals) that help achieve it and a set of superordinate goals it helps achieve. For example, a person's goal to get on a baking show may be connected to a subgoal of learning how to bake and to a superordinate goal of becoming a celebrity.

Importantly, parallel goals in the hierarchy are connected to each other in either facilitatory or inhibitory links. Goals facilitate each other whenever pursuing one advances the other or whenever pursuing one complements others by addressing a life aspect that would otherwise be neglected. For example, the goal of going on a beach vacation can directly energize an exhausted employee, helping them recharge their motivation to work. Hence, pursuing one goal helps another. Alternatively, a vacation can complement the work goal for employees who aspire to both goals: professional success and traveling the world.

Goals are connected by inhibitory links when they directly undermine one another. For example, a person's desire to join a wine club directly conflicts with their goal of improving their health. Alternatively, goals can compete for limited resources such as time, money, and effort. Goal conflict is inherent to human psychology. According to existential philosophy, recognizing human mortality—and the limited time available—enables individuals to prioritize their goals and avoid being sidetracked by less important pursuits (Heidegger, 1927/1962). Without this awareness of finitude, people might become preoccupied with trivialities, endlessly postponing meaningful goals. From this perspective, awareness of limited resources and the resulting goal conflicts is not only an unavoidable reality of life but also a valuable mechanism for identifying and focusing on what truly matters.

The experience of goals as facilitating versus inhibiting each other has emotional and motivational consequences. People report greater happiness and motivation when their goals share facilitatory links. Our research on *goal harmony* finds that the perception of harmony between life goals predicts motivation and well-being (Wang & Fishbach, 2025). This perception results from the framing of goals, which can be situationally modified through a cognitive process of mental integration and acquired through past experiences and social learning. The same two or more personal goals can be mentally represented as being in harmony versus conflict.

To illustrate the effect of mental integration on perceived goal harmony, in some studies, we encouraged people to consider how their goals across diverse life domains (e.g., work, health, and family) either complement or compete with each other. In one study, when participants considered how a work activity also facilitated their leisure goals (i.e., it is a multifinal means), they perceived a greater harmony between work and leisure goals. For example, when participants considered how networking (a means for success at work) could facilitate their leisure goals (expanding one's social circle beyond work), they perceived these goals—career advancement and leisure—as being in harmony. In turn, they reported feeling less torn and more motivated to engage in work compared with participants in a control group, who considered how a work activity is independent of leisure (see Figure 8.1).

Another study manipulated the perceived relationship between two potential goals for helping: concern for others and self-enhancement. These goals often seem conflicting. People see helpers who wish to promote their own reputation as less prosocial (Carlson & Zaki, 2018; Newman & Cain, 2014). The phrase *tainted altruism* captures the idea that helping is less charitable if it is self-interested because, presumably, selfish and selfless goals are in conflict. However, when participants considered how helping others also helps the self—for example, by teaching them valuable skills—they reported more goal harmony and were more willing to help.

Goal harmony is also shaped through social learning. For instance, we find that, on average, men experience less work–family conflict than

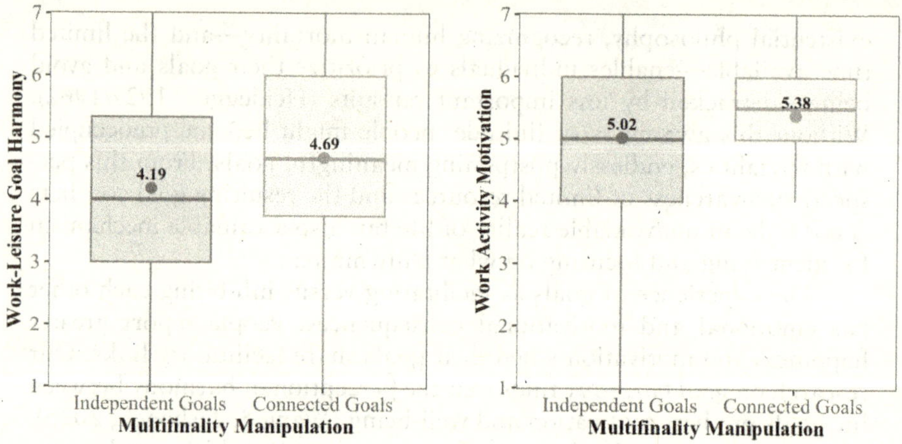

FIGURE 8.1. Harmony and motivation in the connect and control conditions. *Note:* Participants who elaborated on how their work activity facilitated their leisure goal (a multifinality intervention) reported greater perceived harmony and motivation to engage in the work activity than those in the control condition. The bottom and top edges of the boxes represent the first (Q1) and third (Q3) quartiles of data. The horizontal line inside each box indicates the median value of the data. The dots and numbers indicate the mean. From Wang and Fishbach (2025).

women. This difference partly arises because society frames men's family goals around providing financial support, which makes professional success aligned with parenting. In contrast, women are socialized to view family goals as requiring significant time investment, which makes time spent at work feel like time away from family. Culture further influences goal harmony. People in five collectivistic countries reported higher levels of goal harmony compared to those in five individualistic countries—for example, we observed greater harmony in India and China than in the Netherlands and the United States.

The perceived relationships between goals also depend on their level of construal, with greater perceived harmony between more abstract goals (Freitas, Clark, Kim, & Levy, 2009). When using a more abstract construal, a person's various goals complement each other. These goals make a person's life more versatile and psychologically rich. However, when people focus on the concrete aspects of their goals, resource constraints such as limited time and money become more salient. After all, a person can only be in one place, mostly doing one thing at a time. The result is perceived conflict. For example, whereas a busy college student may perceive a conflict between completing academic work and getting enough sleep, that student will more likely perceive harmony between academic success and mental health.

Goals Determine Evaluation and Experience

Goals change the meaning of a stimulus, be it an action, object, idea, or person. When a stimulus is seen as facilitating a goal, it elicits a more positive evaluation (Ferguson & Bargh, 2004). Further, the emotions associated with goal achievement transfer to this stimulus as a function of the goal–means association strength (Fishbach, Shah, & Kruglanski, 2004). These positive evaluations and emotions, in turn, motivate goal pursuit (Custers & Aarts, 2005; Ferguson, 2008).

According to the dilution effect, when a goal is served by multiple means (e.g., actions, objects, people who help), the association between this goal and each means is weaker. The result is that people evaluate each means less positively (Zhang, Fishbach, & Kruglanski, 2007). For example, when participants listed two means for achieving a goal (e.g., running and swimming to keep fit), they perceived the first activity as less enjoyable and less important than when it was the only activity listed (Fishbach et al., 2004).

Other research documented a devaluation of a stimulus that was incompatible with a goal. For example, hungry participants (with a focal goal of eating) rated consumer products unrelated to that need (e.g., shampoo) as less valuable (Brendl, Markman, & Messner, 2003). Goals can even change the visual meaning of stimuli (i.e., what people see). When looking at an ambiguous figure (e.g., an image that is either the letter B or the number 13), participants tended to see the interpretation that assigned them to outcomes they favored (Balcetis & Dunning, 2006), and when thirsty, they saw a bottle of water as closer (Balcetis & Dunning, 2010; see also Landy, Daley, & Balcetis, this volume).

Interpersonal relationships are similarly influenced by the goals they support or obstruct. People in one's life—such as friends, family members, or colleagues—are evaluated more positively when they facilitate a goal and more negatively when they hinder one (Fitzsimons, Finkel, & VanDellen, 2015; Fitzsimons & Fishbach, 2010). This dynamic has several implications: Individuals tend to feel greater gratitude toward helpers while they still need assistance (Converse & Fishbach, 2012) and prefer relationship partners who understand their goals (i.e., those who know them rather than those who are known by them; Schroeder & Fishbach, 2024).

Given that people hold multiple goals, the meaning and experience of any stimulus is a function of the various goals that it facilitates and inhibits. People often report attitude ambivalence: They simultaneously hold strong positive and negative evaluations about the same attitude object (Ito & Cacioppo, 2001; Thompson & Zanna, 1995). Such ambivalence results from having some goals facilitated by that stimulus and others that this stimulus hinders. So, when people express ambivalence about assisted suicide, it is because they simultaneously wish to give others control over their bodies and desire to protect others' lives at all costs. Their ambivalence leads to a more nuanced, simultaneous positive and negative evaluation of the same stimulus.

Ambivalence can undermine motivation and well-being (Kelly, Mansell, & Wood, 2015; Moberly & Dickson, 2018). In one of the earliest experience sampling studies, Emmons and King (1988) found that undergraduates' experiences of goal conflict and ambivalence were associated with negative affect, depression, neuroticism, psychosomatic complaints, and illnesses. Yet later research documented that holding multiple goals and experiencing ambivalence can also foster flexible perspectives (Reich & Wheeler, 2016; Van der Weele, 2013) and enhance resilience (Rothman, Pratt, Rees, & Vogus, 2017).

The simultaneous activation of multiple goals often leads to the experience of mixed emotions, such as bittersweet feelings or excitement tinged with anxiety. These contradictory emotions arise in response to the same stimulus. For instance, leisure activities might evoke pleasurable guilt if a person perceives that enjoying leisure (pleasure) comes at the expense of saving money or working extra hours (guilt; Holbrook & Hirschman, 1982; Dhar & Simonson, 2003).

Similarly, as we will explore next, yielding to temptation frequently results in mixed emotions. People may experience basic emotions (e.g., joy) from fulfilling an immediate desire alongside self-conscious emotions (e.g., shame and guilt) from failing to uphold a higher-priority goal (Moran & Eyal, 2022; Tangney, 1999). These self-conscious emotions play a critical role in regulating behavior. For example, dieters who were first exposed to negative self-conscious emotion words, such as *guilty* and *embarrassed*, subsequently consumed less food (Giner-Sorolla, 2001).

PART II: THE SELF-CONTROL CONFLICT

The self-control conflict is the goal conflict that has captured most of the attention in psychological research. It involves an immediate desire (i.e., temptation) that is in opposition to a high-priority goal that aligns with a person's long-term interests (Baumeister & Heatherton, 1996; Hofmann, Friese, & Strack, 2009; Loewenstein, 1996; Mischel, Shoda, & Rodriguez, 1989; Trope & Fishbach, 2000). According to Fujita et al.

(2024; see also Carnevale & Fujita, this volume), self-control conflicts occur whenever contractive concerns (immediate, local considerations) clash with expansive concerns (broader, long-term priorities). Although we agree with this perspective, we are salient on what makes one desire a "goal" while the other is a "temptation." What matters is that the individual feels they should pursue the high-priority goal but wants to pursue the low-priority one.

Exercising self-control changes the meaning of the high-priority goal, the low-priority desire, or both. The result of exercising self-control is that two opposing forces with similar motivational pull—a goal and a temptation—get further apart, with the motivation to adhere to the goal getting significantly stronger than the motivation to give in to temptation. For example, instead of wanting to eat the cake (a temptation) and have it too (the high-priority goal), the motivation to save the cake for future cravings becomes significantly stronger than the temptation to have it all right now.

Research on *counteractive control* has explored the process by which temptations trigger the mental processes that reduce their appeal (Fishbach & Trope, 2005; Trope & Fishbach, 2000). In one illustrative study (Myrseth, Fishbach, & Trope, 2009), gym-goers were offered a choice between a health bar and a chocolate bar. Almost everybody chose the health bar because these were all health-conscious people. But how much more appealing was the health bar compared with the chocolate bar? It depended on the timing of asking the question. Before making the choice, participants rated the health bar as much more appealing than the chocolate bar. However, those who rated the options only after choosing rated the health bar and chocolate bar as equally appealing. By considering the positive aspects of goal-related stimuli and the negative aspects of temptation, gym-goers changed the meaning of pursuing a goal versus giving in to temptation so that it was more attractive to adhere to the goal (Fishbach, Zhang, & Trope, 2010).

Another counteractive response involves bringing to mind goal-related thoughts and inhibiting thoughts about temptations (Fishbach, Friedman, & Kruglanski, 2003). People secure their goals by making them more accessible and by inhibiting thoughts of temptations. We assume these implicit responses are instrumental because successful self-regulators are more likely to engage in these processes of changing the meaning of goals and temptations than less successful ones (Papies, Stroebe, & Aarts, 2008).

People also change the meaning of goals and temptations by reflecting on the cool (i.e., less arousing or unappetizing), abstract features of temptations and by adopting a more abstract mindset, which emphasizes the benefit of goals and the costs of temptations (Fujita, Trope,

Liberman, & Levin-Sagi, 2006; Fujita & Han, 2009; Kross, Ayduk, & Mischel, 2005; Metcalfe & Mischel, 1999). Self-control operations even change expectations. People set high-performance standards to motivate themselves (Locke & Latham, 1990; Wright & Brehm, 1989). So, when facing temptation, people set even more ambitious expectations for themselves. They engage in counteractive optimism: stating optimistic predictions of future engagement with goals and disengagement from temptations (Zhang & Fishbach, 2010). These optimistic predictions motivate behavior because once a target is set (e.g., finishing that project by the end of the week), people are motivated to meet it (Atkinson & Feather, 1966; Brehm & Self, 1989; Heath, Larrick, & Wu, 1999; Locke & Latham, 1990).

For example, when college students were first asked to estimate how much time they would likely spend on leisure on the day of the experiment, they subsequently planned to allocate more time to studying that same day (counteractive optimism). However, when students were first asked to estimate the time they would spend studying, they seemed to recognize that time is a finite resource: More time spent studying would mean less time available for leisure. As a result, when the question about studying was presented first, they planned to spend less time on leisure (Zhang & Fishbach, 2010).

These shifts in the meaning of goals and temptations influence action. For instance, the decision to cooperate in social dilemmas often requires self-control. People may assign higher priority to cooperation, believing it fits better with their moral values, and yet they may feel tempted to compete for an immediate benefit. Sheldon and Fishbach (2011) found that participants cooperated more when they were reminded in advance of the temptation to compete. The mental shifts in goal representation enabled their cooperation.

PART III: TWO ROUTES TO SUCCESS: IDENTIFYING SELF-CONTROL CONFLICT VERSUS FINDING GOAL HARMONY

In 2013, Lance Armstrong, a celebrated cyclist, admitted to doping but justified it by stating he believed this practice was widespread among elite cyclists. He did not think he got an unfair advantage, and hence, he did not experience a self control conflict over using performance-enhancing drugs. By his logic, his goals to win and to do so ethically were aligned.

The experience of self-control conflict depends on the framing of goals. Giving in to a momentary desire may provide a refreshing temporary break, or it can even facilitate the overriding goal. When the immediate goal complements the higher-priority goal, these motivations are in harmony, and there is no self-control conflict. The person would seek to balance between the goals (vs. highlight the more important goal; Fishbach, Dhar, & Zhang, 2006), engage with each one in moderation (vs. abstain from the low-priority goal; Le, Scholer, & Fujita, 2024), or identify compromise (Simonson, 1989).

These are all forms of *mixed solutions* that are meant to satisfy all goals, and we contrast them with *extreme solutions* that favor one goal over the other (Shaddy, Fishbach, & Simonson, 2021). Seeking mixed solutions is appropriate if the goals are in harmony or if the goals are conflicting yet equally important. Seeking extreme solutions is a better solution if the goals pose a self-control conflict.

Identifying a goal as a temptation—something that conflicts with a higher-priority goal—is a prerequisite for exercising self-control. Self-control thus requires that the person must first identify a temptation before they battle it (Fishbach & Converse, 2011). Many potential temptations are not identified as such. These potential temptations often have negligible cost when engaged in moderation; after all, one cigarette will not kill you. Alternatively, the person might not realize that they should hold an overriding goal in the first place. It is hard for people in their 20s to envision life after retirement, making it hard to see the long-term harm of neglecting to save (Hershfield et al., 2011). To identify a conflict, a person ought to consider a broader array of time, space, people, and possibilities (Fujita, Trope, & Liberman, 2024). Further, the person needs to believe that within this broad frame, pursuing one (immediate) goal comes at the expense of another.

Although recognizing conflict is a prerequisite for exercising self-control, it is not a necessary condition or the only path for advancing long-term interests. Self-control is used to overcome temptation; however, it is not always the most effective route to success. In fact, self-control can occasionally fail to support high-priority goals and may even undermine them. This can happen either because alternative approaches to pursuing high-priority goals exist that do not require sacrificing immediate desires or because self-control efforts themselves may fail.

Decades of research on intrinsic motivation have found that adherence to professional, academic, and health goals is more likely when individuals pursue related activities as an end in themselves (Cameron & Pierce, 1994; Deci, 1975; Fishbach & Woolley, 2022). The long-term and short-term interests collide, at least to some extent (e.g., even the most intrinsically motivated professional might enjoy time off). People who perceive conflict and exercise self-control miss out on the intrinsic route of successfully pursuing long-term interests in ways that are also immediately gratifying. A person may fail to identify the immediate benefits of adhering to a goal, believing, for example, that studying is boring, exercising is painful, and healthy food is bland. Not realizing that studying can be fascinating, exercising is fun, and healthy food can be delicious, the person perceives conflict and exercises self-control instead of choosing multifinal means that satisfy both immediate- and long-term interests.

Both identifying conflict and recognizing harmony between high- and low-priority goals can, in principle, be instrumental in pursuing high-priority goals. In addition, perceived conflict and perceived harmony may each also undermine these goals. We provide examples for each of these scenarios in Table 8.1. We next provide detailed research examples of when perceiving harmony versus conflict is beneficial for long-term regulatory success.

Example 1: Perceiving Harmony between Health and Taste Promotes Healthy Eating

The perception of conflict between health and taste provides an illustrative case of how perceiving a conflict changes the meaning of a goal—in this case, healthy food consumption. Indeed, although health and taste correlate positively in nature (e.g., toxic foods usually taste bad), which is critical for the survival of our species, many people perceive health and taste as conflicting goals (Kunz, Haasova, Pivecka, Schmidt, & Florack, 2023). This is partially the outcome of modern Western food production, characterized by food abundance and using additives that improve taste while undermining health (e.g., in ultra-processed foods). This is also partially the outcome of selection bias (i.e., the foods in one's pantry pose a healthy–taste trade-off), as well as the cognitive representation of food: Foods perceived as low on the taste goal are seen as particularly effective for health. The representation of foods follows the principle of

TABLE 8.1. Example of Scenarios Where Identifying Conflict versus Harmony Is Beneficial versus Undermining of Self-Regulatory Success

	Self-Regulatory Success	Self-Regulatory Failure
Identifying Goal Conflict	Identifying smoking as undermining lung health promotes long-term health	Viewing parenting as competing with career pursuits undermines long term mental health
Identifying Goal Harmony	Believing that healthy food is tasty promotes a healthy diet	Believing that cheating on school assignments aligns with learning undermines long-term academic success.

counterfinality: A means viewed as hindering one goal seems more effective for another (Kruglanski et al., 2015).

The result of perceiving goal conflict is the common belief that food labeled as healthy is less tasty (Cornil & Chandon, 2016; Mai & Hoffmann, 2015; Raghunathan, Naylor, & Hoyer, 2006). Merely emphasizing a food's healthiness reduces its perceived flavor and the likelihood of being chosen (Maimaran & Fishbach, 2014; Turnwald et al., 2019; Wansink & Chandon, 2006). Indeed, children as young as 3 years old inferred that food that made them smart or strong did not taste good. When they heard a story about a girl who had carrots and was then able to count to 100, they ate fewer carrots than when they heard a control story (Maimaran & Fishbach, 2014).

Beyond consumption, the representation of food changes when people perceive conflict. In Maimaran and Fishbach's studies, children who learned that food offers health benefits rated it less tasty: They said it was more like an onion than ice cream. Other research (Turnwald & Fishbach, 2024b) has found that people in the United States mentally represent healthier foods in their least tasty form: unseasoned, unbaked, and generally less prepared. One study had participants consider unhealthy versus healthier versions of the same food (e.g., "cauliflower-crust pizza" vs. "wheat-crust pizza" and "whole-wheat pasta" vs. "white pasta") and indicate for each food whether what comes to mind is a prepared or unprepared dish. For example, they indicated what first comes to mind when reading "whole-wheat pasta": (1) a photo of cooked pasta with sauce or (2) dry pasta sticks. As shown in Figure 8.2, participants mentally represented healthier (vs. unhealthy) versions of foods in a less prepared form; they consistently chose the unprepared image for the healthier food and the prepared version for the unhealthy food. Because many people perceive a health–taste conflict, what comes to mind when reading "veggie burger" is a frozen patty, whereas what comes to mind when reading "beef burger" is a sizzling patty in a bun with toppings.

If the perception of goal conflict informs the mental representation of food, we should expect those who perceive greater health–taste conflict to have different representations than those who perceive less conflict. Indeed, the tendency to represent healthier food as less prepared consistently emerges in the United States but did not replicate in India, where the traditional cuisine features cooked and seasoned vegetables, and there is potentially less social learning that health and taste conflict. Further, individual differences matter. Americans who reported greater perceived health–taste conflict were more likely to mentally represent healthy foods in less prepared forms.

The perception of goal conflict also shapes the emotional tone people associate with goals and temptations. When individuals perceive

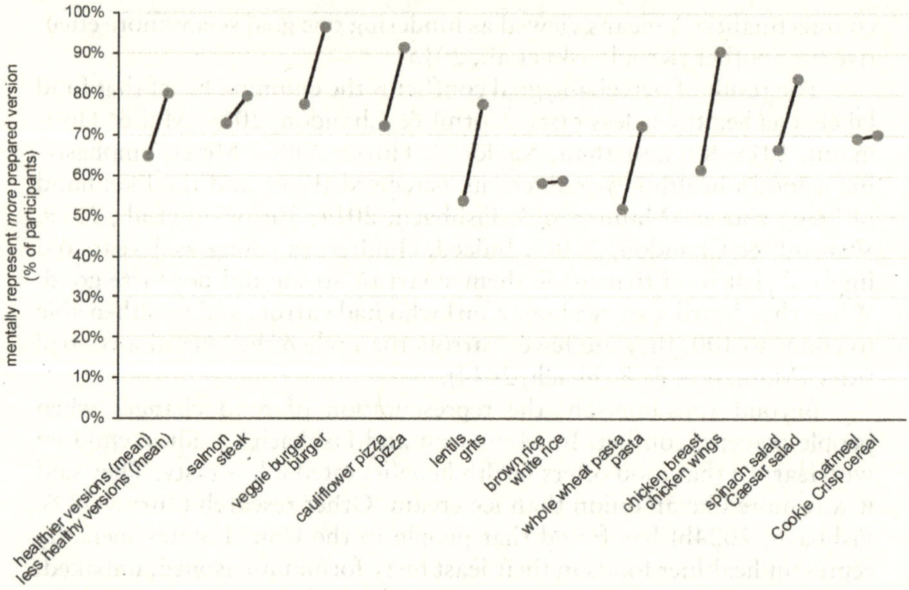

FIGURE 8.2. Participants thought of healthier versions of foods as less prepared than unhealthy versions of similarly matched foods. Note that plot depicts the percentage of participants who indicated that they think of a given food in its more prepared state. Circles represent the percentage for a given food, and lines connect the healthier (left) and unhealthy (right) versions of each similarly matched food pair. From Turnwald and Fishbach (2024b).

a health–taste conflict, they tend to highlight the cool, nonemotional benefits of eating healthily rather than its immediate emotional benefits. This self-control–driven representation diminishes the intrinsic appeal of healthy eating—specifically, making it seem less tasty. Indeed, when analyzing the emotionality of thousands of recipe descriptions from Allrecipes.com, Yelp reviews, and celebrity Instagram posts, Turnwald and Fishbach (2024a) found that people use nonaffective language to persuade others to eat healthy foods while reserving their emotions to convince others to consume unhealthy foods. A typical healthy recipe would state, "Taste great with hardly any fat!"; in contrast, a recipe not tagged as healthy would state, "Prepare to become ADDICTED to this yummy dish." Although nonaffective features might readily come to mind when discussing healthy food, those who post these recipes would have been more persuasive had they included emotionality in their healthy recipes.

The perception of conflict can undermine health if it discourages individuals from choosing healthy food that is also tasty. Further, when healthy eating is framed as requiring self-control, individuals may perceive the cost as too high and give up. In fact, describing food as delicious increases consumption, partly because it reduces the perception of goal conflict and the associated costs of adherence. Healthy food consumption rises when it does not require sacrificing taste (Turnwald et al., 2019).

A similar dynamic is observed in other domains. For instance, communication with greater emotional content has been shown to predict voting behavior, possibly by aligning immediate gratification with long-term benefits (Lavine, Thomsen, Zanna, & Borgida, 1998). People are more likely to stick to high-priority goals when they perceive immediate benefits in pursuing them.

Overall, whereas perceiving goal conflict activates self-control, perceiving goal harmony often leads to adhering to important goals by evoking intrinsic motivation. When individuals perceive health–taste harmony (as opposed to conflict or independence), they are more likely to choose healthier food. Beyond food, if people view exercising as conflicting with comfort, they tend to imagine workouts devoid of enjoyable features. They do not envision playing sports, dancing, or watching a movie on the treadmill. Additionally, when studying is seen as conflicting with interest, people are more likely to envision it as a rote memorization of boring text rather than a creative and exploratory activity.

Example 2: Perceiving Conflict Increases Patience in Intertemporal Choice

Intertemporal choices are decisions between rewards that vary by magnitude and time: The person decides between a larger-later reward and a smaller-sooner reward. The person who chooses the larger-later reward is said to be patient. When presented with a choice between getting $100 today and $110 next month, the patient person will decide to wait, whereas an impatient person will opt for the $100 today.

The perception of conflict is key to being patient and, ultimately, achieving long-term goals. Indeed, those who are impatient in monetary trade-off tasks tend to exhibit more addictive behaviors (e.g., smoking, alcohol, substance abuse; MacKillop et al., 2011), exercise less, and have a higher body mass index (BMI; Chabris, Laibson, Morris, Schuldt, & Taubinsky, 2008), and they report relationship infidelity (Reimers, Maylor, Stewart, & Chater, 2009) and poorer financial health (Meier & Sprenger, 2012). What is less clear is whether these individuals cannot adhere to long-term interests or do not wish to do so.

Some early research on patience assumed that if a person can wait, they will—that a conflict is always identified. Those who did not wait were thought to have poor willpower (Frederick & Loewenstein, 2002; Mischel & Ayduk, 2002). For example, in research on the delay-of-gratification paradigm (i.e., the "marshmallow test"), Walter Mischel and his colleagues suggested that a cool representation of a marshmallow (e.g., as a cloud) helps children resist it in favor of the two marshmallows that will arrive later. However, this self-control strategy—decreasing the appeal of a marshmallow through mental imagery—can only be enacted if the child believes that one marshmallow implies not getting two later, which is clearly not the reality in every household.

Patience requires that one desires to wait in the first place. If a person does not perceive a conflict between immediate desires and long-term interests, they are likely to choose the immediate reward without attempting to resist. For instance, a child who values the larger-later reward less (e.g., they only moderately like marshmallows) or who has low trust in the promise that forgoing smaller-sooner reward will pay off (e.g., they believe adults often forget their promises, marshmallows run out, etc.) will opt for the immediate option without experiencing an internal conflict.

Performance on the delay-of-gratification test—like patience in monetary trade-offs—has long been associated with later-life success. Children who waited longer tended to make healthier financial, educational, and medical choices in adulthood (Mischel et al., 1989; Mischel & Ebbesen, 1970). However, a recent reanalysis of the longitudinal results suggests that what the test measures is not the ability to wait (willpower) but rather the desire to wait—specifically, the recognition of a conflict. Although the original study found that the amount of time children waited predicted later cognitive and social achievements, the reanalysis revealed that this advantage could be entirely attributed to whether children decided to wait—specifically, whether they waited longer than 20 seconds (Watts, Duncan, & Quan, 2018). For instance, it made no difference whether children waited 15 minutes versus 10 minutes—a difference potentially reflecting their ability to wait—but it mattered whether they chose to wait 60 seconds versus 10 seconds. Because the act of waiting begins with the decision to wait, which would take at least a few seconds, the variation between children likely captures the decision itself rather than the subsequent ability to follow through.

What factors predict whether someone would identify a goal conflict in an intertemporal choice and conclude that they ought to try to wait? One such factor is the magnitude of the rewards. People are more likely to identify a goal conflict (and wait) when the stakes are higher. For example, the *magnitude effect* (Thaler, 1981) refers to the tendency to choose to wait for larger magnitudes of money (e.g., people are more likely to wait for $100 in 6 months over $80 today compared with $10 in 6 months over $8 today). Subjective value similarly promotes conflict identification. Most people choose to wait for a large portion of their favorite coffee or chocolate in 1 month over receiving a smaller sample today. But few choose to wait a month for a larger portion of an "okay" coffee or chocolate (Roberts, Shaddy, & Fishbach, 2020).

Although it may seem obvious that increasing the value of a larger-later reward enhances patience—one might wait longer for three artisan chocolates than for two—the magnitude effect and research on subjective value explore a different effect: Greater patience is observed when both the smaller-sooner and the larger-later rewards become more valuable. Because the smaller-sooner option becomes even more tempting under these conditions (i.e., it is less "smaller"), the increased patience reflects heightened conflict identification.

Interestingly, though, although an increase in the appeal of the rewards will make it easier to identify a conflict, it will make it harder to resolve the conflict. When the stakes are higher, people are more likely to decide to wait but find it harder to wait. To explore these opposite effects of reward value, Roberts and Fishbach (2024) had participants evaluate different bonus amounts. Some rated how impatient they would feel, whereas others rated how likely they were to wait 3 months for the bonuses instead of receiving half of that amount immediately (e.g., waiting for $10 instead of $5 immediately, or $1,000 instead of $500 immediately). As shown in Figure 8.3, as the rewards became more valuable, participants were more likely to wait but reported they would struggle more.

Another factor that enhances conflict identification is trust in rewards. After all, waiting involves risk. People are more likely to choose to wait when they trust that larger-later rewards will be delivered (McGuire & Kable, 2013). So, when community trust in the government increased in Bangladesh, residents made more patient monetary choices (Jachimowicz, Chafik, Munrat, Prabhu, & Weber, 2017). Although increased trust in delayed benefits does not make waiting easier, it makes it feel more worthwhile.

As we discussed, once a conflict is identified, individuals recruit self-control. Conflict identification is thus a prerequisite for self-control, including a more positive evaluation of and preference for larger-later rewards over smaller-sooner ones. For instance, individuals who exercise self-control might decide to make their choice in advance to increase patience. According to the *common difference effect*, preferences between two delayed outcomes switch when both delays are incremented by a given constant amount (Loewenstein & Prelec, 1992; Thaler, 1981). A person would be tempted to choose $100 now over $120 next month but be less tempted to choose $100 next year over $120 in 13 months,

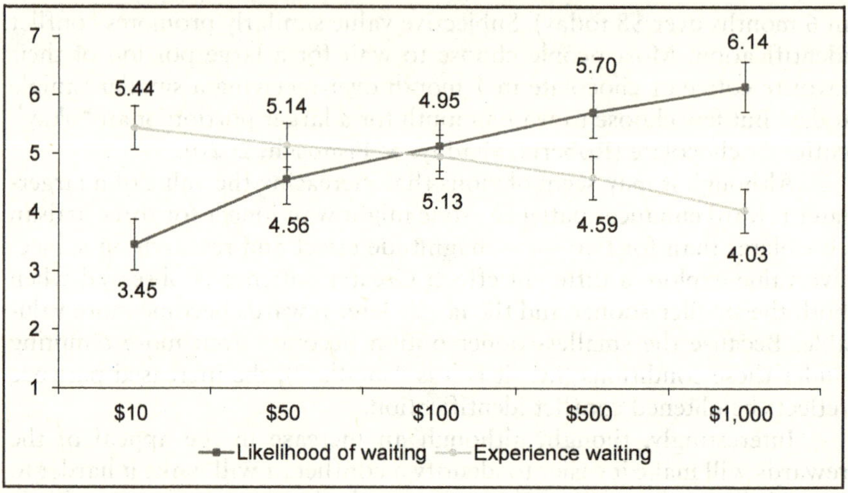

FIGURE 8.3. Participants' choice to wait (likelihood of waiting) and positive experience while waiting (experience waiting) for the amount indicated in 3 months instead of receiving half of that amount sooner. Note that error bars represent 95% confidence intervals. Participants made more patient choices for larger magnitudes of money, even though they anticipated feeling less patient waiting for larger magnitudes of money. From Roberts and Fishbach (2024).

even though the only difference between these two trade-offs is a constant delay of 1 year. By making their decision ahead of time, individuals can avoid reversing their preference for the larger-later reward when a smaller-sooner option becomes immediately available.

The smaller-sooner option becomes even less appealing when a person waits before making an intertemporal choice. The *wait-to-choose* self-control technique (Dai & Fishbach, 2014; Imas, Kuhn, & Mironova, 2022) introduces a delay between learning about the rewards trade-off and the point of decision making. When individuals waited to choose, they demonstrated greater patience compared with choosing immediately, even when the options were closer in time. Waiting increases the perceived value of both the smaller-sooner and larger-later rewards, thereby amplifying the difference between them. This technique was inadvertently applied in the United States in 2008, when the distribution dates for stimulus payments were determined by the last two digits of recipients' Social Security numbers, effectively creating a random assignment. Individuals who experienced a longer wait for their stimulus payments were more likely to make patient financial decisions, saving more of the money rather than spending it immediately (Thakral & Tô, 2022).

Another self-control strategy involves reducing the emotional toll of waiting. People seek closure: They are eager to complete a goal and receive the reward partly because they want to take it off their minds. Indeed, people value goal completion so much that they would sometimes choose a lower-reward task over a higher-reward task if it allows them to complete it sooner (Converse, Tsang, & Hennecke, 2023; Ruan, Polman, & Tanner, 2024). Closure generates utility (Roberts, Imas, & Fishbach, 2023). By reducing the need for closure, people can increase the likelihood of choosing the larger-later rewards.

To conclude, some people will not wait; others cannot wait. Those in the former group exhibit impatience because they do not perceive pursuing immediate desires as conflicting with their long-term interests—or they prioritize the immediate goal. They do not recognize a conflict, and as a result, they do not exercise self-control to reinterpret the stimuli in ways that support waiting. In contrast, those in the latter group are impatient because they cannot resist the pull of immediate gratification. These individuals recognize the conflict but fail to overcome the temptation of the immediate reward.

CONCLUSIONS

Goals shape the meaning of the stimuli associated with them. This chapter explores how the relationship between goals as either facilitating or inhibiting each other shapes the meaning of related stimuli. Whether goals are in harmony or conflict and whether an individual prioritizes one goal over another or tries to attend to both determine the meaning ascribed to the stimuli and action choice.

We argue that both perceived goal harmony and conflict can support the pursuit of long-term interests. However, our examples for these scenarios are primarily anecdotal. Previous research found that perceiving harmony between health and taste promotes healthy eating because the individual identifies healthy foods that are tasty, whereas perceiving a conflict between smaller-sooner and larger-later rewards aids in achieving larger rewards in intertemporal choice.

Future research could identify principles that determine when perceptions of harmony versus conflict are most beneficial. For example, it may be that perceiving harmony at the level of overarching goals while recognizing conflict at the level of specific activities (or means) is crucial for motivating adherence to high-priority goals. Effective self-regulation might involve framing saving and spending as complementary goals while acknowledging the conflict between a tropical vacation this winter and a dwindling bank account. For now, we can determine that exploring the relationships between goals offers a promising avenue for addressing how goals shape the meaning assigned to social and nonsocial environments, as well as how individuals go on pursuing their goals.

REFERENCES

Atkinson, J., & Feather, N. (1966). *A theory of achievement motivation*. Wiley.

Balcetis, E., & Dunning, D. (2006). See what you want to see: Motivational influences on visual perception. *Journal of Personality and Social Psychology, 91*(4), 612–625.

Balcetis, E., & Dunning, D. (2010). Wishful seeing: Motivational influences on visual perception of the physical environment. In E. Balcetis & G. D. Lassiter (Eds.), *Social psychology of visual perception* (pp. 77–101). Psychology Press.

Baumeister, R. F., & Heatherton, T. F. (1996). Self-regulation failure: An overview. *Psychological Inquiry, 7*(1), 1–15.

Berrios, R., Totterdell, P., & Kellett, S. (2015). Investigating goal conflict as a source of mixed emotions. *Cognition and Emotion, 29*(4), 755–763.

Brehm, J. W., & Self, E. A. (1989). The intensity of motivation. *Annual Review of Psychology, 40*, 109–131.

Brendl, C. M., Markman, A. B., & Messner, C. (2003). The devaluation effect: Activating a need devalues unrelated objects. *Journal of Consumer Research, 29*(4), 463–473.

Cacioppo, J. T., Gardner, W. L., & Berntson, G. G. (1997). Beyond bipolar conceptualizations and measures: The case of attitudes and evaluative space. *Personality and Social Psychology Review, 1*(1), 3–25.

Cameron, J., & Pierce, W. D. (1994). Reinforcement, reward, and intrinsic motivation: A meta-analysis. *Review of Educational Research, 64*(3), 363–423.

Carlson, R. W., & Zaki, J. (2018). Good deeds gone bad: Lay theories of altruism and selfishness. *Journal of Experimental Social Psychology, 75*, 36–40.

Chabris, C. F., Laibson, D., Morris, C. L., Schuldt, J. P., & Taubinsky, D. (2008). Individual laboratory-measured discount rates predict field behavior. *Journal of Risk and Uncertainty, 37*(2), 237–269.

Converse, B. A., & Fishbach, A. (2012). Instrumentality boosts appreciation: Helpers are more appreciated while they are useful. *Psychological Science, 23*(6), 560–566.

Converse, B. A., Tsang, S., & Hennecke, M. (2023). The value of mere completion. *Journal of Experimental Psychology: General, 152*(11), 3021–3036.

Cornil, Y., & Chandon, P. (2016). Pleasure as an ally of healthy eating? Contrasting visceral and Epicurean eating pleasure and their association with portion size preferences and wellbeing. *Appetite, 104*, 52–59.

Custers, R., & Aarts, H. (2005). Positive affect as implicit motivator: On the nonconscious operation of behavioral goals. *Journal of Personality and Social Psychology, 89*(2), 129–142.

Dai, X., & Fishbach, A. (2014). How nonconsumption shapes desire. *Journal of Consumer Research, 41*(4), 936–952.

Deci, E. L. (1975). *Intrinsic motivation.* Plenum.

Dhar, R., & Simonson, I. (2003). The effect of forced choice on choice. *Journal of Marketing Research, 40*(2), 146–160.

Emmons, R. A., & King, L. A. (1988). Conflict among personal strivings: Immediate and long-term implications for psychological and physical well-being. *Journal of Personality and Social Psychology, 54*(6), 1040–1048.

Ferguson, M. J. (2008). On becoming ready to pursue a goal you don't know you have: Effects of nonconscious goals on evaluative readiness. *Journal of Personality and Social Psychology, 95*(6), 1268–1294.

Ferguson, M. J., & Bargh, J. A. (2004). Liking is for doing: The effects of goal pursuit on automatic evaluation. *Journal of Personality and Social Psychology, 87*(5), 557–572.

Fishbach, A., & Converse, B. A. (2011). Identifying and battling temptation. In K. D. Vohs & R. F. Baumeister (Eds.), *Handbook of self-regulation: Research, theory, and applications* (2nd ed., pp. 244–260). Guilford Press.

Fishbach, A., Dhar, R., & Zhang, Y. (2006). Subgoals as substitutes or complements: The role of goal accessibility. *Journal of Personality and Social Psychology, 91*(2), 232–242.

Fishbach, A., Friedman, R. S., & Kruglanski, A. W. (2003). Leading us not into temptation: Momentary allurements elicit overriding goal activation. *Journal of Personality and Social Psychology, 84*(2), 296.

Fishbach, A., Shah, J. Y., & Kruglanski, A. W. (2004). Emotional transfer in goal systems. *Journal of Experimental Social Psychology, 40*(6), 723–738.

Fishbach, A., & Trope, Y. (2005). The substitutability of external control and self-control. *Journal of Experimental Social Psychology, 41*(3), 256–270.

Fishbach, A., & Woolley, K. (2022). The structure of intrinsic motivation. *Annual Review of Organizational Psychology and Organizational Behavior, 9*(1), 339–363.

Fishbach, A., Zhang, Y., & Trope, Y. (2010). Counteractive evaluation: Asymmetric shifts in the implicit value of conflicting motivations. *Journal of Experimental Social Psychology, 46*(1), 29–38.

Fitzsimons, G. M., Finkel, E. J., & VanDellen, M. R. (2015). Transactive goal dynamics. *Psychological Review, 122*(4), 648–673.

Fitzsimons, G. M., & Fishbach, A. (2010). Shifting closeness: Interpersonal effects of personal goal progress. *Journal of Personality and Social Psychology, 98*(4), 535–549.

Frederick, S., & Loewenstein, G. (2002). Time discounting and time preference: A critical review. *Journal of Economic Literature, 40*(2), 351–401.

Freitas, A. L., Clark, S. L., Kim, J. Y., & Levy, S. R. (2009). Action-construal levels and perceived conflict among ongoing goals: Implications for positive affect. *Journal of Research in Personality, 43*(5), 938–941.

Fujita, K., & Han, H. A. (2009). Moving beyond deliberative control of impulses: The effect of construal levels on evaluative associations in self-control conflicts. *Psychological Science, 20*(7), 799–804.

Fujita, K., Trope, Y., & Liberman, N. (2024). Understanding self-control as a problem of regulatory scope. *Psychological Review, 132*(1), 50–75.

Fujita, K., Trope, Y., Liberman, N., & Levin-Sagi, M. (2006). Construal levels and self-control. *Journal of Personality and Social Psychology, 90*(3), 351–367.

Giner-Sorolla, R. (2001). Guilty pleasures and grim necessities: Affective attitudes in dilemmas of self-control. *Journal of Personality and Social Psychology, 80*(2), 206–221.

Heath, C., Larrick, R. P., & Wu, G. (1999). Goals as reference points. *Cognitive Psychology, 38*(1), 79–109.

Heidegger, M. (1927/1962). *Being and time* (J. Macquarrie & E. Robinson, Trans.). Blackwell. (Original work published 1927)

Hershfield, H. E., Goldstein, D. G., Sharpe, W. F., Fox, J., Yeykelis, L., Carstensen, L. L., et al. (2011). Increasing saving behavior through age-progressed renderings of the future self. *Journal of Marketing Research, 48*(Suppl.), S23–S37.

Hofmann, W., Friese, M., & Strack, F. (2009). Impulse and self-control from a dual-systems perspective. *Perspectives on Psychological Science, 4*(2), 162–176.

Holbrook, M. B., & Hirschman, E. C. (1982). The experiential aspects of consumption: Consumer fantasies, feelings, and fun. *Journal of Consumer Research, 9*(2), 132–140.

Imas, A., Kuhn, M. A., & Mironova, V. (2022). Waiting to choose: The role of deliberation in intertemporal choice. *American Economic Journal: Microeconomics, 14*(3), 414–440.

Ito, T. A., & Cacioppo, J. T. (2001). Affect and attitudes: A social neuroscience approach. In J. P. Forgas (Ed.), *The handbook of affect and social cognition* (pp. 50–74). Erlbaum.

Jachimowicz, J. M., Chafik, S., Munrat, S., Prabhu, J. C., & Weber, E. U. (2017). Community trust reduces myopic decisions of low-income individuals. *Proceedings of the National Academy of Sciences, 114*(21), 5401–5406.

Kelly, R. E., Mansell, W., & Wood, A. M. (2015). Goal conflict and well-being: A review and hierarchical model of goal conflict, ambivalence, self-discrepancy and self-concordance. *Personality and Individual Differences, 85*, 212–229.

Kross, E., Ayduk, O., & Mischel, W. (2005). When asking "why" does not hurt: Distinguishing rumination from reflective processing of negative emotions. *Psychological Science, 16*(9), 709–715.

Kruglanski, A., Chernikova, M., Babush, M., Dugas, M., & Schumpe, B. M. (2015). The architecture of goal systems: Multifinality, equifinality, and counterfinality in means–end relations. In A. J. Elliot (Ed.), *Advances in motivation science* (Vol. 2, pp. 69–98). Elsevier.

Kruglanski, A., Shah, J., Fishbach, A., Friedman, R., Chun, W. Y., & Sleeth-Keppler, D. (2002). A theory of goal systems. *Advances in Experimental Social Psychology, 34*, 331–378.

Kunz, S., Haasova, S., Pivecka, N., Schmidt, J., & Florack, A. (2023). Food is all around: How contexts create misbeliefs about the health–taste relationship. *Psychological Science, 34*(5), 568–580.

Lavine, H., Thomsen, C. J., Zanna, M. P., & Borgida, E. (1998). On the primacy of affect in the determination of attitudes and behavior: The moderating role of affective-cognitive ambivalence. *Journal of Experimental Social Psychology, 34*(4), 398–421.

Locke, E. A., & Latham, G. P. (1990). *A theory of goal setting & task performance* (pp. xviii, 413). Prentice Hall.

Loewenstein, G. (1996). Out of control: Visceral influences on behavior. *Organizational Behavior and Human Decision Processes, 65*(3), 272–292.

Loewenstein, G., & Prelec, D. (1992). Anomalies in intertemporal choice: Evidence and an interpretation. *Quarterly Journal of Economics, 107*(2), 573–597.

MacKillop, J., Amlung, M. T., Few, L. R., Ray, L. A., Sweet, L. H., & Munafò, M. R. (2011). Delayed reward discounting and addictive behavior: A meta-analysis. *Psychopharmacology, 216*(3), 305–321.

Mai, R., & Hoffmann, S. (2015). How to combat the unhealthy = tasty intuition: The influencing role of health consciousness. *Journal of Public Policy & Marketing, 34*(1), 63–83.

Maimaran, M., & Fishbach, A. (2014). If it's useful and you know it, do you eat? Preschoolers refrain from instrumental food. *Journal of Consumer Research, 41*(3), 642–655.

McGuire, J. T., & Kable, J. W. (2013). Rational temporal predictions can underlie apparent failures to delay gratification. *Psychological Review, 120*(2), 395–410.

Meier, S., & Sprenger, C. D. (2012). Time discounting predicts creditworthiness. *Psychological Science, 23*(1), 56–58.

Mejía, S. T., & Hooker, K. (2017). Mixed emotions within the context of goal pursuit. *Current Opinion in Behavioral Sciences, 15*, 46–50.

Metcalfe, J., & Mischel, W. (1999). A hot/cool-system analysis of delay of gratification: Dynamics of willpower. *Psychological Review, 106*(1), 3–19.

Mischel, W., & Ayduk, O. (2002). Self-regulation in a cognitive–affective personality system: Attentional control in the service of the self. *Self and Identity, 1*(2), 113–120.

Mischel, W., & Ebbesen, E. B. (1970). Attention in delay of gratification. *Journal of Personality and Social Psychology, 16*(2), 329–337.

Mischel, W., Shoda, Y., & Rodriguez, M. L. (1989). Delay of gratification in children. *Science, 244*(4907), 933–938.

Moberly, N. J., & Dickson, J. M. (2018). Goal conflict, ambivalence and psychological distress: Concurrent and longitudinal relationships. *Personality and Individual Differences, 129*, 38–42.

Moran, T., & Eyal, T. (2022). Emotion regulation by psychological distance and level of abstraction: Two meta-analyses. *Personality and Social Psychology Review, 26*(2), 112–159.

Myrseth, K. O. R., Fishbach, A., & Trope, Y. (2009). Counteractive self-control: When making temptation available makes temptation less tempting. *Psychological Science, 20*(2), 159–163.

Newman, G. E., & Cain, D. M. (2014). Tainted altruism: When doing some good is evaluated as worse than doing no good at all. *Psychological Science, 25*(3), 648–655.

Papies, E. K., Stroebe, W., & Aarts, H. (2008). The allure of forbidden food: On the role of attention in self-regulation. *Journal of Experimental Social Psychology, 44*(5), 1283–1292.

Raghunathan, R., Naylor, R. W., & Hoyer, W. D. (2006). The unhealthy = tasty intuition and its effects on taste inferences, enjoyment, and choice of food products. *Journal of Marketing, 70*(4), 170–184.

Reich, T., & Wheeler, S. C. (2016). The good and bad of ambivalence: Desiring ambivalence under outcome uncertainty. *Journal of Personality and Social Psychology, 110*(4), 493–508.

Reimers, S., Maylor, E. A., Stewart, N., & Chater, N. (2009). Associations between a one-shot delay discounting measure and age, income, education and real-world impulsive behavior. *Personality and Individual Differences, 47*(8), 973–978.

Roberts, A., & Fishbach, A. (2024). *Can't wait or won't wait? The two barriers to patience* [Working paper]. University of Texas, Austin.

Roberts, A., Shaddy, F., & Fishbach, A. (2020). Love is patient: People are more willing to wait for things they like. *Journal of Experimental Psychology: General, 150*(7), 1423–1437.

Roberts, A. R., Imas, A., & Fishbach, A. (2023). Can't wait to pay: The desire for goal closure increases impatience for costs. *Journal of Personality and Social Psychology, 126*(6), 1019–1035.

Rothman, N., Pratt, M., Rees, L., & Vogus, T. (2017). Understanding the dual nature of ambivalence: Why and when ambivalence leads to good and bad outcomes. *Academy of Management Annals, 11*(1), 33–72.

Ruan, B., Polman, E., & Tanner, R. J. (2024). The one-away effect: The pursuit of mere completion. *Journal of Consumer Research, 50*(5), 945–961.

Schroeder, J., & Fishbach, A. (2024). Feeling known predicts relationship satisfaction. *Journal of Experimental Social Psychology, 111*, 1–15.

Shaddy, F., Fishbach, A., & Simonson, I. (2021). Trade-offs in choice. *Annual Review of Psychology, 72*(1), 181–206.

Sheldon, O. J., & Fishbach, A. (2011). Resisting the temptation to compete: Self-control promotes cooperation in mixed-motive interactions. *Journal of Experimental Social Psychology, 47*(2), 403–410.

Simonson, I. (1989). Choice based on reasons: The case of attraction and compromise effects. *Journal of Consumer Research, 16*(2), 158.

Tangney, J. P. (1999). The self-conscious emotions: Shame, guilt, embarrassment and pride. In T. Dalgleish & M. J. Power (Eds.), *Handbook of cognition and emotion* (pp. 541–568). Wiley.

Thakral, N., & Tô, L. (2022). *Anticipation and consumption* [Working paper]. Boston University.

Thaler, R. (1981). Some empirical evidence on dynamic inconsistency. *Economics Letters, 8*(3), 201–207.

Thompson, M. M., & Zanna, M. P. (1995). The conflicted individual:

Personality-based and domain-specific antecedents of ambivalent social attitudes. *Journal of Personality, 63*(2), 259–288.

Trope, Y., & Fishbach, A. (2000). Counteractive self-control in overcoming temptation. *Journal of Personality and Social Psychology, 79*(4), 493–506.

Turnwald, B., Bertoldo, J. D., Perry, M. A., Policastro, P., Timmons, M., Bosso, C., et al. (2019). Increasing vegetable intake by emphasizing tasty and enjoyable attributes: A randomized controlled multisite intervention for taste-focused labeling. *Psychological Science, 30*(11), 1603–1615.

Turnwald, B., & Fishbach, A. (2024a). Intuitive advertisers: Emotionality in communication about unhealthy food. *Health Psychology, 43*(3), 184–193.

Turnwald, B., & Fishbach, A. (2024b). Thinking of food: The mental representation of healthy foods as unprepared, *Appetite, 200*, 107510.

Turnwald, B. P., Bertoldo, J. D., Perry, M. A., Policastro, P., Timmons, M., Bosso, C., et al. (2019). Increasing vegetable intake by emphasizing tasty and enjoyable attributes: A randomized controlled multisite intervention for taste-focused labeling. *Psychological Science, 30*(11), 1603–1615.

Van der Weele, C. N. (2013). Meat and the benefits of ambivalence. In H. Röcklinsberg & P. Sandin (Eds.), *The ethics of consumption: The citizen, the market and the law* (pp. 290–295). Academic Publishers.

Wang, J. & Fishbach, A. (2025). Goal harmony. *Journal of Personality and Social Psychology*. Advance online publication. *https://doi.org/10.1037/pspa0000452*

Wansink, B., & Chandon, P. (2006). Can "low-fat" nutrition labels lead to obesity? *Journal of Marketing Research, 43*(4), 605–617.

Watts, T. W., Duncan, G. J., & Quan, H. (2018). Revisiting the marshmallow test: A conceptual replication investigating links between early delay of gratification and later outcomes. *Psychological Science, 29*(7), 1159–1177.

Wright, R. A., & Brehm, J. W. (1989). Energization and goal attractiveness. In L. A. Pervin (Ed.), *Goal concepts in personality and social psychology* (pp. 169–210). Erlbaum.

Zhang, Y., & Fishbach, A. (2010). Counteracting obstacles with optimistic predictions. *Journal of Experimental Psychology: General, 139*(1), 16–31.

Zhang, Y., Fishbach, A., & Kruglanski, A. (2007). The dilution model: How additional goals undermine the perceived instrumentality of a shared path. *Journal of Personality and Social Psychology, 92*(3), 389–401.

CHAPTER 9

On Control Readiness

The Constant Interplay between Conflict and Control

Tali Kleiman

The importance of cognitive control to human functioning cannot be overstated. It is a basic, fundamental, and crucial cognitive function that enables individuals to achieve their goals. Cognitive control is activated by your cognitive system both when you are adding sugar, not salt, to your morning coffee and when you are persistently working on a long-term work project. This is the case for all individuals and across the vast range of goals, from the most trivial to those of utmost significance. This is especially the case when obstacles or distractions conflict with the individual's goals. Given that such cases are far from being a rare occurrence, it is not surprising that questions pertaining to the operation of cognitive control and its interaction with conflict have received much theoretical and empirical attention across domains in psychological research.

This chapter presents the idea of control readiness, the motivational take on the interplay between conflict and control. It addresses basic terminology, introduces the principles of adaptive control, and explains how adaptive control describes the interplay between conflict and control, all through the lens of control readiness. The chapter concludes with a discussion of how research on control readiness contributes to the understanding of conflict resolution and control while connecting it to other conceptualizations.

SOME DEFINITIONS OF SOME CONCEPTS ON THE WAY TO CONTROL READINESS

Conflict can be defined as "the simultaneous activation of incompatible, and competing, representations" (Botvinick, Braver, Barch, Carter, & Cohen, 2001, p. 630). *Cognitive control* is a fundamental cognitive function responsible for the coordination of one's attention and actions in ways that are consistent with one's goals (Botvinick et al., 2001; Levy, Enisman, Perry, & Kleiman, 2023; Miller & Cohen, 2001).[1] This is especially true in ambiguous or conflicting situations, in which cognitive control is recruited to focus solely on decision-relevant information, to carefully consider alternative courses of action, or to merely force oneself to reach a decision. Thus, control is essential, but it is also costly. *Adaptive control* (sometimes referred to as *conflict adaptation* or *control learning*; Chiu & Egner, 2019; Schmidt, 2013; see Braem et al. [2019] for a review) refers to the dynamic modulations of cognitive control, which enable an effective adaptation to the ever-changing environment while considering the inherent cost of control implementation and the need to allocate it wisely based on its expected contribution to goal attainment (Shenhav, Botvinick, & Cohen, 2013).

CONTROL READINESS AND THE ROLE OF MEANING WITHIN IT

Control readiness (Kleiman, Hassin, & Trope, 2014) is inspired by Jerome Bruner's take on perceptual readiness, whereby "readiness in the sense that we are using it is not a luxury, but a necessity for smooth adjustment" (Bruner, 1957, p. 149). Control readiness denotes adaptive control that is domain general rather than domain specific. Crucially, the domain generality is enabled because the cognitive system seeks to fulfill a meaningful purpose. Thus far, adaptive control has mostly been studied and documented within domains, where reencountering the same type of conflict facilitates control activation. However, control adjustments across domains, or instances where control is adjusted across different types of conflict, have been much less studied, and effects have rarely been found. The logic underlying the idea of control readiness is

[1]Cognitive control is thought to operate in two distinct modes (Braver, 2012). *Proactive control* is anticipatory in nature, whereby goal-relevant information is constantly maintained. Conversely, *reactive control* is a transient, stimulus-driven mode, whereby goal-relevant information is reactivated anew when needed.

that one important moderator could be the extent to which the cognitive system is "motivated" to resolve the conflict. Namely, control adaptation across domains, whereby the activation of control on one domain can facilitate the implementation of control in another, depends on the meaning that the cognitive system infuses into the outcome of the control activation. Infusing meaning makes cognitive control, a core cognitive function, more flexible.

A TWO-STAGE MODEL: DETECTING CONFLICT AND IMPLEMENTING CONTROL

The dominant accounts for achieving goals in an environment proliferated with distracting stimuli adopt a two-stage model. Theories in both cognitive neuroscience and social cognition propose that to achieve a desired goal in the face of distractions, one first needs to identify a conflict between one's goal and potential distractions.[2] Once a conflict is identified, control processes are set in motion to secure goal attainment. Achieving one's goal therefore depends on (1) conflict identification and (2) control activation (Botvinick et al., 2001; Myrseth & Fishbach, 2009; Wegner, 2009). These two processes are thought to be supported by different brain regions: the anterior cingulate cortex (ACC) and the prefrontal cortex (PFC) for conflict detection and control implementation, respectively (Kerns et al., 2004). Failure to achieve a goal can thus be a product of either failure to identify the conflict or insufficient activation of control.

FROM CONFLICT TO CONTROL AND BACK AGAIN

The ongoing, constant interplay between conflict and control, as depicted in the two-stage conflict adaptation model (Botvinick et al., 2001) described in the previous section, leads to two related theoretical

[2]I use the terms *goal* (or *target*) and *distractors* because these are the terms that are most commonly used in the cognitive control literature from which the paradigms and a substantial part of the theoretical thinking of the work described in this chapter draws. Other research uses other terms, for example, *temptations*; *impulses*; and *smaller, concrete, immediate rewards versus larger, abstract, delayed, remote rewards or goals*. Naming a construct undoubtedly infuses meaning into it and creates associations that then persist in research traditions. However, I believe that the essence lies in how these constructs are thought to operate within a psychological process (see Fujita, 2011). I elaborate on this point in the Take-Home Messages and Additional Thoughts section at the end of this chapter.

predictions. The first is that the detection of conflict and the consequent activation of control to resolve it make the resolution of a subsequent immediate conflict less costly. This prediction is empirically manifested in the sequential congruency effect (Gratton, Coles, & Donchin, 1992). The second prediction is that the cost of control activation to resolve conflicts reduces as the frequency of conflicts in the environment increases. This prediction is empirically manifested in the proportion congruent effect (PCE; e.g., Gratton et al., 1992; Lindsay & Jacoby, 1994; Logan, 1980). The following section describes how the cost of activating control is conceptualized and measured via congruency effects. The two predictions are elaborated on, with an emphasis on how these basic cognitive principles that have been traditionally studied in the "hardcore" cognitive and cognitive neuroscience literature are applied to social cognition research. This synthesis of principles, ideas, and paradigms contributes to both fields, helps in distilling common and distinct features, explains discrepancies in empirical findings, aids in understanding boundary conditions, and when taken together, facilitates the understanding of the core psychological concepts of conflict and control.

The Cost of Control Activation: The Congruency Effect

As noted earlier, the activation of cognitive control is costly. The hallmark empirical demonstration of the cost of the activation and implementation of cognitive control is the congruency effect, which is mostly studied within stimulus–response compatibility (SRC) tasks (Kornblum, Hasbroucq, & Osman, 1990). In these types of tasks, the participant's goal is to quickly and accurately respond to a relevant target stimulus. The target's "environment," however, also contains goal-irrelevant stimuli, or distractors, which are also assigned a response. The response to these distractors can be either compatible (congruent) with the response required to achieve the goal or incompatible (incongruent) with it. The congruency effect is the robust (often very large) effect whereby incongruent trials take longer to resolve than congruent trials. This is the case across various paradigms that manipulate incongruency in various ways. For example, in the Stroop task, incongruency stems from a conflict between the responses assigned to the meaning versus the color in which the word is written; in the flanker task (Eriksen & Eriksen, 1974), incongruency stems from a conflict between the responses assigned to a central target and the stimuli spatially flanking it; and in the Simon task (Simon, 1990), the incongruency stems from a conflict between the target location and the location of its assigned response (for a comprehensive overview and a taxonomy of SRC tasks, see Kornblum et al. [1990]). Crucially, the size of the congruency effect is used as an indicator of the taxation on the cognitive system in resolving conflicts. Larger congruency effects denote a greater cost.

Sequential Conflict-Activated Control Adaption

Sequential control adaption (or conflict adaptation), also known as the *congruency sequence effect* (CSE) or the *Gratton effect* (Gratton et al., 1992), is the empirical observation whereby congruency effects are smaller on trial *n* if trial *n* – 1 is incongruent rather than congruent (see Figure 9.1 for a schematic depiction). Put differently, the cost of resolving the present conflict is smaller when it is preceded by a conflict situation rather than a no-conflict situation. The essence of the Gratton effect is that individuals are more efficient in activating and implementing cognitive control after having experienced conflict, which in turn leads to improved performance in subsequent trials that involve similar conflicts. The seminal Gratton effect, which is almost a pure manifestation of the two-stage model of the interplay between conflict and control, has received ample empirical investigation and support (see Egner [2007, 2008] for reviews). Vast empirical support notwithstanding, the idea also instigated lively debates on the underlying mechanisms and boundary conditions of the sequential conflict-driven control adaptation (listing all of the proposed theories and accounts is beyond the scope of the present chapter; for a review, see Braem, Abrahamse, Duthoo, & Notebaert [2014]).

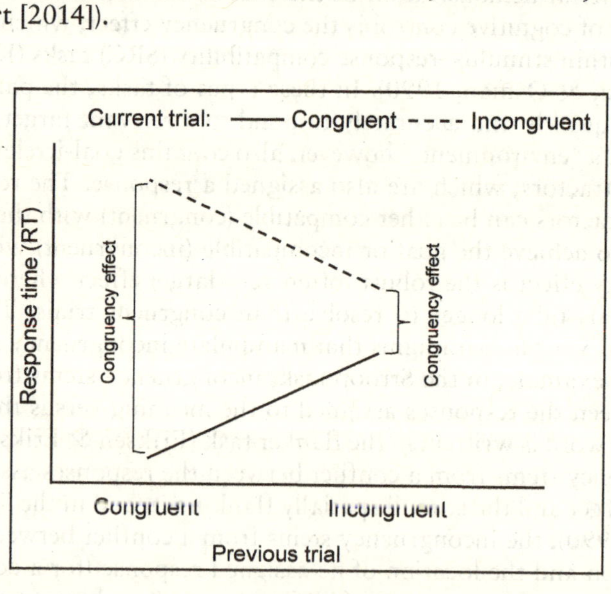

FIGURE 9.1. A schematic of the congruency sequence effect.

Nevertheless, there are two central issues emerging from the debate on the nature of sequential control adaptation that are of particular interest and relevance to the concept of control readiness. One issue pertains to the question of whether the sequential adaptation is driven by conflict monitoring and ensuing control activation, as the original model suggested (Botvinick et al., 2001), or rather by associative or learning processes that are orthogonal to control processes (e.g., Hommel, Proctor, & Vu, 2004; Schmidt, 2013). This issue is of particular relevance to the second prediction related to expectancy-based control adaptation (the PCE), which is discussed in the next section. The second issue pertains to the question of whether conflict-driven control adjustments are domain general or domain specific (Braem et al., 2019; Egner, 2008). The domain-specific view, which undoubtedly is still the dominant view, posits that control is adjusted only when the same type of conflict is encountered. Very concretely, this means that encountering an incongruent Stroop trial will only facilitate control activation and conflict resolution in a subsequent Stroop trial, but not if the subsequent trial is a flanker task trial. The underlying logic is that conflicts vary with respect to the levels of stimulus and response representations (Egner, 2008; see, however, Becker et al. [2024] for a framework that aims at reconciling these discrepancies). The domain-general view posits that control recruited by one type of conflict can and will affect conflict resolution for another type of conflict. Interestingly, in reading the original conflict adaptation model article (Botvinick et al., 2001), it does not seem to preclude the possibility that conflict adaptation is domain general. Although the domain-general view is held by a rather small minority, it did receive some empirical support (e.g., Freitas, Bahar, Yang, & Banai, 2007; Kan et al., 2013; Linzarini, Houdé, & Borst, 2015; Strümer Seiss, & Leuthold, 2005). Braem and colleagues (2014) have tried to reconcile the discrepant findings by proposing a U-shaped pattern whereby conflict dis(similarity) determines conflict adaptation. When conflicts are highly similar, adaptation occurs akin to the manner in which domain-specific proponents think of conflict adaptation. When conflicts are sufficiently dissimilar, they can be simultaneously maintained in working memory without interfering with each other. However, when there is only some degree of dis(similarity) between conflicts, interference precludes the adaptation of control across conflicts.

My colleagues and I (Kleiman et al., 2014) proposed a different type of explanation. Our reasoning was that thus far, conflict (or control) adaptation studies have almost exclusively used classic SRC tasks or cognitive variations thereof. The stimuli in such tasks are arguably "meaningless" (e.g., letters, numbers, or shapes). I do not mean "meaningless" in a derogatory sense but rather that participants do not have any affect or motivation associated with these stimuli.[3] In such cases, the cognitive system does not have an internally induced motivation to resolve these conflicts one way or the other. In other words, the cognitive system "cares" less, so the integration of processing stages or procedures is less likely. However, when the stimuli are infused with meaning—for example, social meaning—the cognitive system is more motivated, so "getting help" to resolve the conflict from other, currently active processes is more likely. This is the essence of control readiness.

We thus set out to test this idea (Kleiman et al., 2014). In a first study, we examined whether the activation of gender stereotypes that associate women with weakness and men with strength (e.g., Banaji & Hardin, 1996; Gawronski, Deutsch, Mbirkou, Seibt, & Strack, 2008) could be reduced via a previous activation of control. Participants thus engaged in two tasks. The first was the Eriksen flanker task (Eriksen & Eriksen, 1974). Participants were shown a vertical string of three letters (e.g., SHS) and were asked to respond to the middle, target letter. On congruent (no-conflict) trials, the three-letter string was composed of the same letter (e.g., HHH). This essentially means that both the target and the distractors are mapped to the same response; hence, no conflict arises, and control processes are not set in motion. On incongruent (conflict) trials, the middle (target) letter and the distracting letters are mapped to different responses (e.g., SHS), so a response conflict arises, and control processes are activated to resolve the conflict and achieve the goal (e.g., pressing the "H" key). The flanker task thus served as the control readiness vessel via which control was activated and operating. The second task was a gender flanker task in which participants were presented with prototypical male or female names (e.g., David, Karen), with a strength- or a weakness-related word both above and below the name. Participants had to indicate whether the name was a female or a male name by pressing one of two designated keys. This setup created stereotypically congruent trials, in which the name and the trait were stereotypically consistent (e.g., the name Karen surrounded by the trait "fragile"), and stereotypically inconsistent trials, in which the name and the trait pointed to different responses (e.g., the name Karen surrounded by the trait "forceful"). The gender flanker task thus served as a test of the control readiness outcome, whereby control readiness should reduce

[3]This setup, of course, has many advantages, the chief one being the ability to look at basic, "pure" cognitive processes, to the extent that cognitive processes can be purely captured (this, I believe, also explains the very large effects found when using SRC tasks and, in comparison, the often smaller effects when adding components; for a somewhat similar argument regarding priming and replicability is social versus non-social psychological research, see Sherman and Rivers (2020, 2021a, 2021b).

the activation of the stereotype. And indeed, on gender flanker trials that followed Eriksen flanker congruent trials, we found the modal gender stereotypes activation pattern. Participants were slower in correctly responding to a name when it was surrounded by gender-incongruent stereotypical traits than when it was surrounded by gender-congruent stereotypical traits. However, gender flanker trials that followed incongruent Eriksen flanker trials did not succumb to this pattern. We found no difference in response time to names regardless of whether they were surrounded by stereotypically congruent or incongruent traits. In a second study, we examined racial stereotypes and employed a sequential priming task rather than a spatial priming task. Specifically, we used the Weapon Identification Task (WIT; Payne, 2001). The WIT is a sequential priming task that measures implicit racial bias. Participants in this task are typically quicker to identify guns and slower to identify hand tools when they follow Black face primes compared with White face primes. This response pattern is thought to reflect an automatic activation of a stereotype associating Black individuals with violence. Indeed, WIT trials that followed congruent Eriksen flanker trials exhibited this exact pattern. However, we found no evidence for implicit stereotyping as measured by the WIT in WIT trials that followed incongruent Eriksen flanker trials. From the control readiness perspective, these findings suggest that when individuals need to activate control in order to achieve a meaningful goal (e.g., stop or inhibit stereotype activation), they will use whatever resources are available to them in the immediate context, resources that might otherwise not have been used.

In another article, my colleagues and I (Kleiman, Trope, & Amodio, 2016) tested the impact of control readiness on overt and covert attention. As was the case in the studies described previously, participants performed alternating trials of two tasks. The first used the classic Stroop task as a means of manipulating control readiness via congruent versus incongruent trials. The second task was an attention task that varied between the studies. To gauge overt attention, we used a dot-probe task in which participants had to respond to the location (left or right) of a dot on a screen. Crucially, before the dot appeared on the screen, participants saw two pictures on the left and right sides of the screen. One of the pictures depicted what is typically considered to be a healthy snack (e.g., carrot sticks), whereas the other picture depicted what is typically considered to be an unhealthy snack (e.g., potato chips). In a second study, to gauge covert attention, we used a variation of the emotional Stroop task, in which words denoting healthy foods (e.g., cucumber) and unhealthy foods (e.g., fries) were presented in blue or red ink. In both studies, we computed a "health focus score" for each participant whereby higher health focus scores indicated greater relative attention toward healthy versus unhealthy snacks, a pattern arguably consistent with having a health goal. At the end of both studies, we asked participants to indicate their height and weight so that we could calculate a body mass index (BMI) score. We used the BMI score as a proxy for health goal importance and motivation.[4] In both studies, we found that activating control at time $n - 1$ modulated attention to food cues at time n in a manner consistent with the individual's goal. Thus, we gained support for the idea of control readiness, whereby conflict-activated control can transfer across different contexts and tasks and whose application depends on the importance of the goal. More concretely, control readiness, via the preactivation of control, would allow one to both shift their overt gaze from temptations threatening the attainment of their goal (overt attention) or mentally shift their attention (covert attention).

As noted earlier, the domain-specific camp is much larger than the domain-general camp. Moreover, there is probably as much to be understood about sequential control adaptation as is already known. Nevertheless, adopting a social cognitive perspective in examining a basic cognitive procedure sheds new light on this debate, with the idea of control readiness now in the mix.

Proportion Congruency—Expectancy-Based Control Adaptation

The typical paradigm to study expectancy-based control adaptation varies the proportion of incongruent to congruent trials in a task block. The size of congruency effects is then compared between the blocks. For example, participants are tasked with performing the Stroop task. In some blocks, 50% of the trials are incongruent. In other blocks, 75% of the trials are incongruent. Congruency effects are then calculated for each type of block and are compared. The robust PCE (e.g., Botvinick et al., 2001; Braem et al., 2019; Kane & Engle, 2003; Lindsay & Jacoby, 1994; Logan & Zbrodoff, 1979; MacLeod, 1991) is the observation that congruency effects are smaller in blocks where the proportion of incongruent trials is larger. The adaptive control perspective's interpretation of this effect is that the cost of activating control in order to deal with conflict resolution decreases as the proportion of conflict in the environment increases.

As is the case with sequential control adaptation, research on expectancy-based control adaptation has focused almost solely on SRC tasks. However, the conflicts used in SRC tasks have a very particular

[4]The study was conducted more than 10 years ago, and we likely would not have used BMI to operationalize goal importance if the study were conducted today.

set of characteristics and are arguably quite far from faithfully representing the vast range of conflicts. First, conflicts in SRC tasks have a single, objectively correct solution, which is set by the task rules. For example, in a Stroop task, adhering to the instructions to respond to the ink color means that the only correct response to the word *red* written in blue ink is "blue." Second, conflicts in SRC tasks are manipulated in a binary manner, conflict versus no conflict (congruent vs. incongruent trials). However, a more nuanced and accurate way to represent conflicts would be using a continuum because various conflicts vary in intensity, and the same conflict can vary in intensity depending on the context. Finally, and perhaps most importantly, recall that the basic premise underlying this research is that the cost of dealing with conflict is reduced as the frequency of conflict in the environment increases. However, the frequency of conflict in the environment has thus far been externally manipulated by the experimenter (e.g., 75% incongruent trials) and was the same for all participants. This method has implicitly neglected individual differences in the degree of experienced conflict by implicitly assuming that an "objective," externally induced proportion of conflict is uniformly experienced across individuals.

In a recent series of studies, my colleagues and I (Levy, Hart, & Kleiman, 2025) aimed at extending the notion of expectancy-based control adaptation beyond binary conflict situations and conflict with a single objectively correct solution while assessing and taking into account individual differences in experienced conflict. In order to achieve our aim, we first selected tasks in which the degree of conflict is continuous and in which conflict resolution depends on personal biases or preferences. This is the case for social categorization tasks in which faces representing the stereotypical edges of a category (e.g., gender, race) are morphed so that a spectrum is created on which lie categorically ambiguous stimuli (faces; Freeman, 2014; Freeman, Pauker, & Sanchez, 2016; Krosch & Amodio, 2014). Participants have to categorize the faces into one of two categories (e.g., male or female). This categorization process is easier (faster) for faces lying at the edges of the spectrum (e.g., 100% male face) and gets more difficult (slower) as the ambiguity level increases (e.g., a morph of 70% male face with a 30% female face). For each participant, a point of subjective equality (PSE), the point at which the participant is equally likely to categorize the face into one of the two categories, is calculated. Gradual increases in conflict level, and conflict resolution that is based on subjective preferences, characterize intertemporal choice tasks as well. In these tasks, participants have to choose between an immediate, smaller reward and a delayed, larger one (e.g., Kable & Glimcher, 2007; Lin, Saunders, Hutcherson, & Inzlicht, 2018). Here, too, an indifference point (PSE) can be calculated to denote equal likelihood in choosing the immediate and delayed rewards.

In both tasks (social categorization and intertemporal choice), a psychometric curve depicting each participant's categorizations or choices can be extracted from the pattern of their responses. My colleagues and I (Levy et al., 2025) propose to use the steepness of the psychometric curve as an indicator of the individually experienced proportion of conflict (IEPC). Very briefly, the underlying logic is as follows: Participants with steep psychometric curves should experience conflict only in a narrow window of manipulated conflict levels and perceive other conflicts as easy to resolve. Conversely, participants with gradual psychometric curves should experience conflict in a wider window of conflict levels and perceive only a small subset of conflicts, those with more clear-cut solutions (e.g., a 90%–10% morph) as easy to resolve. Using the language of the original PCE studies, the proportion of conflict trials out of the entire pool of trials is larger for participants with gradual, rather than steep, psychometric curves.

For both social categorization and intertemporal choice, we found that participants who experienced a larger proportion of conflict had a smaller effect of conflict intensity on conflict resolution time. Put differently, participants who experienced more conflict incurred smaller costs in conflict resolution. This was the case for individually experienced conflict, independent of the "objective," in an experimentally manipulated amount.

Recall that one of the pertinent issues in the debate regarding the nature of conflict-activated adaptive control concerns the question of whether the observed empirical effects of reduced cost for conflict resolution (i.e., shorter response times) as a function of context (either the previous trial or the proportion of conflict in the environment) is due to control adjustment processes or rather due to other control-unrelated processes. Specifically, some researchers suggest that the PCE can be explained by a process of learning stimulus–response contingencies (see Schmidt [2013, 2019] for reviews), so incongruent stimulus–response associations (e.g., the correct response is "blue" when the word presented is *red* in the Stroop task) are more frequent in blocks where the proportion of incongruent trials is larger. In emphasizing the importance of individual differences in the experience of conflict in the environment, we can take sides in this debate in favor of the adaptive control-based account. Because we did not manipulate the proportion of conflict trials but instead measured the proportion of individually experienced conflict, all participants (i.e., both high- and low-conflict participants) performed the exact same task. This essentially means that the difference between high- and low-conflict participants in conflict resolution cost (response time) very likely stems from conflict-activated adaptive control.

TAKE-HOME MESSAGES AND SOME ADDITIONAL THOUGHTS

The idea of control readiness is profoundly inspired by and heavily relies on the notion of adaptive control. Cognitive control, which is arguably inherently adaptive, allows individuals flexibility in the service of goal attainment in an ever-changing and stimulus-prolific environment. Control readiness is the idea that cognitive control is domain general rather than domain specific. But perhaps more important is the unique explanation that the concept of control readiness offers as to why control adjustments could be, should be, and—given certain circumstances—are domain general. As was elaborated on in this chapter, the dominant view in the cognitive control literature states that conflict-triggered control adjustments are domain specific. Nevertheless, there has been some empirical evidence within this domain of research suggesting that such adjustments can be domain general. Braem and colleagues (2014) have suggested that domain-general control adjustments occur when the conflict activating the control and the conflict that should subsequently benefit from control activation are different enough to not occupy the same space in working memory. Thus, their explanation relies on procedural task resolution (dis)similarity. The control readiness explanation relies on motivation. It suggests that when the cognitive system "cares" enough about resolving the conflict in accordance with the individual's goals, it is motivated to seek and find "help" and thus is more efficient in using it. Arguably, not being (or appearing) prejudiced by using stereotypes lies further down the continuum of things the cognitive system cares about than resolving a Stroop trial. The idea of motivation affecting basic cognitive processes is, of course, not new to psychological theorizing and research. This is the case for motivated perception (Cole & Balcetis, 2021), motivated information processing (Klayman, 1995), and even motivation to use self-control (Werner & Milyavskaya, 2019), to name just a few examples.

Another notable point that emerges from the research on control readiness is that the resolution of conflicts and the activation of control go beyond mere effortful impulse inhibition (Fujita, 2011). Indeed, the very definition of the successful activation of control pertains to diverting attention away from distractors (which can manifest as impulses or temptations), but even more importantly to directing attention toward the target (Botvinick et al., 2001; which can be manifested as a higher-order goal). Moreover, as elaborately discussed earlier, research suggests that more conflict in the environment actually results in less effort in resolving it, which goes against the notion of effortful inhibition as a sole solution.

Relatedly, not all conflicts have a hierarchical structure (e.g., a goal and an impulse or a temptation; or a longer- vs. shorter-term goal). Some conflicts might be considered to have a non-hierarchical structure, and they entail a choice between equally desired (or undesired) options. In such cases, effective conflict resolution is simply making a decision, and here as well, the flexible nature of control allows it. Indeed, in a recent article, my colleagues and I (Levy et al., 2023) examined the neural underpinnings of motivational conflicts (i.e., approach–approach and avoidance–avoidance conflicts; Enisman, Levy, & Kleiman, 2024; Levy et al., 2023; Lewin, 1931; Miller, 1944). We found that higher midfrontal theta power (a reliable neural conflict marker) was linked to shorter decision (conflict resolution) times on a single-trial basis. This finding is discrepant with the modal finding in SRC tasks, whereby trials with high midfrontal theta power are linked to longer decision times (Cohen & Cavanagh, 2011). We found this discrepancy to be interesting and informative because, we argued, it nicely demonstrates the flexible nature of cognitive control. In SRC tasks, where there is a single objectively correct response, one's goal is to select it. Thus, control is activated to avoid the incorrect response and consider the alternative, correct response (Kaiser, Iliopoulos, Steinmassl, & Schütz-Bosbach, 2022). Conversely, motivational conflicts do not have an objectively correct response, and the primary goal is simply to make a decision (rather than deferring it). In such cases, control is activated to facilitate—namely, to speed—decision making.

Taken together, what I believe to be unique to the idea of control readiness is that it implies that motivation (1) facilitates procedural flexibility (rather than rigidity); (2) in recruiting the resources to do so, assigns them "correctly"; and (3) does so without an explicit instruction to do so. This is, at the end of the day, greasing the wheels of a basic cognitive process by infusing meaning into it.

REFERENCES

Banaji, M. R., & Hardin, C. D. (1996). Automatic stereotyping. *Psychological Science, 7*(3), 136–141.

Becker, D., Bijleveld, E., Braem, S., Fröber, K., Götz, F. J., Kleiman, T., et al. (2024). An integrative framework of conflict and control. *Trends in Cognitive Sciences, 28*(8), 757–768.

Botvinick, M. M., Braver, T. S., Barch, D. M., Carter, C. S., & Cohen, J. D. (2001). Conflict monitoring and cognitive control. *Psychological Review, 108*(3), 624–652.

Braem, S., Abrahamse, E. L., Duthoo, W., & Notebaert, W. (2014). What determines the specificity of conflict adaptation? A review, critical analysis, and proposed synthesis. *Frontiers in Psychology, 5*, Article 1134.

Braem, S., Bugg, J. M., Schmidt, J. R., Crump, M. J. C., Weissman, D. H., Notebaert, W., et al. (2019). Measuring adaptive control in conflict tasks. *Trends in Cognitive Sciences, 23*(9), 769–783.

Braver, T. S. (2012). The variable nature of cognitive control: A dual mechanisms framework. *Trends in Cognitive Sciences, 16*(2), 106–113.

Bruner, J. S. (1957). On perceptual readiness. *Psychological Review, 64*(2), 123–152.

Chiu, Y.-C., & Egner, T. (2019). Cortical and subcortical contributions to context-control learning. *Neuroscience & Biobehavioral Reviews, 99*, 33–41.

Cohen, M., & Cavanagh, J. F. (2011). Single-trial regression elucidates the role of prefrontal theta oscillations in response conflict. *Frontiers in Psychology, 2*.

Cole, S., & Balcetis, E. (2021). Motivated perception for self-regulation: How visual experience serves and is served by goals. In B. Gawronski (Ed.), *Advances in experimental social psychology* (Vol. 64, pp. 129–186). Elsevier.

Egner, T. (2007). Congruency sequence effects and cognitive control. *Cognitive, Affective, & Behavioral Neuroscience, 7*(4), 380–390.

Egner, T. (2008). Multiple conflict-driven control mechanisms in the human brain. *Trends in Cognitive Sciences, 12*(10), 374–380.

Enisman, M., Levy, A., & Kleiman, T. (2024). Hand movement trajectories illustrate the mechanism underlying Kurt Lewin's distinction between approach–approach and avoidance–avoidance motivational conflicts. *Journal of Personality and Social Psychology, 127*(2), 239–258.

Eriksen, B. A., & Eriksen, C. W. (1974). Effects of noise letters upon the identification of a target letter in a nonsearch task. *Perception & Psychophysics, 16*(1), 143–149.

Freeman, J. B. (2014). Abrupt category shifts during real-time person perception. *Psychonomic Bulletin & Review, 21*(1), 85–92.

Freeman, J. B., Pauker, K., & Sanchez, D. T. (2016). A perceptual pathway to Bias: Interracial exposure reduces abrupt shifts in real-time race perception that predict mixed-race bias. *Psychological Science, 27*(4), 502–517.

Freitas, A. L., Bahar, M., Yang, S., & Banai, R. (2007). Contextual adjustments in cognitive control across tasks. *Psychological Science, 18*(12), 1040–1043.

Fujita, K. (2011). On conceptualizing self-control as more than the effortful inhibition of impulses. *Personality and Social Psychology Review, 15*(4), 352–366.

Gawronski, B., Deutsch, R., Mbirkou, S., Seibt, B., & Strack, F. (2008). When "just say no" is not enough: Affirmation versus negation training and the reduction of automatic stereotype activation. *Journal of Experimental Social Psychology, 44*(2), 370–377.

Gratton, G., Coles, M. G. H., & Donchin, E. (1992). Optimizing the use of information: Strategic control of activation of responses. *Journal of Experimental Psychology: General, 121*(4), 480–506.

Hommel, B., Proctor, R. W., & Vu, K.-P. L. (2004). A feature-integration account of sequential effects in the Simon task. *Psychological Research, 68*(1), 1–17.

Kable, J. W., & Glimcher, P. W. (2007). The neural correlates of subjective value during intertemporal choice. *Nature Neuroscience, 10*(12), 1625–1633.

Kaiser, J., Iliopoulos, P., Steinmassl, K., & Schütz-Bosbach, S. (2022). Preparing for success: Neural frontal theta and posterior alpha dynamics during action preparation predict flexible resolution of cognitive conflicts. *Journal of Cognitive Neuroscience, 34*(6), 1070–1089.

Kan, I. P., Teubner-Rhodes, S., Drummey, A. B., Nutile, L., Krupa, L., & Novick, J. M. (2013). To adapt or not to adapt: The question of domain-general cognitive control. *Cognition, 129*(3), 637–651.

Kane, M. J., & Engle, R. W. (2003). Working-memory capacity and the control of attention: The contributions of goal neglect, response competition, and task set to Stroop interference. *Journal of Experimental Psychology: General, 132*(1), 47–70.

Kerns, J. G., Cohen, J. D., MacDonald, A. W., Cho, R. Y., Stenger, V. A., & Carter, C. S. (2004). Anterior cingulate conflict monitoring and adjustments in control. *Science, 303*(5660), 1023–1026.

Klayman, J. (1995). Varieties of confirmation bias. In K. D. Federmeier (Ed.), *Psychology of learning and motivation* (Vol. 32, pp. 385–418). Elsevier.

Kleiman, T., Hassin, R. R., & Trope, Y. (2014). The control-freak mind: Stereotypical biases are eliminated following conflict-activated cognitive control. *Journal of Experimental Psychology: General, 143*(2), 498–503.

Kleiman, T., Trope, Y., & Amodio, D. M. (2016). Cognitive control modulates attention to food cues: Support for the control readiness model of self-control. *Brain and Cognition, 110*, 94–101.

Kornblum, S., Hasbroucq, T., & Osman, A. (1990). Dimensional overlap: Cognitive basis for stimulus-response compatibility—A model and taxonomy. *Psychological Review, 97*(2), 253–270.

Krosch, A. R., & Amodio, D. M. (2014). Economic scarcity alters the perception of race. *Proceedings of the National Academy of Sciences, 111*(25), 9079–9084.

Levy, A., Enisman, M., Perry, A., & Kleiman, T. (2023). Midfrontal theta as an index of conflict strength in approach–approach *vs* avoidance–avoidance conflicts. *Social Cognitive and Affective Neuroscience, 18*(1), nsad038.

Levy, A., Hart, Y., & Kleiman, T. (2025). *Individual differences in the proportion of experienced conflict affect adaptive control in subjective decisions* [Manuscript in preparation].

Lewin, K. (1931). Environmental forces in child behavior and development. In *A handbook of child psychology* (pp. 94–127). Clark University Press.

Lin, H., Saunders, B., Hutcherson, C. A., & Inzlicht, M. (2018). Midfrontal theta and pupil dilation parametrically track subjective conflict (but also surprise) during intertemporal choice. *NeuroImage, 172*, 838–852.

Lindsay, D. S., & Jacoby, L. L. (1994). Stroop process dissociations: The relationship between facilitation and interference. *Journal of Experimental Psychology: Human Perception and Performance, 20*(2), 219–234.

Linzarini, A., Houdé, O., & Borst, G. (2015). When Stroop helps Piaget: An inter-task positive priming paradigm in 9-year-old children. *Journal of Experimental Child Psychology, 139*, 71–82.

Logan, G. D. (1980). Attention and automaticity in Stroop and priming tasks: Theory and data. *Cognitive Psychology, 12*(4), 523–553.

Logan, G. D., & Zbrodoff, N. J. (1979). When it helps to be misled: Facilitative effects of increasing the frequency of conflicting stimuli in a Stroop-like task. *Memory & Cognition, 7*(3), 166–174.

MacLeod, C. M. (1991). Half a century of research on the Stroop effect: An integrative review. *Psychological Bulletin, 109*(2), 163–203.

Miller, E. K., & Cohen, J. D. (2001). An integrative theory of prefrontal cortex function. *Annual Review of Neuroscience, 24*(1), 167–202.

Miller, N. E. (1944). Experimental studies of conflict. In J. M. Hunt (Ed.), *Personality and the behavior disorders* (pp. 431–465). Ronald Press.

Myrseth, K. O. R., & Fishbach, A. (2009). Self-control: A function of knowing when and how to exercise restraint. *Current Directions in Psychological Science, 18*(4), 247–252.

Payne, B. K. (2001). Prejudice and perception: The role of automatic and controlled processes in misperceiving a weapon. *Journal of Personality and Social Psychology, 81*(2), 181–192.

Schmidt, J. R. (2013). Questioning conflict adaptation: Proportion congruent and Gratton effects reconsidered. *Psychonomic Bulletin & Review, 20*(4), 615–630.

Schmidt, J. R. (2019). Evidence against conflict monitoring and adaptation: An updated review. *Psychonomic Bulletin & Review, 26*(3), 753–771.

Shenhav, A., Botvinick, M. M., & Cohen, J. D. (2013). The expected value of control: An integrative theory of anterior cingulate cortex function. *Neuron, 79*(2), 217–240.

Sherman, J. W., & Rivers, A. M. (2020). Social priming: Time to ditch a dubious term? *Nature, 579*(7797), 29–29.

Sherman, J. W., & Rivers, A. M. (2021a). A final word on train wrecks. *Psychological Inquiry, 32*(1), 49–52.

Sherman, J. W., & Rivers, A. M. (2021b). There's nothing social about social priming: Derailing the "train wreck." *Psychological Inquiry, 32*(1), 1–11.

Simon, J. R. (1990). The effects of an irrelevant directional cue on human information processing. In R. W. Proctor & T. G. Reeve (Eds.), *Advances in psychology* (Vol. 65, pp. 31–86). Elsevier.

Stürmer, B., Seiss, E., & Leuthold, H. (2005). Executive control in the Simon task: A dual-task examination of response priming and its suppression. *European Journal of Cognitive Psychology, 17*(5), 590–618.

Wegner, D. M. (2009). How to think, say, or do precisely the worst thing for any occasion. *Science, 325*(5936), 48–50.

Werner, K. M., & Milyavskaya, M. (2019). Motivation and self-regulation: The role of want-to motivation in the processes underlying self-regulation and self-control. *Social and Personality Psychology Compass, 13*(1), e12425.

CHAPTER 10

What People Understand about Expanding and Contracting Regulatory Scope

Jessica J. Carnevale and Kentaro Fujita

The central theme of this book is the psychological quest for meaning: the notion that people are not passive sensors but instead organisms that actively seek to understand their social worlds in a purposeful manner. The present chapter describes one way in which people's motivations and goals shape this understanding. Goals can inspire structure and a sense of purpose in thoughts, feelings, and behavior—an important form of meaning making (see Fishbach & Wang, this volume; Liberman, this volume). In this chapter, we discuss a different way that goals may influence meaning making: specifically, by affecting how people regulate both the quantity and quality of motivational states to attain goals—that is, metamotivation (e.g., Fujita, Le, Scholer, & Miele, 2024; Miele & Scholer, 2018; Miele, Scholer, & Fujita, 2020; Scholer, Miele, Murayama, & Fujita, 2018). We highlight some of the strategic efforts people engage in to create meaning to instantiate motivational states that they believe facilitate goal-directed performance. Ultimately, this work highlights the central role that meaning making may play in determining the questions of who, when, and why some succeed and others fail in their pursuit of goals.

METAMOTIVATION

Self-regulation research traditionally focuses on how people monitor and modulate their thoughts, feelings, and behaviors to attain valued goals (e.g., Mann, de Ridder, & Fujita, 2013). The metamotivation approach, however, is unique in that it focuses on the regulation of motivational states, with the assumption that motivations are the source and impetus for most thoughts, feelings, and behaviors (e.g., Fujita, Le, et al., 2024; Miele & Scholer, 2018; Miele et al., 2020; Scholer et al., 2018). The term *metamotivation* does not refer to motivations about motivations in the same way that the term *metacognition* is sometimes informally understood as "thoughts about thoughts." Instead, it draws from research proposing that psychological processes can be described as operating at the meta-level and object level: Meta-level processes monitor and modify other psychological processes that operate at the object level (Nelson & Narens, 1990). Metamotivation processes can be cognitive, affective, motivational, and so forth; the key is that they target motivational states as the object of regulation. The thesis of this chapter is that one way in which people instantiate motivational states that support and sustain goal pursuit is via meaning making. Specifically, we suggest that people engage in strategic forms of subjective representation or construal to reify motivational states conducive to successful goal-directed performance (Fujita, Le, et al., 2024). Through this meaning-making process, people not only regulate how much motivation they experience but also what kind. To support this argument, we describe research primarily conducted within the context of construal-level theory (CLT; Liberman & Trope, 2008; Trope & Liberman, 2010; Trope, Ledgerwood, Liberman, & Fujita, 2021), focusing on how regulatory scope sensitizes people to contractive versus expansive motivational concerns.

REGULATORY SCOPE

Life requires people to "zoom in" and "zoom out" to make good decisions and act in accordance with valued goals. At times, tasks demand that we immerse ourselves in the immediate present and be responsive to local demands and contingencies. Metaphorically, these tasks require a narrow, high-precision lens that sensitizes us to our current environment, allowing us to tailor our behavior to specific circumstances—as is required when we must be vigilant for errors when proofreading or throwing darts. At other times, tasks demand that we expand beyond the "here and now" and consider more distant times, places, people, and possibilities. Metaphorically, these tasks require a broad, wide-angle lens that makes us more responsive to contingencies beyond our direct experience—as is required when we must motivate ourselves to forgo the allure of our favorite indulgent foods to advance our weight-loss goals. Effective goal-directed behavior requires that people zoom in and zoom out as called for by the tasks at hand.

Recent formulations of CLT (Trope et al., 2021) refer to this zooming in and zooming out as the modulation of regulatory scope. Regulatory scope can be defined as the range of considerations one contemplates and responds to in goal-directed decision making and behavior. People contract scope when they consider the narrower, more focal set of concerns relevant to their present circumstances; by contrast, they expand scope when they consider a broader, more diffuse set of concerns that may require thinking about more distant times, places, people, and possibilities.

To be clear, neither contracting nor expanding regulatory scope is superior or leads to more effective outcomes than the other. Both entail important trade-offs. Zooming in allows one to immerse themselves in the present but trades off responsiveness to the bigger picture. Zooming out allows one to step back and take in the larger scene but at the expense of the immersive details facilitated by contraction. In our complex worlds, people must be able to flexibly expand and contract in response to task demands and read the environmental cues that signal which scope will serve them best. Such skillful and flexible modulation of expansive versus contractive scope is a key challenge for self-regulation as people face a wide array of regulatory challenges that require targeted strategies for success.

CONSTRUAL LEVEL AS A MENTAL TOOL

One of the key epistemic challenges in modulating scope is dealing with heterogeneity. Addressing concerns that extend beyond immediate circumstances (i.e., expanding scope) requires being responsive to a greater number and diversity of possibilities. That is, whereas contracting scope requires one to focus on only those concerns relevant to the here and now, expanding scope requires being responsive not only to the concerns of the current environment but also those that are more remote. Because one's cognitive system can only attend to so many things at any given time (Miller, 1956), to address this increase in number and variability, CLT proposes that people leverage cognitive abstraction (high-level construal) and concretization (low-level construal) as mental tools. Construals are subjective interpretations of the world; they facilitate imposing meaning in a goal-directed way (Trope & Liberman, 2010; Trope et al., 2021). Construals vary from low-level interpretations of the available information, highlighting the individuating details that make similar objects and instances unique, to high-level interpretations that highlight the unifying features of objects and events (Trope & Liberman, 2003). Formally, *low-level construal* refers to a representational process that highlights the context-specific features that render events idiosyncratic and unique. *High-level construal*, on the other hand, refers to a representational process that focuses on the essential and goal-relevant features that are invariant and common across all possible manifestations of an event.

As an example, consider a dog. Someone engaging in low-level construal might construe this dog as "Lolo," a friend's cute but angry Chihuahua. This concrete representation contracts scope, leading one to be able to tailor one's behavior toward this specific dog—that is, being mindful of one's fingers and toes relative to the dog's teeth. By contrast, someone engaging in high-level construal might construe this same dog as a "pet." This abstract representation may not be tailored to Lolo specifically, but it is one that generalizes to a number of possible entities, providing guidance and expectations as to how to behave around not just a friend's dog but also their cats, rabbits, snakes, and spiders.

In this way, low-level construal allows people to create highly specific representations of their present circumstances and be responsive to local contingencies—thereby contracting scope. By contrast, high-level construal allows people to deal with variability. By leveraging more abstract representations, one can still manage all of the possibilities expanding scope entails. High-level construal is thus a cognitive solution for the epistemic challenges associated with expanding scope.

Metaphorically, one could imagine a lantern that one can lower or raise on a pole (construal level), with corresponding changes to what one can see on the ground (regulatory scope). When the lantern is lowered (i.e., low-level construal), the light shone upon the ground will be more concentrated and intense but also more limited and narrower in diameter (contractive scope). When the lantern is raised (i.e., high-level construal), the light shone upon the ground will be more diffuse yet illuminate greater surface area (expansive scope).

There is extensive empirical evidence for these theoretical assertions (e.g., Soderberg, Callahan, Kochersberger, Amit, & Ledgerwood, 2015; Trope et al., 2021); a thorough review of this literature is beyond the scope of this chapter. Instead, we focus on research specific to the self-regulation domain. We highlight in particular the notion of *task–motivation fit:* Performance should be enhanced to the extent that people match or fit high-level construal with expansive tasks and low-level construal with contractive tasks.

THE ROLE OF CONSTRUAL LEVEL IN SELF-REGULATION

A long tradition suggests that self-regulation cannot be reduced to a single problem or process (e.g., Bonanno & Burton, 2013; Gollwitzer,

1990; Higgins, 2000; Miele, Fujita, & Scholer, 2024). Instead, self-regulation presents multiple challenges that are addressed by distinct solutions. As noted earlier, one way tasks can differ is in the extent to which they require expansion versus contraction of regulatory scope.

Self-control is a self-regulation challenge that requires expansion. *Self-control* can be formally defined as a motivational conflict between the expansive versus contractive implications of a decision (e.g., Fujita, 2011; Fujita, Trope, & Liberman, 2025). It is typically experienced as a choice between larger-later versus smaller-sooner outcomes (e.g., Ainslie, 1975; Fujita, 2011; Mischel, Shoda, & Rodriguez, 1989). Rewards and opportunities in their immediate environment frequently tempt people to act in ways that are contrary to their more expansive concerns. A piece of chocolate cake, for example, tempts dieters to indulge, threatening their weight-loss goals. Expanding regulatory scope allows one to understand the value of immediately available rewards in the context of these broader concerns. It is harder for dieters to indulge in chocolate cake, for example, when they know the repercussions that this decision might have not only for their weight-loss goals but also for other concerns, such as their motivations for self-improvement ("becoming the better me"), health ("reducing risk factors for diabetes and other health issues"), and being a model parent ("exemplifying self-discipline for my kids"), among others. To the extent that self-control requires expanding regulatory scope, performance should be enhanced when people engage in high-level versus low-level construal.

Empirical work supports this hypothesis that high-level construal facilitates self-control (e.g., Fujita & Carnevale, 2012; Fujita et al., 2025). For example, Fujita and Han (2009) experimentally induced expansion versus contraction by manipulating high-level versus low-level construal among female undergraduates and observed that the former were more likely to select an apple over a candy bar (Fujita & Han, 2009; see also Carnevale, Fujita, Han, & Amit, 2015). Similarly, experimentally inducing people to engage in high-level versus low-level construal reduces temporal discounting—the tendency to devalue larger-delayed relative to smaller-immediate rewards (Fujita, Trope, Liberman, & Levin-Sagi, 2006; Malkoc, Zauberman, & Bettman, 2010; Rudzinska-Wojciechowska, 2017; Yi, Stuppy-Sullivan, Pickover, & Landes, 2017; Stillman, Medvedev, & Ferguson, 2017). In sum, self-control—a task that requires expansion—appears to benefit from engaging in high-level rather than low-level construal (see Fujita et al. [2025] for recent review).

Not all self-regulation challenges entail self-control, however (e.g., Nguyen, Carnevale, Scholer, Miele, & Fujita, 2019). Regulating behavior such as shooting a basketball free throw or putting a golf ball, for example, requires physical and emotional regulation but does not entail a conflict between two mutually exclusive goals, as does self-control. Athletes do not want to miss their shots. These challenges instead require behavioral precision—goal-directed performance of an action in response to situational contingencies (Baumeister, 1984; Beilock & Carr, 2004). Given the need to attune to one's immediate environment, behavioral precision should benefit from contractive rather than expansive scope. If this is true, people should perform better on these tasks when engaged in low-level versus high-level construal.

Empirically supporting this prediction, participants induced to low-level versus high-level construal performed better on a stop signal task—a regulatory task that requires vigilant attunement to the immediate environment in order to override a habitual behavioral response (Schmeichel, Vohs, & Duke, 2011). Similarly, participants more focused on the concrete means rather than the abstract ends of a dart-throwing task exhibited superior dart performance (Zimmerman & Kitsantas, 1996, 1997). These findings and others suggest that low-level rather than high-level construal benefits performance on behavioral precision tasks—tasks that require contraction rather than expansion.

METAMOTIVATIONAL KNOWLEDGE ABOUT CONSTRUAL LEVEL AND SCOPE

The studies reviewed previously have little to say about how people create meaning to fulfill their goals; this is because construal level was experimentally induced by researchers. The metamotivational approach takes a different tack by examining how people regulate their own motivational states to achieve goals without experimental induction (Fujita, Le, et al., 2024; Miele & Scholer, 2018; Miele et al., 2020; Scholer et al., 2018). From this perspective, expansive versus contractive regulatory scope can be seen as states that promote sensitivity to broader versus narrower motivational concerns. When presented with expansive tasks, people may engage in efforts to expand regulatory scope—presumably by self-inducing high-level construal; when presented with contractive tasks, people may engage in efforts to contract regulatory scope—presumably by self-inducing low-level construal. That is, to the extent that they are effective self-regulators, we might expect them to construe expansive tasks in high-level terms and contractive tasks in low-level terms. By doing so, they would create task–motivation fit and increase the likelihood of success.

The metamotivational approach suggests that creating task–motivation fit of individuals' own accord requires two types of knowledge by individuals: (1) distinguishing and recognizing when tasks require expansion versus contraction and (2) understanding how to induce themselves into high-level versus low-level construal, respectively. An emerging and growing field of research demonstrates that people do indeed have some understanding of both of these types of knowledge and that such knowledge may affect important real-world outcomes.

The first work in this area explored people's understanding of the role of construal level in self-control. When faced with the self-control challenge of resisting temptation, participants reported that thinking about "why" (a high-level construal) would be a more successful strategy than thinking about "how" (a low-level construal) in facilitating their ability to exert self-control successfully. For example, participants reported that it would be more beneficial for them to think about why rather than how when attempting to restrain themselves from a food-related temptation (MacGregor, Carnevale, Dusthimer, & Fujita, 2017). Subsequent studies examined people's knowledge not only of the benefits of high-level construal for self-control but also of the benefits of low-level construal for behavioral precision. In one study, for example, research participants not only reported that engaging in a preparatory exercise that had them think about "how" versus "why" would be more beneficial for behavioral precision tasks—such as proofreading or playing darts—that require careful attention to contextual details but also that thinking about "why" vs. how would be more useful for self-control tasks, such as choosing between smaller-sooner versus larger-later monetary rewards (Nguyen et al., 2019). Such metamotivational knowledge appears robust in that it extends across task domains (e.g., health, finance, social relationships) and across various experimental operationalizations of construal (e.g., global vs. local processing, generating categories vs. exemplars, and contemplating "why" vs. "how").

These findings indicate that people can distinguish between tasks that require expansion versus contraction. Although this might strike some as trivial, we might instead suggest that this is somewhat surprising. This distinction extends to tasks that may appear superficially similar, such as intertemporal choice tasks versus Stroop tasks. Although a regulatory scope perspective might suggest that these two tasks are distinct, many scientists have used Stroop tasks to try to gain insight into self-control (e.g., Gailliot et al., 2007; Hagger, Wood, Stiff, & Chatzisarantis, 2010; Hofman, Friese, & Strack, 2009; Inzlicht & Gutsell, 2007). Given that many scientists have not distinguished these two tasks, we find it remarkable that lay individuals do. Indeed, their judgments appear more concordant with more recent research suggesting that tasks like Stroop may be distinct from self-control (e.g., Duckworth & Kern, 2011; Eisenberg et al., 2019; Saunders, Milyavskaya, Etz, Randles, & Inzlicht, 2018).

People also seem to recognize various means with which to induce high-level versus low-level construal for expansive versus contractive tasks, respectively. This, too, would appear remarkable, given the diversity of operationalizations of construal level with which they were presented. Rather than reflecting some superficial feature matching, these findings suggest that lay individuals have some deeper (yet perhaps implicit or tacit) insight into the psychological operations that various tasks may entail and their effect on regulatory scope.

One might ask whether these findings extend beyond the Western, college-educated samples that these initial studies included. Research by Nguyen, Togawa, Scholer, and Fujita (2020) indicates that knowledge of how to use construal level to regulate scope may generalize across cultures. Participants in both the United States and Japan were presented with a list of scenarios that previous research indicated require expansion (i.e., self-control), contraction (i.e., behavioral precision), or control condition scenarios. For each scenario, participants were asked how useful it would be for task performance to think about why they would engage in the task (an indicator of high-level knowledge) versus how they would engage in the task (an indicator of low-level knowledge). Both American and Japanese participants recognized that thinking about why benefits high-level tasks, whereas thinking about how benefits low-level tasks. Similarly, American and Japanese participants reported that global processing would facilitate high-level tasks, whereas local processing would facilitate low-level tasks. Taken together, these results provide evidence that individuals across cultures are able to recognize how to match their construals to the task demands.

DEVELOPMENT AND ACQUISITION OF METAMOTIVATIONAL KNOWLEDGE

Emerging research suggests that this metamotivational knowledge of how construals affect regulatory scope is evident even among school-age children and adolescents. Teo, Chen, Fujita, and Scholer (2024) had middle and high school students in Singapore complete assessments of construal-level knowledge similar to those employed by earlier research. Students in grades 6–10 were asked to report whether performance on various expansion (i.e., self-control) and contraction (i.e., behavioral precision) tasks would benefit most from preparatory exercises of thinking about why to do the task versus how to do the task. Consistent with previous research, these young participants reported that thinking about "how" would be most valuable for contractive tasks and thinking about "why" would be most valuable for expansive tasks. These reports, however, varied by participant age. Although all grades reported accurate metamotivational knowledge, the strength of that knowledge increased with each grade level, particularly for knowledge that high-level construal benefits expansive tasks. These results suggest that metamotivational knowledge is still developing during adolescence and that high-level knowledge may develop later than low-level knowledge.

In addition, there was preliminary evidence that socioeconomic status may be associated with knowledge such that students with higher household incomes had significantly higher metamotivational knowledge (both high level and low level) compared with peers from lower-income households. These findings suggest that socioeconomic status may be an important contributor to the development of accurate metamotivational knowledge. Given the correlational nature of these findings, however, future research still needs to determine causality and explore why these differences emerge.

METAMOTIVATIONAL KNOWLEDGE AND PERFORMANCE

Although people appear to have metamotivational knowledge of the benefits of high-level and low-level construal for expanding and contracting scope, respectively, there is significant individual variability in the extent of this knowledge, with some people not fitting construal to task at all. One might ask whether individual differences in this knowledge affect task performance. Do those with accurate knowledge outperform those with less accurate knowledge?

The answer to these questions appears to be yes. Dieters who associated self-control with high-level construal reported lower body mass index, suggesting that they were more successful in their weight-loss efforts (MacGregor et al., 2017). Psychology students in the United States who reported that high-level construal would benefit academic self-control conflicts earned higher final grades in their psychology class than those who did not (MacGregor et al., 2017). In another study (Nguyen, Scholer, Miele, Edwards, & Fujita, 2023), American college students enrolled in an Introduction to Psychology course reported their metamotivational knowledge of the benefits of construal level during weeks 11–15 of the semester, along with known covariates of final grades such as high school grade point average (GPA), amount of academic motivation, academic self-concept, and demographic characteristics. Knowledge of the benefits of both high-level and low-level construal uniquely predicted final course grades, even when controlling for known covariates. These findings are not merely an artifact of White, educated, industrialized, rich, and democratic (WEIRD) sample populations. Singaporean adolescents' metamotivational knowledge predicted their exam performance across multiple classes and subjects while controlling for potential confounds for academic success (e.g., intelligence, prior academic achievement) by statistically adjusting for performance on the previous year's exam in the same subject (Teo et al., 2024). Thus, understanding the benefits of construal level for modulating regulatory scope appears to predict self-regulatory outcomes over and above traditional predictors of success—across different operationalizations of construal level and across Western and Eastern cultures.

DISCUSSION

Taken together, these findings make important contributions to our understanding of how people can use meaning making to advance their goals. In particular, this work reveals how people use construal level strategically to navigate the complex challenges they face in life. First, this line of research demonstrates that people have the knowledge to regulate their own construal level organically and in the absence of any research induction, indicating that construal level as a self-regulation strategy is not an artificial lab phenomenon. Second, individuals evidence a large degree of variability in their metamotivational knowledge, and that variability predicts self-regulation outcomes. This evidence suggests that understanding what people know about construal level may provide insights not only into who succeeds in self-regulation but also when and why.

Third, given the variety of challenges that people face as they attempt to regulate and the many points along that path affected by construal level, the research reviewed suggests novel interventions that could be designed to address specific self-regulatory problems. Although abundant experimental research reveals what works to facilitate versus impair self-regulation, comparatively less is known about what people know about motivation and what they spontaneously do to regulate their motivation. The value of the metamotivational approach described in this chapter is filling in these gaps about what people do on their own to manage their regulation challenges. This approach highlights knowledge of regulation strategies rather than capacity for regulation as the key determinant for successful regulation, and one could imagine the development of education-based interventions that target misbeliefs and flawed knowledge.

We might note parallels between our approach and that of Walter Mischel's classic delay-of-gratification studies (e.g., Mischel, Shoda, &

Rodriguez, 1989). That is, Mischel and colleagues suggested that children's failures of self-regulation may stem from a lack of knowledge of what strategies are effective (as opposed to some deficient cognitive capacity; Mischel & Mischel, 1983; Rodriguez, Mischel, & Shoda, 1989). However, rather than focusing solely on beliefs about what strategies might be effective, our approach also highlights people's more basic understanding of what motivational states are called for by a task and how to instantiate those states. We also provide a broad theoretical framework that predicts and explains why strategies that work for one self-regulation challenge (self-control) may not work for another (behavioral precision). In these ways, the present work builds on and extends this classic work.

At its broadest level, metamotivational research highlights the importance of meaning making in the act of self-regulation. People do not simply passively make sense of the world based on the information that happens to waft past their noses. Rather, people actively and strategically shape their understanding of the tasks, events, and other information around them in a manner that facilitates their ability and motivation to pursue their goals effectively.

IMPLICATIONS

Meaning making through construal level may be important not only for how individuals regulate their own motivational states and goal pursuit but also for how they influence others to do the same. People are often tasked with motivating others to deliver their best performance, whether as managers, teachers, coaches, or parents. Such motivational management includes not only the amount of motivation, by attempting to increase the motivation or effort of another, but also the type of motivation, by attempting to influence someone else to modulate their motivation to fit the task at hand. There is some evidence that having the appropriate metamotivational knowledge may be an important precursor to one's ability to motivate others in the context of regulatory focus theory (Jansen, Miele, Fujita, & Scholer, 2022). Participants with supervisory occupational roles reported knowledge of fit between a promotion/prevention focus and an eager/vigilant task for both themselves and for hypothetical employee reports and prepared these hypothetical subordinates for upcoming eager versus vigilant tasks with promotion- versus prevention-focused exercises, respectively. Taken together, these findings indicate that effective motivators may be those who possess greater knowledge about task–motivation fit. Future research should explore this possibility by examining how beliefs about other types of metamotivational challenges, including construal level, affect the ability to motivate others. Are the most effective managers those who recognize that high-level construal promotes expansive tasks and low-level construal promotes contractive tasks and are therefore able to pass that knowledge on to subordinates, students, mentees, and so forth to facilitate improved outcomes?

This type of metamotivational regulation of others has clear implications for education. Teachers may struggle to convince students to work harder, but perhaps modulating the amount of motivation is less impactful than modulating the type of motivation. Expanding and contracting regulatory scope are not known to differ in terms of their cognitive expenditure. Therefore, intervening to help students better fit their motivation type to the task at hand may improve educational outcomes even if students' amount of effort does not change. One might expect that the most effective teachers are those with not only the requisite metamotivational knowledge of construal task–motivation fit but also the skill to pass this knowledge to their students. It is possible that effective teachers transmit such metamotivational knowledge explicitly through direct training. Alternatively, given that metamotivational knowledge is often tacit rather than explicit, effective metamotivational regulation of others might also take place tacitly. Future research should examine whether teachers with the best student outcomes are those with the highest level of metamotivational knowledge combined with skill at transmitting it. Furthermore, research should examine the means by which effective teachers transmit this knowledge and whether explicit instruction or tacit direction is more meaningful.

Parenting is another role that requires regulating the motivations of others. There is enormous variability across developmental stages, as well as individual differences in the capacity to expand scope. Parents must help their children to develop metamotivational knowledge while working within the constraints of their child's cognitive development. Parents play the most meaningful role in children's self-control development in particular, not only because self-control may be somewhat genetically determined (with a heritability estimate of 60%, according to a recent meta-analysis; Willems, Boesen, Li, Finkenauer, & Bartels, 2019) but also because parents shape children's knowledge of what type of motivation to apply to which tasks, either through explicit instruction or through implicit modeling.

The processes that play out among those charged with regulating others' motivations are highly complex because those individuals must also regulate their own motivations. Children and students are not always open to the lessons their parents and teachers try to impart. The interplay between self and other may not always render clear how expansive or contractive one should be. There may be mismatches, for example, in the scope of regulation one is trying to impart on another versus one's own regulatory state. A harried attempt to shoe a toddler and leave the house on time for an appointment is both an expansive attempt to impart the value of being on time for obligations and a more contractive challenge of enduring an endless parade of delays, diversions, and frustrations as the toddler removes each shoe as soon as it has been put on.

One cannot regulate their own motivational states unless they are also able to monitor them. How do individuals monitor their scope? People may monitor their motivational states by attending to the motivationally relevant emotions that accompany those states (e.g., Miele et al., 2020). For example, confidence may signal high levels of self-efficacy, whereas frustration and hopelessness signal low levels. Such motivationally relevant emotional monitoring may require cognitive skills to disentangle because the same emotion may signal low levels of multiple types of motivation. For example, feelings of boredom or indifference may signal low levels of either promotion value or prevention value.

There is not yet a broad consensus about how individuals monitor their regulatory scope, but one possibility is that they do so by monitoring emotions that are associated with low versus high construal level. Emotions vary in their scope, such that emotions tied to specific singular objects and events are construed at a lower level, whereas emotions that cut across multiple instances of similar objects and events are construed at a higher level (e.g., Moran, Bornstein, & Eyal, 2022). For example, lust, an emotion rooted in the physical here and now, is construed concretely, whereas love, an emotion that can traverse psychological barriers, is construed more concretely (Epstude & Förster, 2011). Even within one emotional construct, it is possible to discern distinctions between low-level and high-level instantiations of that emotion. For example, research differentiates between core disgust and sociomoral disgust (Haidt, Rozin, McCauley, & Imada, 1997; Rozin, Haidt, & McCauley, 2008). Core disgust is elicited by unclean physical objects perceived as physically harmful, such as filthy toilets or festering wounds, and is associated with low-level construal. Sociomoral disgust, by contrast, does not typically involve physical filth and is instead elicited by culturally determined morally objectionable acts or objects and is associated with high-level construal (Moran et al., 2021). Construal level and disgust activate each other bidirectionally such that stimuli that elicit core (vs. sociomoral) disgust are construed at a lower (vs. higher) construal level, and stimuli inducing low-level (vs. high-level) construal elicit more core (vs. sociomoral) disgust. It may be that people monitor their construal level by monitoring whether their current emotional states are those associated with low-level construal (e.g., lust, core disgust, anger) or those associated with high-level construal (e.g., love, sociomoral disgust, hatred).

People with sufficient metamotivational knowledge of the regulatory functions of construal may up- or down-regulate their emotional experience to strategically modulate their regulatory scope via the construal level associated with those emotions. A recent metanalysis (Moran & Eyal, 2022) revealed that high-level (vs. low-level) construal reduces (vs. increases) the emotional intensity of low-level emotions such as anger, but it increases (vs. decreases) the intensity of high-level emotions such as hate. This association between certain emotions and construal level may be bidirectional, such that inducing high-level relative to low-level emotions induces high-level relative to low-level construal. Thus, to expand regulatory scope, people may attempt to intensify their experiences of high-level emotions, whereas to contract regulatory scope, they may attempt to intensify their experiences of low-level emotions. Research has not yet demonstrated that people have this sort of knowledge or that they use this knowledge strategically to achieve such task–motivation fit in this way.

Any attempts to create educational interventions that target people's knowledge about the role of construal level in modulating scope will have to address several critical issues. First, research has yet to articulate a theoretical framework with which to understand which instantiations of construal level may be more or less effective than others. Although the research reviewed herein suggests that people understand that thinking about "why" versus "how" is likely to expand versus contract scope, this operationalization of construal level was one of convenience—it had been used in past research (e.g., Freitas, Gollwitzer, & Trope, 2004; Fujita et al., 2006). Future research might explore the best methods that people can use to self-induce high-level versus low-level construal. Similarly, one might ask whether there are ways to expand and contract regulatory scope via alternative means beyond construal level. That is, it might be more effective for people to directly target regulatory scope rather than construal level to optimize task–motivation fit.

BEYOND REGULATORY SCOPE: REGULATING OTHER MOTIVATIONAL STATES VIA MEANING

This chapter focused on research conducted within the construal-level context. One should not, however, mistakenly assume that the strategic meaning making we have described here is limited to regulatory scope.

Other research inspired by the metamotivation approach highlights other motivational states people target via meaning-making processes to promote goals (for recent reviews, see Fujita, Scholer, & Miele, 2024; Miele et al., 2024). For example, people can pursue their goals out of concerns for advancement (promotion) versus security (prevention; Higgins, 1997), and these distinct motivational orientations promote performance on different tasks (those requiring eagerness vs. vigilance, respectively; Higgins, 2005). Critically, as with construal level and regulatory scope, people appear to have the requisite knowledge to distinguish tasks on the basis of eagerness versus vigilance and to identify means with which to induce promotion versus prevention, respectively (Scholer & Miele, 2016).

The metamotivational approach may also provide novel insights into how people regulate self-defensive motivations that impede goal attainment. Setbacks, failures, and negative feedback, for example, can often lead people to react defensively, leading them to engage in short-term efforts to protect their self-esteem rather than longer-term efforts to assess their shortcomings and grow in ways that support goal pursuit (e.g., Trope & Neter, 1994). For example, people may choose to dismiss information that they are engaging in behaviors that are harmful to their health (e.g., Sherman, Nelson, & Steele, 2000). This response appears to occur as a result of how people construe or understand the negative self-relevant information: Interpreting such events as "useful information" rather than "hurtful or embarrassing news" should reduce defensiveness (e.g., Belding, Naufel, & Fujita, 2015). Recent metamotivation work suggests that although people are generally aware of strategies that might help this meaning-making process (e.g., self-affirmation; Sherman et al., 2000), they may prefer to engage in alternative strategies that do not change the meaning of the negative event (e.g., telling themselves to just "shake it off"; Reeves, Nguyen, Scholer, Fujita, & Spencer, 2023).

Thus, the notion that people may strategically engage in meaning making to promote their goals may extend beyond modulating regulatory scope and be relevant to other self-regulatory challenges. These may include how people regulate intrinsic versus extrinsic motivation (e.g., Converse, Juarez, & Hennecke, 2019; Kuratomi, Johnsen, Kitagami, Hatano, & Murayama, 2023; Murayama, Kitagami, Tanaka, & Raw, 2016; Woolley & Fishbach, 2015), respond to self-discontinuity (see Sedikides & Wildschut, this volume), and pursue achievement goals (Gilbert & Elliot, 2024). In this way, we believe that the research we review serves as an important springboard for understanding the centrality of strategic meaning making in the pursuit of goals.

SUMMARY

In this chapter, we described people's understanding of how to strategically create meaning to advance valued goals. Specifically, we explored how people leverage high-level versus low-level construal to prepare for tasks that require expansions versus contraction. Not only are people sensitive to which tasks require expansion versus contraction, but they also appear to recognize a wide variety of means with which to induce high-level and low-level construal, respectively. This knowledge, moreover, predicts meaningful real-world outcomes. This work thus highlights how people actively construct meaning to pursue their goals: Rather than passively sensing the world around them, people actively engage in constructing a view of the world that helps them achieve their goals. Thus, goals not only inspire people by providing them with purpose and direction—a very important form of meaning making—but also motivate them to engage in meaning making that enhances the ability to carry out these goals effectively.

REFERENCES

Ainslie, G. (1975). Specious reward: A behavioral theory of impulsiveness and impulse control. *Psychological Bulletin, 82*(4), 463–496.

Baumeister, R. F. (1984). Choking under pressure: Self-consciousness and paradoxical effects of incentives on skillful performance. *Journal of Personality and Social Psychology, 46*(3), 610–620.

Beilock, S. L., & Carr, T. H. (2004). From novice to expert performance. In A. M. Williams & N. J. Hodges (Eds.), *Skill acquisition in sport: Research, theory and practice.* Routledge.

Belding, J. N., Naufel, K. Z., & Fujita, K. (2015). Using high-level construal and perceptions of changeability to promote self-change over self-protection motives in response to negative feedback. *Personality and Social Psychology Bulletin, 41*(6), 822–838.

Bonanno, G. A., & Burton, C. L. (2013). Regulatory flexibility: An individual differences perspective on coping and emotion regulation. *Perspectives on Psychological Science, 8*(6), 591–612.

Carnevale, J. J., Fujita, K., Han, H. A., & Amit, E. (2015). Immersion versus transcendence: How pictures and words impact evaluative associations assessed by the Implicit Association Test. *Social Psychological and Personality Science, 6*(1), 92–100.

Converse, B. A., Juarez, L., & Hennecke, M. (2019). Self-control and the reasons behind our goals. *Journal of Personality and Social Psychology, 116*(5), 860–883.

Duckworth, A. L., & Kern, M. L. (2011). A meta-analysis of the convergent validity of self-control measures. *Journal of Research in Personality, 45*(3), 259–268.

Eisenberg, I. W., Bissett, P. G., Zeynep Enkavi, A., Li, J., MacKinnon, D. P., Marsch, L. A., et al. (2019). Uncovering the structure of self-regulation through data-driven ontology discovery. *Nature Communications, 10*(1), 2319.

Epstude, K., & Förster, J. (2011). Seeing love, or seeing lust: How people interpret ambiguous romantic situations. *Journal of Experimental Social Psychology, 47*(5), 1017–1020.

Freitas, A. L, Gollwitzer, P., & Trope, Y. (2004). The influence of abstract and concrete mindsets on anticipating and guiding others' self-regulatory efforts. *Journal of Experimental Social Psychology, 40*(6), 739–752.

Fujita, K. (2011). On conceptualizing self-control as more than the effortful inhibition of impulses. *Personality and Social Psychology Review, 15*(4), 352–366.

Fujita, K., & Carnevale, J. J. (2012). Transcending temptation through abstraction: The role of construal level in self-control. *Current Directions in Psychological Science, 21*(4), 248–252.

Fujita, K., & Han, H. A. (2009). Moving beyond deliberative control of impulses: The effect of construal levels on evaluative associations in self-control conflicts. *Psychological Science, 20*(7), 799–804.

Fujita, K., Le, P. Q., Scholer, A. A., & Miele, D. B. (2024). The metamotivation approach: Insights into the regulation of motivation and beyond. *Social and Personality Psychology Compass, 18*(2), Article e12937.

Fujita, K., Scholer, A. A., & Miele, D. B. (2024). Metamotivation: The regulation of motivation in self-control. *Current Opinion in Psychology, 60*, Article 101883.

Fujita, K., Trope, Y., & Liberman, N. (2025). Understanding self-control as a problem of regulatory scope. *Psychological Review, 132*(1), 50–75.

Fujita, K., Trope, Y., Liberman, N., & Levin-Sagi, M. (2006). Construal levels and self-control. *Journal of Personality and Social Psychology, 90*(3), 351–367.

Gailliot, M. T., Baumeister, R. F., DeWall, C. N., Maner, J. K., Plant, E. A., Tice, D. M., et al. (2007). Self-control relies on glucose as a limited energy source: Willpower is more than a metaphor. *Journal of Personality and Social Psychology, 92*(2), 325–336.

Gilbert, K. M., & Elliot, A. J. (2024). Metamotivational task knowledge of performance-approach and performance-avoidance achievement goals. *Current Psychology, 43*(41), 32288–32302.

Gollwitzer, P. M. (1990). Action phases and mind-sets. In E. T. Higgins & R. M. Sorrentino (Eds.), *Handbook of motivation and cognition: Foundations of social behavior* (pp. 53–92). Guilford Press.

Hagger, M. S., Wood, C., Stiff, C., & Chatzisarantis, N. L. D. (2010). Ego depletion and the strength model of self-control: A meta-analysis. *Psychological Bulletin, 136*(4), 495–525.

Haidt, J., Rozin, P., McCauley, C., & Imada, S. (1997). Body, psyche, and culture: The relationship between disgust and morality. *Psychology and Developing Societies, 9*(1), 107–131.

Higgins, E. T. (1997). Beyond pleasure and pain. *American Psychologist, 52*(12), 1280–1300.

Higgins, E. T. (2000). Making a good decision: Value from fit. *American Psychologist, 55*(11), 1217–1230.

Higgins, E. T. (2005). Value from regulatory fit. *Current Directions in Psychological Science, 14*(4), 209–213.

Hofmann, W., Friese, M., & Strack, F. (2009). Impulse and self-control from a dual-systems perspective. *Perspectives on Psychological Science, 4*(2), 162–176.

Inzlicht, M., & Gutsell, J. N. (2007). Running on empty: Neural signals for self-control failure. *Psychological Science, 18*(11), 933–937.

Jansen, E. J., Miele, D. B., Fujita, K., & Scholer, A. A. (2022). Managing the motivation of others: Do managers recognize how to manage regulatory focus in subordinates? *Motivation Science, 8*(4), 330–345.

Kuratomi, K., Johnsen, L., Kitagami, S., Hatano, A., & Murayama, K. (2023). People underestimate their capability to motivate themselves without performance-based extrinsic incentives. *Motivation & Emotion, 47*(4), 509–523.

Liberman, N., & Trope, Y. (2008). The psychology of transcending the here and now. *Science, 322*(5905), 1201–1205.

MacGregor, K. E., Carnevale, J. J., Dusthimer, N. E., & Fujita, K. (2017). Knowledge of the self-control benefits of high-level versus low-level construal. *Journal of Personality and Social Psychology, 112*(4), 607–620.

Malkoc, S. A., Zauberman, G., & Bettman, J. R. (2010). Unstuck from the concrete: Carryover effects of abstract mindsets in intertemporal preferences. *Organizational Behavior and Human Decision Processes, 113*(2), 112–126.

Mann, T., de Ridder, D., & Fujita, K. (2013). Self-regulation of health behavior: Social psychological approaches to goal setting and goal striving. *Health Psychology, 32*(5), 487–498.

Miele, D. B., Fujita, K., & Scholer, A. A. (2024). The role of metamotivational knowledge in the regulation of motivation. *Motivation Science, 10*(3), 197–209.

Miele, D. B., & Scholer, A. A. (2018). The role of metamotivational monitoring in motivation regulation. *Educational Psychologist, 53*(1), 1–21.

Miele, D. B., Scholer, A. A., & Fujita, K. (2020). Metamotivation: Emerging research on the regulation of motivational states. In A. J. Elliot (Ed.), *Advances in Motivation Science* (Vol. 7, pp. 1–42). Elsevier.

Miller, G. A. (1956). The magical number seven, plus or minus two: Some limits on our capacity for processing information. *Psychological Review, 63*(2), 81–97.

Mischel, H. N., & Mischel, W. (1983). The development of children's knowledge of self-control strategies. *Child Development, 54*(3), 603–619.

Mischel, W., Shoda, Y., & Rodriguez, M. L. (1989). Delay of gratification in children. *Science, 244*(4907), 933–938.

Moran, T., Bornstein, O., & Eyal, T. (2021). The level of construal involved in the elicitation of core versus moral disgust. *Emotion, 21*(2), 391–404.

Moran, T., & Eyal, T. (2022). Emotion regulation by psychological distance and level of abstraction: Two meta-analyses. *Personality and Social Psychology Review, 26*(2), 112–159.

Murayama, K., Kitagami, S., Tanaka, A., & Raw, J. A. L. (2016). People's naiveté about how extrinsic rewards influence intrinsic motivation. *Motivation Science, 2*(3), 138–142.

Nelson, T. O., & Narens, L. (1990). Metamemory: A theoretical framework and new findings. In G. H. Bower (Ed.), *Psychology of learning and motivation* (pp. 125–173). Academic Press.

Nguyen, T., Carnevale, J. J., Scholer, A. A., Miele, D. B., & Fujita, K. (2019). Metamotivational knowledge of the role of high-level and low-level construal in goal-relevant task performance. *Journal of Personality and Social Psychology, 117*(5), 876–899.

Nguyen, T., Scholer, A. A., Miele, D. B., Edwards, M. C., & Fujita, K. (2023). Predicting academic performance with an assessment of students' knowledge of the benefits of high-level and low-level construal. *Social Psychological and Personality Science, 14*(2), 195–206.

Nguyen, T., Togawa, T., Scholer, A. A., & Fujita, K. (2020). A cross-cultural investigation of metamotivational knowledge of construal level in the United States and Japan. *Motivation Science, 6*(4), 386–400.

Reeves, S. L., Nguyen, T., Scholer, A. A., Fujita, K., & Spencer, S. J. (2023). Examining beliefs about the benefits of self-affirmation for mitigating self-threat. *Personality and Social Psychology Bulletin, 49*(11), 1615–1632.

Rodriguez, M. L., Mischel, W., & Shoda, Y. (1989). Cognitive person variables in the delay of gratification of older children at risk. *Journal of Personality and Social Psychology, 57*(2), 358–367.

Rozin, P., Haidt, J., & McCauley, C. R. (2008). Disgust. In M. Lewis, J. M. Haviland-Jones, & L. F. Barrett (Eds.), *Handbook of emotions* (3rd ed., pp. 757–776). Guilford Press.

Rudzinska-Wojciechowska, J. (2017). If you want to save, focus on the forest rather than on trees. The effects of shifts in levels of construal on saving decisions. *PLOS ONE, 12*(5), e0178283.

Saunders, B., Milyavskaya, M., Etz, A., Randles, D., & Inzlicht, M. (2018). Reported self-control is not meaningfully associated with inhibition-related executive function: A Bayesian analysis. *Collabra: Psychology, 4*(1), 39.

Schmeichel, B. J., Vohs, K. D., & Duke, S. C. (2011). Self-control at high and low levels of mental construal. *Social Psychological and Personality Science, 2*(2), 182–189.

Scholer, A. A., & Miele, D. B. (2016). The role of metamotivation in creating task-motivation fit. *Motivation Science, 2*(3), 171–197.

Scholer, A. A., Miele, D. B., Murayama, K., & Fujita, K. (2018). New directions in self-regulation: The role of metamotivational beliefs. *Current Directions in Psychological Science, 27*(6), 437–442.

Sherman, D. A. K., Nelson, L. D., & Steele, C. M. (2000). Do messages about health risks threaten the self? Increasing the acceptance of threatening health messages via self-affirmation. *Personality and Social Psychology Bulletin, 26*(9), 1046–1058.

Soderberg, C. K., Callahan, S. P., Kochersberger, A. O., Amit, E., & Ledgerwood, A. (2015). The effects of psychological distance on abstraction: Two meta-analyses. *Psychological Bulletin, 141*(3), 525–548.

Stillman, P. E., Medvedev, D., & Ferguson, M. J. (2017). Resisting temptation: Tracking how self-control conflicts are successfully resolved in real time. *Psychological Science, 28*(9), 1240–1258.

Teo, Q. K., Chen, P, Fujita, K., & Scholer, A. A. (2024). *Metamotivational knowledge of construal level predicts academic performance* [Manuscript submitted for publication].

Trope, Y., Ledgerwood, A., Liberman, N., & Fujita, K. (2021). Regulatory scope and its mental and social supports. *Perspectives on Psychological Science, 16*(2), 204–224.

Trope, Y., & Liberman, N. (2003). Temporal construal. *Psychological Review, 110*(3), 403–421.

Trope, Y., & Liberman, N. (2010). Construal-level theory of psychological distance. *Psychological Review, 117*(2), 440–463.

Trope, Y., & Neter, E. (1994). Reconciling competing motives in self-evaluation: The role of self-control in feedback seeking. *Journal of Personality and Social Psychology, 66*(4), 646–657.

Willems, Y. E., Boesen, N., Li, J., Finkenauer, C., & Bartels, M. (2019). The heritability of self-control: A meta-analysis. *Neuroscience & Biobehavioral Reviews, 100*, 324–334.

Woolley, K., & Fishbach, A. (2015). The experience matters more than you think: People value intrinsic incentives more inside than outside an activity. *Journal of Personality and Social Psychology, 109*(6), 968–982.

Yi, R., Stuppy-Sullivan, A., Pickover, A., & Landes, R. D. (2017). Impact of construal level manipulations on delay discounting. *PLOS ONE, 12*(5), e0177240.

Zimmerman, B. J., & Kitsantas, A. (1996). Self-regulated learning of a motoric skill: The role of goal setting and self-monitoring. *Journal of Applied Sport Psychology, 8*(1), 60–75.

Zimmerman, B. J., & Kitsantas, A. (1997). Developmental phases in self-regulation: Shifting from process goals to outcome goals. *Journal of Educational Psychology, 89*(1), 29–36

PART III

CREATING MEANING IN LIFE

CHAPTER 11

Changing Views of Implicit Cognition and Conscious Thinking

Melissa J. Ferguson and Ran R. Hassin

Meaning making is a process that begins with early perception, where a collection of conscious experiences are given a name—the sea, a beer, a pink elephant—and goes all the way up the hierarchy of high-level cognitive processing to narratives. In other words, meaning making entails the stories we tell ourselves about who we are, where we come from, what our norms and values are, and what it is that we aspire to (Trope, this volume). The dominant view has it that meaning making is an active and largely conscious process. It involves conscious thinking about the nature of our environment and ourselves in it. This chapter challenges this view.

This chapter is composed of two sections. The sections deal with general views on non-conscious processes and implicit cognition, on the one hand, and the complementary side of conscious thinking, on the other. Both sections challenge accepted views of the dual nature of the mind *vis-à-vis* what came to be known as two modes of operation (implicit vs. explicit, conscious vs. non-conscious, automatic vs. controlled, etc.; see Sherman, Gawronski, & Trope, 2014). For ease of communication, we will refer to those as *implicit* versus *explicit* cognition, although we fully acknowledge the richness of the dual-process approach and the variation in the models. While the two sections diverge in terms of methods and style, and although they focus on different mental capacities, together they make a strong argument: The division of labor is not what it seems to be.

Both sections develop new ideas regarding the characteristics of these processes, and the division of labor between them. We do all that from a unique angle that has rarely been considered in these areas of our science, that of meaning making. We ponder what these ideas imply for meaning making in various aspects of life: The first section examines meaning making via difficult decisions. The second does this by challenging the accepted view of the functions and capabilities of implicit social cognition.

MEANING MAKING, CONSCIOUSNESS, AND TRANSFORMATIONAL DECISIONS

The Nature of Conscious Thinking

Imagine sitting on the beach, beer in hand, letting your mind wander as you wait for your friend. You watch some dogs joyfully play with their human companions, small children build sandcastles with their parents, and even young lovers on a stroll. The water is perfectly blue, if a tad too warm, as you discovered a few minutes ago. Glimpses of memories come and go: a conversation you had with a friend while driving yesterday; a painting you saw in a gallery last month; the bizarre guy who offered you a shot of tequila at a jazz show last week; the call from your child this morning complaining about the public transportation in their college town. You take another sip from your beer and lean back, waiting for sunset to begin.

What is it that we want in life? What is crucially important, so much so that it cannot be compromised? What comes next? Episodes like this beach afternoon help us figure out our lives, navigate them, and form narratives that define who we are.

The view we discuss in this section of the chapter is based on a view developed by two young social psychologists—Asael Sklar, a professor at Reichman University, and Rasha Kardosh, a professor at Hebrew University. Together, they developed an approach to consciousness that takes seriously core insights of social cognition, while proposing a view that is both trivial and completely new. They call this view the *minimalist approach* (Sklar, Kardosh, & Hassin, 2021).

The minimalist approach can be about our place in life (how did we get here?), a meaningful decision we make (should I have intervened later, or maybe earlier?), or our goals for the future (what is it that I want to achieve?). Although some thoughts are conscious, the work of structuring that stream of consciousness tends not to be conscious. In fact, our argument is that the work of building the stream of consciousness, of weaving thoughts, is *never* conscious, because no cognitive process is. Some contents are conscious, yet processes are not. Because thinking is inherent to meaning making, if one wants to understand meaning making, one must turn their attention to non-conscious mechanisms that shape our thinking.

To illustrate our central argument, here's a case described by one of the founders of cognitive science, Endel Tulving. Tulving (1985, p. 4) described a conversation with patient N. N., who had difficulties with memory and the ability to imagine the future.

> E. T.: "Let's try the question again about the future. What will you be doing tomorrow?"
>
> (*There is a 15-second pause.*)
>
> N. N.: Smiles faintly, then says, "I don't know."
>
> E. T.: "Do you remember the question?"
>
> N. N.: "About what I'll be doing tomorrow?"
>
> E. T.: "Yes. How would you describe your state of mind when you try to think about it?"
>
> (*A 5-second pause.*)
>
> N. N.: "Blank, I guess."

Tulving uses this conversation as an example of deficits in autonoetic consciousness—conscious episodes that involve the self. At a more general level, though, this discussion illustrates a problem we know all too well: when words, sentences, or answers refuse to come to mind. This problem highlights a key component—in fact, the central component—of our argument in this part of the chapter. The argument is simple, and on the face of it, it seems true—although we know thoughts and emotions are happening in our heads, as it were, we don't know, or know very little, about how to will them into being. They simply appear.

Meaningful Decisions

Before we go on to discuss conscious experiences in meaning making, we want to take a moment to think about meaningful decisions. Meaningful decisions are important to meaning making in at least two very different ways. One, they may lead to big changes in life courses, and hence in the meaning we ascribe to our lives. And two, one of these changes may involve how we think about, and create, meaning. (Admittedly, there is a bonus goal here: We want to bring a largely philosophical discussion into the realm of social cognitive psychology.)

Decisions, especially difficult ones, have the potential to change life narratives, and move us from one path to another. This is especially true for the kind of decisions that philosopher Edna Ullmann-Margalit (2006) called *opting* (see also Paul, 2014). Opting is a unique subset of very difficult decisions, because these decisions will lead to changes in core aspects of who we are. In other words, in opting, the decision is likely to change one's norms, goals, habits, and view of life. The person who makes the decision is not exactly the person who will live to experience its consequences.

Assume that something big happened: You were offered a new job in a new state; you consider having your first child; a loved one is very sick and can no longer be on their own. And now you need to make a decision: Are you taking the new job and moving, or are you sticking with the job you already have and like? Are you upending life as you know it to have a child, or not? Are you going to become a caregiver for your loved one, or not?

We all intimately know opting situations, and it is easy to recognize that they have the potential to change who we are. They are decisions that have the potential to create a "sharp discontinuity" between Present Me and Future Me. Ullman-Margalit (2006) stresses that opting cases are decisions that are irrevocable; they are points of no return. "When one opts, one is embarking upon a road that is one way only, leaving burning bridges behind" (p. 159).

Decision theories suggest that when we make decisions, we should weigh the (subjective) value of costs against those of benefits, but in opting we simply can't do it well enough, argues Ullmann-Margalit (2006). Given that Future Me will enjoy different things, have different goals, and value different norms, and given that Present Me doesn't know what these will be, Present Me cannot appreciate the meaning of the decision for Future Me.

Note the chasm that separates regular, even "heavy," decisions, and opting. In the former, one can, in principle, compute the subjective value of a decision. In decisions under uncertainty, the risk is implicit in the decision itself. The subjective value of option A is S1, that of option B is S2, and a mean, or some other function, gives us the decision's subjective value. But if Present Me does not know Future Me's values, norms, and goals, or what makes Future Me happy or sad, how can one compute subjective value? We all want to make well-reasoned decisions, but without so much as an inkling about the subjective values of benefits and costs for our future selves, we simply can't. Hence, Present Me cannot make a rational choice, and we, as observers, cannot estimate how rational one's decision is, argues Ullmann-Margalit (2006).

If we cannot consider rationality, then, how does thinking about these core, seminal issues evolve? How are thoughts formed when one is opting?

Thinking in Decisions

Let's pretend we believe that a choice is determined by a set of conscious arguments and feelings that we shall denote AF_{1-n}. (We have learned enough in cognitive and social psychology to know that there is no list, and that the quasi-list is really a hodge-podge. It may include information we deem relevant, hunches, emotions, and feelings such as fluency. But let's put that mess aside for a moment because it is not the focus of our argument here.) Think about a case of opting that happened to you, and think about your AF_{1-n}.

To develop the minimalist approach, Sklar et al. (2021) introduced what they called *microanalysis*, an analytic thinking tool in which one zooms in on a desired process, moves to slo-mo mode, and closely follows the developments. In the following paragraphs, we will illustrate microanalysis and its working parts.

So, how did you come up with the set AF_{1-n}? Think of the first argument that came to mind. Now, employ microanalysis, zoom in, and move slowly with time. How did you move from the last moment in time in which the argument did not consciously occur to you yet, to the first moment it did? What happened in this minimal temporal interval? One option, that we raise here, if only to reject, is that the list of arguments is nothing but a random selection from the words or thoughts that happened to cross your non-conscious mind. This option is off for many reasons, but it is sufficient to note that we understand enough about memory to know that this is not how it works. Moreover, the list, as it occurred to you, does not appear to be completely random. After all, arguments and feelings are usually somehow related to the question at hand.

The next option is that when we begin the thought process, various relevant (proto-) arguments become non-consciously available and accessible, and these become prioritized for conscious awareness. This option makes more sense, because the thoughts that you will end up thinking will be relevant to the topic at hand. Still, this option assumes that the arguments are stored in memory. Although this is likely to be true for daily decisions we make, such as what to eat for dinner, it is less likely for new decisions, or for opting decisions (at least when we begin the process).

The last option is that no arguments have been stored in memory, and no process of prioritization occurs. Rather, our minds develop and construct them on the fly, as we sit there on the beach to think. Note, that although conscious prompts and an intention to consider might be crucial to the process, this option assumes that the work of developing arguments is done non-consciously.

Taken together, the options we just surveyed suggest a simple conclusion. Either the work of choosing arguments and prioritizing them is done non-consciously, or the work of developing them is done this way. So, although consciousness seems to be accompanying the the process, it doesn't seem to have a big role in these core aspects of "thinking while opting."

The conclusion that consciousness doesn't contribute much to the development of thoughts still leaves it with a potentially very significant role in decision making: translating the thoughts into a decision by integrating the arguments. One of the most prominent theories of consciousness argues, indeed, that consciousness is the integration of information (Tononi & Koch, 2015).

But this move to rescue consciousness would not work much better. To see why this is the case, assume that the evaluations of each of the conscious arguments and feelings use one metric (e.g., they have a common currency), that we consciously compute a set of weights, (W_{i-n}), and that we can consciously use these weights to weigh the arguments and make a choice.

And now let's use microanalysis to examine how weights come to mind. The same procedure we applied to the arguments can now be applied to the weights. Are they randomly retrieved from memory? One would hope that this is not the case, because then our decisions would be random. Are they chosen from a set of good-enough values? If so, this means that the work of computing these values and evaluating them is achieved non-consciously. Are all of them computed non-consciously and then just become conscious?

You get the point. The analytic process we introduced earlier, microanalysis, can be applied regressively and *ad infinitum*. At the end of the process, microanalysis will get you to a point where contents become conscious because of the non-conscious processes that preceded them. But if we get there after a few rounds, then maybe, as Dennett recommended, we do not need all of them. Maybe we can stop after the first round and seriously consider the implication—that cognitive processes are always non-conscious, and that the transition from one thought to another, also known as *thinking*, is done by non-conscious processes. The thoughts themselves may indeed become conscious.

This analysis leaves open the idea that conscious intention and attention are needed as triggers for thinking. The activation of intention and attention (e.g., "Why don't I go grab a cup of coffee and think about this problem that bothers me?") can itself be traced via microanalysis to a non-conscious source. Yet, it might well be the case that without conscious commitment, the process is less likely to take place.

Thinking in Meaningful Decisions

As the rich and wonderful contributions in this volume illustrate, meaning making is a multifactor, multilayered, process (e.g., Trope, this volume). It begins as early as perception does, and it ends with the narratives we tell ourselves about our lives. This section of the chapter is somewhat in the middle. We are interested in meaning making through opting. When we opt, we get to decide on a change from Current Me to Future Me, knowing that if we opt, we change course. Future Me will be different from Current Me; values will not be identical, priorities will shift, emotions, and emotional reactions, will be altered, and relationships with others will change. To extend the logic of Ullmann-Margalit (2006), opting is not only a case in which you decide on your future self; it is also a case in which you decide on many other futures—you will be different, and hence your (social) environment will have to be different.

Extreme examples often serve as wonderful illustrations, but they may come at the cost of generalization. There may be something unique about a specific example that is not true in the general case. Nevertheless, let's imagine what might be a really difficult decision: getting divorced.

Not all decisions to divorce are difficult. Some are, or at least should be, easy. But some are really difficult. Perhaps you have been living with your spouse for three decades. You have known them since high school. You have kids, and you are a very close-knit nuclear family. You spend a lot of time together. Your families are meshed. You share the same friends. And more importantly, you still think warm thoughts of them: They are smart and funny, and a great parent. They understand you better than anyone. All things considered, they are a wonderful human being.

But, as sometimes happens in life, things don't work for you guys. You have grown apart. Spending time together is not as fun as it used to be, you find each other less amusing, and your attention tends to switch out. You are less curious about each other. Routine has taken hold, and you are bothered by the predictability of it all. You might sometimes think the idea of spending the rest of your life together sounds warm and safe, and is the right thing to do. But it is not exciting, it does not open new challenges, new avenues to renew yourself; and it is not something you look forward to.

Perhaps you have been in this situation, or a dear friend has. Perhaps you've only seen this in a movie or read it in a book; in a most mundane occurrence, a wonderful relationship has simply run its course.

Deciding to quit, to begin a new life, is definitely a case of opting. Your life as you know it will be in upheaval, and many others in your life will be affected. And although formally the decision can be undone, it cannot, really. Even if you two end up getting back together, it won't be getting back to what you had.

So, how does thinking go in this kind of situation? Assume, for example, that you find yourself thinking, *Shall I leave?* And then the next thought that occurs to you is, *Let's imagine how daily life will look*, followed by a *gloomy image of you sitting at the breakfast table all by yourself*, and a thought about *how wonderful it could have been to talk to your spouse right now.* This chain of visualizations/thoughts is what we usually call *thinking.* And we usually think of thinking as a conscious act. But if we use microanalysis, if we zoom in and move slowly, we can see that the transition from one thought to another, from an image to words, is not something we consciously do, it is something that our non-conscious processes do for us.

But imagine a different stream of thoughts. You find yourself thinking, *Shall I leave?* And the next thought that occurs to you is of you *enjoying yourself and a drink on the balcony of a small house on a nearby pond.* This image is followed by the verbal thought, *But what about the kids?* This thought is immediately followed by the thought, *They are adults. They have their own families. They'll be all right.*

It is easy to imagine that this train of thought is more likely to increase the likelihood of leaving than the one that just preceded it. And again, microanalysis shows that although you consciously experienced the visuals and thoughts, chaining them is not something you consciously did, it is something that your non-conscious processes did for you.

Now let's push this example a little more. Say that at some point, you tell yourself, *I have to get control of my thoughts, and think about the things that do not easily come to mind.* You decide to search for them. This is definitely a case where the Conscious You takes control of the process and changes its course.

Or is it? How did the thought that you should think other thoughts come to you?

Oh, you say, *you are right, the thought just appeared there in my consciousness, but I consciously weighed the pros and cons and decided to go with it.*

Perhaps, but the minimalist approach asks: How did you come up with the weights?

And this can go on, *ad infinitum*, or at least until we decide to stop.

So, Where Does This All Leave Us?

So, where does all this leave us? The work of weaving thoughts, which is just a fancy way to talk about thinking, is done by our non-conscious processes, not by consciousness. Conscious thinking, we argue, is a misnomer: What we call *conscious thinking* is indeed a conscious experience, but it is composed of conscious contents and non-conscious processes that move us between one thought and another (Sklar, Kardosh, & Hassin, 2021).

In a seminal article that appeared in *Psychological Review*, David Navon (1984) argued that the notion of "resources" is somewhat circular and not very useful. Yet, after having made this strong and convincing argument, Navon goes on to say that he knows that he, and others, will continue to use the notion of resources "out of linguistic preference" (p. 232).

We believe the same is true for the misnomer *conscious thinking* because it reflects the deep intuition we all share that thinking is a conscious process. We suspect that we, and all of you, will still continue to use it, but we hope that the current discussion will add a mental asterisk.

The implications for meaning making are straightforward, and we believe they are more promising than merely adding a mental asterisk. To understand meaning making in general, and meaning making via opting more specifically, we must examine how and why mental content becomes conscious—how information is processed, prepared, and prioritized for conscious experience. How does the invisible needle that threads conscious thought truly function?

Luckily, we do not have to start from scratch. Many areas of social cognition have already done so by studying accessibility, availability, and high-level priming (Barnes, 2017). Similarly, many areas of cognitive science have explored the role of associations and other forms of priming. In other domains in life, practitioners of meditation also focus on observing how thoughts and ideas arise, highlighting points that align with our discussion: that thoughts are not consciously created but rather consciously experienced.

The next section of this chapter brings together tools and insights from across these areas, and harnesses them to develop new research that will enhance our understanding of the broader issue of meaning making.

HOW CAN DUMB ASSOCIATIVE THINKING ENABLE MEANING MAKING?

At first (or even second) glance, the possibility posed by the first section of this chapter—that non-conscious processes prompt, integrate, and assemble all the constituents of cognition that enable meaning making—seems remote. After all, the traditional view of implicit or automatic cognition, including non-conscious thought, is that it consists of fast but seemingly "dumb" associative thinking (e.g., Cao & Banaji,

2016; Cunningham, Zelazo, Packer, & Van Bavel, 2007; Gawronski & Bodenhausen, 2006; Gregg, Seibt, & Banaji, 2006; Rydell & McConnell, 2006; Smith & DeCoster, 2000; Strack & Deutsch, 2004; Wilson, Lindsey, & Schooler, 2000), in some cases barely capable of figuring out the semantic meaning of two words at once (e.g., "green bread"; Greenwald, 1992; cf. Hassin, 2013; Hassin & Sklar, 2014). In this section, we zoom out and consider arguments and frameworks for the implicit mind beyond solely non-conscious processes. In doing so, we raise the possibility that a broader array of implicit processes—beyond non-conscious ones—is likely involved in meaning making. We review the traditional (and in many corners, still currently held) accounts of the implicit mind, and then we briefly review recent findings that challenge this view. We argue that these new findings lend weight to the ideas in the first section. We end with identifying limitations and the need for continued theoretical development and measure refinement.

However, before we get there, we must detour into some brief history and commentary on the term *implicit*. We begin by addressing some definitional issues. You may be wondering how we use terms such as the *implicit mind*. In line with prior conceptualizations (De Houwer, Teige-Mocigemba, Spruyt, & Moors, 2009; Gawronski, De Houwer, & Sherman, 2020; Moors, 2013, 2016), we define the implicit mind as the set of cognitive processes and content that is captured by indirect measures with certain processing constraints, and is thus assumed to operate relatively more automatically than the processes and content captured by direct measures such as the self-report, with its much looser processing constraints. In turn, the *explicit mind* reflects all the content that appears on direct measures, and all the processes that are assumed to require or be described as relatively slower, more intentional, more controllable, and/or more conscious than whatever is captured by indirect measures.

There are important theoretical debates still ongoing about what aspects of automaticity matter for which processes and phenomena, as well as about how and whether indirect and direct measures successfully capture the relatively independent dimensions of consciousness, intentionality, efficiency, controllability, and speed (e.g., Corneille & Hütter, 2020; Gawronski, 2009; Gawronski et al., 2020; Moors, 2013). At the end of this chapter, we return to the current theoretical and methodological landscape.

Putting aside the conceptual messiness inherent in the dichotomy of the implicit versus explicit mind (Bargh, 1994; Melnikoff & Bargh, 2018), we nevertheless use this binary in this section mostly as a rhetorical device to make clear that many types of reasoning, attribution, and evaluation (of life events, surprises, etc.) previously assumed to be exclusively "explicit" in meaning making can actually show up on indirect measures, suggesting that assumptions about meaning making residing primarily or solely in the explicit mind are likely wrong.

Beyond definitional issues, it is worth noting that we are in a new era of scientific debate about what exists in the mind *other* than what people report feeling, thinking, doing, and knowing (i.e., on self-reports). Throughout the 1970s, 1980s, and 1990s, researchers documented various ways to measure human cognition indirectly (without asking them). This happened via priming paradigms, implicit learning, subliminal perception, lexical decision tasks, Stroop tasks, and so forth. This ushered in an explosion of research throughout the last decade of the 1900s and the first decade of the 2000s on the many ways in which social cognition operates outside of conscious guidance and knowledge and contributes to our daily experiences (e.g., see Hassin, Uleman, & Bargh, 2005).

Then two major things happened. First, the replication crisis in psychology began and cast doubt on what we thought we knew about the implicit mind (e.g., see Gelman, 2015; Ioannidis, 2005; Nosek et al., 2022). The failures to replicate well-established lines of implicit mind research meant that lots of assumptions had to be rethought, reconsidered, and retested (e.g., see Cesario, 2014; Sherman & Rivers, 2020). This ushered in considerable skepticism about the methods, measures, and theoretical claims used to study the implicit mind. Today, there exists extensive and lively (and sometimes deeply critical) debate about the nature of the implicit mind, including its conceptualization, measurement, and value (e.g., Corneille & Hütter, 2020; Gawronski et al., 2020). We consider this an exciting, ongoing conversation, and we view recent findings on implicit cognition as compelling for addressing these issues. Although outside the purview of this chapter, in the final section, we try to address how our account is related to these ongoing debates.

Second, alongside this wave of skepticism and replication, the findings from research using best practices have *continued to proliferate* and have shed considerable light on the nature of the implicit mind—what it is, what it is not, what it can do, and what questions remain. These findings—conducted with stronger and better practices, transparency, and replicability—contribute directly to our current view of the implicit mind. In this section, we try to summarize some of these new findings and argue on the basis of these results that the implicit mind is integral to making meaning out of our lives and experiences.

The Fast-but-Dumb Implicit Mind

Many of the theories of mind that were dominant in the 1990s and early 2000s consisted of dual-mode approaches. These theories continue to be extremely generative and are reviewed elsewhere (e.g., Chaiken & Trope, 1999; Sherman et al., 2014), but the main tenets are that the mind can be roughly decomposed into two kinds of systems, processes, and/or types of representations. One mode is characterized as relatively automatic, with some combination of the features of efficiency, non-consciousness, uncontrollability, and unintentionality (e.g., De Houwer et al., 2009; Moors, 2013, 2016). The other is characterized as relatively more controlled, existing on opposite ends of the continua of those processing features. Beyond these features of how a process might unfold (e.g., its efficiency, its consciousness), there are also assumptions about the actual *processing* in terms of how information is combined, integrated, and transformed (e.g., see Moors, 2013, 2016; Sherman, 2006). In terms of processes, many theories (in social cognition) advocated that the main process in the implicit mind is associative, which means that it operates on the basis of simple associations or connections between stimuli based exclusively or mostly on temporal or spatial contiguity (e.g., see Bouton, 2016; Domjan, 2010; Hebb, 1949; Smith & DeCoster, 2000).

What can the implicit mind accomplish from the perspective of these dual-mode theories? It can do a lot. Because of its speed, efficiency, and spontaneity, it is assumed to help populate all perception and cognition and to work mostly seamlessly with the explicit mind (e.g., Kahneman, 2011; Sloman, 1996; Smith & DeCoster, 2000). Nothing that the explicit mind accomplishes can be done without the implicit mind, and in many ways, it is an ill-posed problem to assume that they are separate. For the purposes of this chapter, however, we emphasize that dual-mode theories assume they should be separated, and that the implicit mind is integral to basic functioning.

But the implicit mind is also considered to be severely limited. From the dual-mode perspective, there are two major weaknesses that would seem to render it incapable of contributing to meaning making. We consider what we call the "old bias" and the "simple bias." What are these claims?

Old Bias. First, many theories have argued that the implicit (vs. explicit) mind is harder to change and stuck in initial learning, even when new information is perceived to be persuasive (Cao & Banaji, 2016; Gawronski & Bodenhausen, 2006; Gregg et al., 2006; Petty et al., 2006; Rydell & McConnell, 2006; Smith & DeCoster, 2000; Strack & Deutsch, 2004; Wilson et al., 2000). This suggests a learning bias in which older information is weighted (considerably) more heavily than new. How might a learning bias of this sort affect meaning making? Given that meaning making is often prompted by the attempt to reconcile new experiences with expectations (based on priors), we might assume that the implicit mind would be ill-suited for such reconciliation.

The old-school claims were that this kind of integration was only possible when people had the cognitive resources, time, intentionality, awareness, and control to do so (see also Oizumi, Tsuchiya, & Amari, 2016; Tononi, Boly, Massimini, & Koch, 2016). Thus, when people are faced with new and surprising events, facts, or experiences (that might prompt meaning making), these dual-mode accounts (and some accounts of consciousness) would assume that the explicit mind must be the first part of the mind to grapple with them. In time, and with much practice navigating the new reality, the implicit mind will eventually catch up, fumbling and bumbling along in the rear-view mirror, dragging our past self to its new version. By this view, the explicit mind is the "first responder" to unexpected events and experiences.

For example, research on person perception and impression formation showed that when learning counterattitudinal information about a group, people were able to explicitly incorporate that information and adjust their feelings accordingly. After finding out that the group that seemed to be helpful and kind had actually acted in extremely immoral ways, participants markedly shifted their reported attitudes. Implicitly, however, people in these studies seemed to be stuck in the initial information, unable to integrate the newer information, and thereby missing what seemed to be critical corrective information about others (e.g., Gregg et al., 2006; McConnell, Rydell, Strain, & Mackie, 2008).

From this traditional view, the implicit mind might be viewed as simply constituting the mental scaffolding along which our conscious minds recruit bits and pieces and then forge them together effortfully and consciously into meaning and narrative. In this way, the implicit mind is assumed to serve in a supporting role, providing the contents that the conscious mind integrates in order to make sense of our lives and worlds. Not only does the implicit mind pass along bits and pieces of past learning and memory, but it does so unscrupulously, leaving the explicit (and, purportedly, conscious) mind to forge a narrative of meaning that makes sense and aligns with reality.

For the person who experiences a life-changing event, and needs to make sense of it, the implicit mind is a drag, whereas the explicit mind is actively and often flexibly grappling with all the ways in which the new information and choices—including opting—might affect the person's sense of self, identity, and life circumstances. From the dual-mode account, then, the activity underlying meaning making is predominantly driven by the explicit mind.

Simple Bias. The second major limitation of the implicit mind according to dual-mode theories is that it has been assumed to be unable to process or represent relational information (e.g., Gawronski & Bodenhausen, 2006; Gendler, 2008; Lieberman, Gaunt, Gilbert, & Trope,

2002; Rydell & McConnell, 2006; Smith & DeCoster, 2000; Strack & Deutsch, 2004; see also Cao & Banaji, 2016). This means, for example, that implicit impressions are insensitive to the truth value of information (e.g., Deutsch, Gawronski, & Strack, 2006; Hu, Gawronski, & Balas, 2017; Moran & Bar-Anan, 2013). More specifically, when these implicit impressions are being formed, they can be sensitive to the truth value of the evidence (Moran, Bar-Anan, & Nosek, 2017; Smith, De Houwer, & Nosek, 2013), but they are less so after they have been formed (Gregg et al., 2006). As one example, some work showed that participants' implicit attitudes toward novel targets were insensitive to the truth value of the information and reacted the same way to information that had been characterized as false versus true (Peters & Gawronski, 2011). People's explicit attitudes toward the targets, however, flipped in valence when they were told that the information they had learned was in fact false.

Why would this dissociation happen? Why would implicit reactions (impressions, attitudes, etc.) be insensitive to the nature of new information and its relation to old information (whether it is truth value, causality, or negation)? The primary explanation has been that associative processes are assumed to underlie the implicit impressions and are assumed to be incapable of reflecting causal and propositional information. For example, some early work showed that implicit attitudes were insensitive to whether a target individual was responsible for an aversive event or happened to be merely spatially and temporally contiguous to an aversive event (see Kurdi, Morehouse, & Dunham [2023] for a review). Other work showed that implicit attitudes did not seem to reflect the attribution of events, such as negative acts. This work suggests that associative processes—and thus, *ex hypothesi*, the implicit mind—are incapable of building a story that has logical and causal structure and is sensitive to the kinds of information needed to form a meaningful narrative.

Other work suggested that people would be implicitly affected by information that they explicitly said they did not believe, suggesting that the implicit mind is unable to adjudicate between truth and falsity, suggesting that it contributes to a delusional view of reality. As an example, when we tell you that vaccines do not cause autism, your associative processes would in fact strengthen the link between autism and vaccines, and it is only your propositional (and conscious, controlled, intentional, and resource-heavy) processes that would be able to incorporate the negation. If we asked you what we just said, you would be able to tell us, but if we gave you an Implicit Association Test (IAT), you might show enhanced associative strength between vaccines and autism (Gawronski, Brannon, & Ng, 2022).

How is the simple bias an issue for meaning making? A central theme of meaning making is that people attempt to align the world around them with prior knowledge—in essence, reality testing and tuning. The old-school view is that the implicit mind is not capable of contributing to this kind of mental work. The implicit mind cannot possibly help (much less lead) the weaving together of stories about the self, about our lives, in a logical, coherent manner that would provide guidance for decisions such as opting.

This view of the implicit mind involves extensive theorizing, and the theories that fall under the rubric of dual mode have lots of differences. But, in their adoption of dual modes and their characterization of the implicit mode, they are similar in that their view of the implicit mind is one that contributes to meaning in a largely elemental, piecemeal fashion. This is not a trivial task—after all, the implicit mind allows for the lightning-fast recognition of the numerous objects, words, images, sights, and sounds all around us that constitute the colorful background of our conscious experience. However, it is not the driver of *making sense* of this fabric. None of these theories would claim that people would be able to spin a meaningful tale of their lives using only the implicit mind. They assume that the explicit mind (System 2), using conscious deliberative processing, is needed for making meaning. Most theories assume that the explicit mind uses propositional processes alongside associative processing (or input). From this view, only propositional processing is able to assess validity and truth information, causal reasoning, and logical analysis, and it is assumed to underlie all forms of higher-order thinking and reasoning.

The Fast-and-Smart Implicit Mind

The old bias and the simple bias would render the implicit mind remarkably ill-suited to contribute to meaning making. However, newer work casts doubt on these claims. We briefly review some of these findings here, but they are reviewed extensively elsewhere (e.g., see Ferguson, Mann, Cone, & Shen, 2019; Kurdi & Charlesworth, 2023). There are multiple reasons why older work suggested conclusions that do not align with newer work, and we discuss these potential reasons in each of the following sections.

Old Bias Revisited

Recent findings provide a new interpretation of the former dissociations in impression updating that have been used as evidence for the old bias (for reviews, see Ferguson et al., 2019; Kurdi & Charlesworth, 2023). This new work shows that when new evidence about a person is seen as diagnostic of the person (or group, or nonhuman agent; Surdel et al., 2024), people quickly update both their explicit and implicit impressions—and in ways that appear to be somewhat durable. For example, after participants had formed an initial impression of a novel target person based on extensive learning, they learned one additional piece of information that was counterattitudinal (vs. consistent). Those who had learned about the single new piece of counterevidence reversed both their implicit and explicit attitudes about the person (e.g., Brannon & Gawronski, 2017; Cone & Ferguson, 2015; De Houwer, 2014; Mann, Kurdi, & Banaji, 2020; Mann & Ferguson, 2015, 2017; Mann, Cone, Heggeseth, & Ferguson, 2019; Shen, Mann, & Ferguson, 2020; Shen & Ferguson, 2021; Van Dessel, Ye, & De Houwer, 2019; Wyer, 2016).

This reversal of implicit impressions can also happen with known targets (Van Dessel et al., 2019). For example, although most participants held a positive implicit and explicit impression of Gandhi, after they learned new negative information about how he treated his wife (i.e., withholding lifesaving medication for her, but later taking it himself), they flipped their impressions to negative. As another example, in one study, although most participants initially showed negative impressions of a big-game hunter, they significantly revised their implicit and explicit impressions of the hunter after listening to a *RadioLab* podcast excerpt about how the big-game hunter might cause some good things to happen (Kurdi, Mann, & Ferguson, 2022).

These findings show that the implicit mind can change easily—and possibly efficiently and durably (see Cone, Flaharty, & Ferguson, 2021; Shen & Ferguson, 2021)—at least when it comes to surprises that are seen as signaling something predictive about the target. In other words, when new surprising information about a person is interpreted as relatively informative about how that person is likely to act in future scenarios (e.g., the cause is seen as dispositional rather than situational), implicit impressions are quickly modified.

Why do these new findings not align with the older findings? The newer work suggests an alternative interpretation for why the older work found dissociations between implicit and explicit impressions. Namely, implicit impressions were not updated easily because the new evidence presented to them was actually quite weak in terms of evidence strength. It just so happened that in many of those studies that showed a dissociation, the new counterattitudinal information was on average not that believable or diagnostic. Beyond the discovery that implicit impressions will change easily in response to strong new (surprising) evidence, in line with classic work on persuasion (e.g., Albarracín & Johnson, 2019; Briñol & Petty, 2012), the real question is why explicit impressions seemed to change regardless of evidence strength. (That question is beyond this chapter, although see Ferguson, Mann, Cone, & Shen [2025].)

What do these newer findings imply for the role of the implicit mind in meaning making? They suggest that when people are grappling with a turn of events that is unprecedented, and serious (the events are not just surprising but seen as important, consequential, and diagnostic), the implicit mind will adjust and can reflect these quick turns of events, and the altered feelings, beliefs, and identities that come along with such changes. Given the argument in the first section, these findings suggest that the implicit mind (and possibly including non-conscious processes, although see the Limitations and Next Steps section later in the chapter) may be quite capable of flexibly adjusting in light of the new facts on the ground. Far from being a drag that cannot adjust to new realities, these findings in person perception and impression updating are aligned with the idea that implicit processes are the driver behind making sense of surprises and finding the meaning in them, so long as those changes are seen as reliable, accurate, and reflective of likely future outcomes.

Simple Bias Revisited

There is now considerable evidence that the implicit mind can reflect relational information between stimuli (for reviews, see Kurdi & Dunham, 2020; Kurdi et al., 2023). This includes causal attributions. For example, in a study by Cone and Ferguson (2015), after participants developed a positive impression of a target person, they learned a single piece of extremely negative information. However, that information was either about him (the target was responsible for the horrible behavior) or was mentioned in the same sentence as another person who was responsible for the behavior (a coach at the target's old high school). According to the traditional view of dumb associative processes, the temporal and spatial contiguity of the extremely negative information should get attached to the target even in the case in which he was not responsible. However, this did not happen. Only those who learned that he was causally responsible for the negative information changed their implicit impressions to negative, and those in the coach condition did not budge. This shows sensitivity to causal attribution.

There are multiple other lines of work showing that implicit impressions reflect causal relations. For example, Kurdi, Morris, and Cushman (2022) and Kurdi, Krosch, and Ferguson (2020) showed that people's implicit impressions were sensitive to the causal nature of a connection between two stimuli. People showed sensitivity to the difference between an actor's bad intentions regarding an action versus simply the negative outcome (Kurdi et al., 2020), suggesting that people did differentiate (in terms of their implicit attitudes) toward an actor who accidentally caused a bad outcome versus intentionally caused it. Another article showed that people's implicit attitudes were sensitive to whether one stimulus caused a bad outcome versus simply being simultaneously present with a bad outcome (Kurdi et al., 2022). Using a learning paradigm where participants learned about how different stimuli (geometric shapes) would affect a machine and its output of a reward, participants did show more positive impressions of the stimuli that were seen as causing the reward versus just co-occurring with it. Interestingly, there were some limitations in people's implicit impressions being able to reflect causal analysis that required consolidation of past experiences. For instance, in one of the experiments, the authors tested whether participants' implicit attitudes would reflect a reevaluation of the causal status of a given stimulus after learning distal information about its relationships with other stimuli, and they found that they did not.

This sensitivity to the nature of relations between stimuli extends to truth detection. When people learned that two fictional groups had changed the nature of their moral character (with one becoming violent over time and the other becoming more virtuous over time), only those who *believed* that the groups could actually change their moral fiber in this way (i.e., thought it was a possibility) showed updating of their implicit impressions (Cone, Flaharty, & Ferguson, 2019). This means that the believability of the new information matters. In other work, when new information was presented as reliable, versus as gossip, people's implicit impressions updated significantly more in response to the reliable versus gossipy information (see also Shen et al., 2020).

Why the disconnect between older work and these newer findings? There are many reasons, including differences in stimuli (strength, type), designs, and measures across the different bodies of research. And, there are still many questions to test about the relational sensitivity of the implicit mind—these newer findings constitute an emerging (but not complete) proof of concept that assumptions about the simple bias of the implicit mind are not true. Additional research will need to figure out exactly how the implicit and explicit minds are different or similar in their capacities for relational, logical, and causal thinking. These new findings that challenge the simple bias also help to explain the puzzle of why older research suggested that the implicit mind is inescapably stuck in former experiences and knowledge. Without the capacity to assess truth value or causal connections, it made no sense why the implicit mind did not seem responsive to counterattitudinal information (and explicit responses did). The answer was that that new information was weak in evidence strength and was assessed as not relevant.

How do these findings address meaning making? Any narrative needs structure and coherence, so the previously assumed simple bias of the implicit mind meant that such processes were precluded. These new findings open the door to the possibility that as we connect events, time, people, and places, building narratives and meaning replete with relational structure, the implicit mind has the capacity to undergird such cognition. The $64,000 question is to what extent the implicit mind needs certain features or processes that are traditionally considered to be part of the explicit mind in order to do this work.

Limitations and Next Steps

The purpose of this section is to highlight how our broad understanding of the implicit mind has changed considerably over the last 10 years, in particular with regard to what we term the *old bias* and the *simple bias*. This shift is relevant to the argument offered in the first section: that meaning making is driven by non-conscious processes. The new view of the implicit mind is more aligned with the argument that non-conscious processes can selectively connect bits of information in sophisticated ways, flexibly integrating past knowledge and experiences with surprising new ones. However, we make these claims in the relatively short space of this chapter, so we cannot give appropriate attention to many limitations and needed next steps. We nod at some of these before we close.

Theory. Recent findings like the ones we reviewed here challenge former dual-mode theories. But there is not yet a comprehensive theoretical framework that has replaced the dual-mode account. Such an account would have to explain, for example, when and why certain dissociations emerge between implicit and explicit responses, why and when implicit and explicit responses differentially or similarly predict other behaviors, and how the division of the mind (whether via systems, processes, or representational format) aligns with recent cognitive science views of organizational schemes that question the simplicity of two categories (of systems, modes of processing, representations, etc.; see Cisek & Hayden, 2022; Cisek & Green, 2024; see also Carlston & Smith, 1996).

Beyond this critical need for continued theoretical development and refinement on the implicit-versus-explicit dichotomy, our argument in this chapter is that theories of meaning making could incorporate a much larger role of the implicit and/or non-conscious processes we discuss here. However, we also acknowledge some serious alignment issues between the first section and the current section. The first section argues for the functionality of non-conscious processes in particular, but the research we've reviewed in this section addresses the implicit mind more generally. And, in fact, much of this work (against the old bias and the simple bias) used indirect measures that were not designed to assess lack of awareness, but rather principally unintentionality and speed (see Kurdi et al., 2022). Therefore, it remains an open question whether the updating and relational sophistication we review here provide support for non-conscious processes in particular. That remains to be tested.

Caution is also warranted in assuming that this work speaks to the characteristics and functionality of the learning *process* itself, versus the outputs that reflect that learning. There is a large literature on implicit learning (in language, and other domains), but none of the research we review here uses or studies a learning process that is itself implicit. Instead, the implicit mind, as we have defined it, refers to the output captured on indirect measures. This raises the possibility that these outputs—which show updating, flexibility, truth value, and so on—are dependent on a careful, conscious, reasoning process that occurs beforehand. This, too, requires additional testing.

Measures

Because of space constraints here, we do not discuss the different types of indirect measures, and the assumptions and implications of each. The evidence of the updating and relational sophistication has been replicated on the three most commonly used indirect measures (the IAT, the affect misattribution procedure [AMP], and evaluative priming), but the majority of the work has used the AMP, which has been argued to measure unintentional impressions (e.g., see Hughes et al., 2023; Kurdi et al., 2024). There are some differences between these measures (Van Dessel, Cummins, Hughes, Kasran, Cathelyn, & Moran, 2020), and there are many remaining questions about the particular constraints of each and what it might mean that the measures do not always align.

We have also glossed over possible reasons for why there may have been and continue to be dissociations between output on direct and indirect measures. The predominant dual-mode interpretation is that output is different because the processes and content underlying these sets of measures are different (because of the processing constraints on direct vs. indirect). However, direct and indirect measures differ in many ways (structurally) that might explain dissociations, and more work needs to be conducted to identify the reason(s) for any dissociation, and whether it is something related to the purported implicit versus explicit mind in terms of processing characteristics or underlying content/systems (e.g., see Béna, Melnikoff, Mierop, & Corneille, 2022; Ferguson et al., 2019; Payne, Burkley, & Stokes, 2008; Payne et al., 2013; Surdel & Ferguson, 2025). What some of the new work shows is that the previous explanation for the dissociations—that the mental architecture of whatever aspects of the mind contributed to those findings does not allow for fast updating or relational analysis—must be dismissed.

CONCLUSIONS

How do humans make meaning out of their experiences and lives? In the psychological sciences, this question drives a large, heterogeneous body of work that covers many phenomena, including narratives, reasoning, attributions, identities, emotions, memory, and more. How do we grapple with—and make meaning out of—the unexpected events and experiences that are an inevitable part of life? We focused on the broad assumption that meaning making mostly involves relatively explicit processes. On the contrary, we argue here that relatively more automatic, or implicit, processes reflect the updating, flexibility, and causal and logical analysis that surely are required for meaning making. In doing so, we hope to expand the predominant understanding of meaning making from a solely deliberative, conscious, and intentional act of sense making to a much richer cognitive feat likely involving many implicit processes.

REFERENCES

Albarracín, D., & Johnson, B. T. (2019). *Handbook of attitudes: basic principles* (2nd ed). Routledge.

Bargh, J. A. (1994). The four horsemen of automaticity: Awareness, intention, efficiency, and control in social cognition. In R. S. Wyer, Jr. & T. K. Srull (Eds.), *Handbook of social cognition: Basic processes; Applications* (2nd ed., pp. 1–40). Lawrence Erlbaum Associates.

Bargh, J. A. (2017). *Before you know it: The unconscious reasons why we do what we do.* Atria Books.

Béna, J., Melnikoff, D. E., Mierop, A., & Corneille, O. (2022). Revisiting dissociation hypotheses with a structural fit approach: The case of the prepared reflex framework. *Journal of Experimental Social Psychology, 100,* 1–12.

Brannon, S. M., & Gawronski, B. (2017). A second chance for first impressions? Exploring the context-(in)dependent updating of implicit evaluations. *Social Psychological and Personality Science, 8*(3), 275–283.

Bouton, M. E. (2016). *Learning and behavior: A contemporary synthesis* (2nd edition). Sinauer Associates.

Briñol, P., & Petty, R. E. (2012). The history of attitudes and persuasion research. In A. Kruglanski & W. Stroebe (Eds.), *Handbook of the history of social psychology* (pp. 285–320). Psychology Press.

Cesario, J. (2014). Priming, replication, and the hardest science. *Perspectives on Psychological Science, 9*(1), 40–48.

Cao, J., & Banaji, M. R. (2016). The base rate principle and the fairness principle in social judgment. *Proceedings of the National Academy of Sciences of the United States of America, 113*(27), 7475–7480.

Carlston, D. E., & Smith, E. R. (1996). Principles of mental representation. In E. T. Higgins & A. W. Kruglanski (Eds.), *Social psychology: Handbook of basic principles* (pp. 184–210). Guilford Press.

Chaiken, S., & Trope, Y. (Eds.). (1999). *Dual-process theories in social psychology.* Guilford Press.

Carlston, D. E., & Smith, E. R. (1996). Principles of mental representation. In E. T. Higgins & A. W. Kruglanski (Eds.), *Social psychology: Handbook of basic principles* (pp. 184–210). Guilford Press.

Cisek, P., & Green, A. M. (2024). Toward a neuroscience of natural behavior. *Current Opinion in Neurobiology, 86*, 102859.

Cisek, P., & Hayden, B. Y. (2022). Neuroscience needs evolution. *Philosophical Transactions of the Royal Society of London. Series B, Biological Sciences, 377*(1844), 20200518.

Cone, J., & Ferguson, M. J. (2015). He did what? The role of diagnosticity in revising implicit evaluations. *Journal of Personality and Social Psychology, 108*(1), 37–57.

Cone, J., Flaharty, K., & Ferguson, M. J. (2019). Believability of evidence matters for correcting social impressions. *Proceedings of the National Academy of Sciences of the United States of America, 116*(20), 9802–9807.

Cone, J., Flaharty, K., & Ferguson, M. J. (2021). The long-term effects of new evidence on implicit impressions of other people. *Psychological Science, 32*(2), 173–188.

Corneille, O., & Hütter, M. (2020). Implicit? What do you mean? A comprehensive review of the delusive implicitness construct in attitude research. *Personality and Social Psychological Review, 24*(3), 212–232.

Cunningham, W. A., Zelazo, P. D., Packer, D. J., & Van Bavel, J. J. (2007). The iterative reprocessing model: A multilevel framework for attitudes and evaluation. *Social Cognition, 25*, 736–760.

De Houwer, J. (2014). A propositional model of implicit evaluation. *Social and Personality Psychology Compass, 8*(7), 342–353.

De Houwer, J., Teige-Mocigemba, S., Spruyt, A., & Moors, A. (2009). Implicit measures: A normative analysis and review. *Psychological Bulletin, 135*(3), 347–368.

Deutsch, R., Gawronski, B., & Strack, F. (2006). At the boundaries of automaticity: Negation as reflective operation. *Journal of Personality and Social Psychology, 91*(3), 385–405.

Domjan, M. (2010). *The principles of learning and behavior* (6th edition.). Nelson Education.

Ferguson, M. J., Mann, T. C., Cone, J., & Shen, X. (2019). When and how implicit impressions can be updated. *Current Directions in Psychological Science, 28*(4), 331–336.

Ferguson, M. J., Mann, T. C., Cone, J., & Shen, X. (2025). *Rethinking dual-mode theories: On the role of pragmatics and evidence strength* [Unpublished manuscript].

Gawronski, B. (2009). Ten frequently asked questions about implicit measures and their frequently supposed, but not entirely correct answers. *Canadian Psychology, 50*(3), 141–150.

Gawronski, B., & Bodenhausen, G. V. (2006). Associative and propositional processes in evaluation: an integrative review of implicit and explicit attitude change. *Psychological Bulletin, 132*(5), 692–731.

Gawronski, B., Brannon, S. M., & Ng, N. L. (2022). Debunking misinformation about a causal link between vaccines and autism: Two preregistered tests of dual-process versus single-process predictions (with conflicting results). *Social Cognition, 40*(6), 580–599.

Gawronski, B., De Houwer, J., & Sherman, J. W. (2020). Twenty-five years of research using implicit measures. *Social Cognition*, 38(Suppl.), s1–s25.

Gelman, A. (2015). The connection between varying treatment effects and the crisis of unreplicable research: A Bayesian perspective. *Journal of Management, 41*(2), 632–643.

Greenwald, A. G. (1992). New Look 3: Unconscious cognition reclaimed. *American Psychologist, 47*(6), 766–779.

Gregg, A. P., Seibt, B., & Banaji, M. R. (2006). Easier done than undone: Asymmetry in the malleability of implicit preferences. *Journal of Personality and Social Psychology, 90*(1), 1–20.

Hassin, R. R. (2013). Yes it can: On the functional abilities of the human unconscious. *Perspectives on Psychological Science, 8*(2), 195–207.

Hassin, R. R., & Sklar, A. Y. (2014). The human unconscious—A functional perspective. In J. W. Sherman, B. Gawronski, & Y. Trope (Eds.), *Dual-process theories of the social mind* (pp. 299–313). Guilford Press.

Hassin, R. R., Uleman, J. S., & Bargh, J. A. (2005). *The new unconscious.* Oxford University Press.

Hebb, D. O. (1949). *The organization of behavior: A neuropsychological theory.* Wiley.

Hu, X., Gawronski, B., & Balas, R. (2017). Propositional versus dual-process accounts of evaluative conditioning: I. The effects of co-occurrence and relational information on implicit and explicit evaluations. *Personality and Social Psychology Bulletin, 43*(1), 17–32.

Hughes, S., Cummins, J., & Hussey, I. (2023). Effects on the affect misattribution procedure are strongly moderated by influence awareness. *Behavior Research Methods, 55*(4), 1558–1586.

Ioannidis, J. (2005). Why most published research findings are false. *PLoS Medicine, 2*(8), e124.

Kahneman, D. (2011). *Thinking, fast and slow.* Farrar, Straus and Giroux.

Kurdi, B., & Charlesworth, T. E. S. (2023). A 3D framework of implicit attitude change. *Trends in Cognitive Sciences, 27*(8), 745–758.

Kurdi, B., & Dunham, Y. (2020). Propositional accounts of implicit evaluation: Taking stock and looking ahead. *Social Cognition, 38*(Suppl.), s42–s67.

Kurdi, B., Krosch, A. R., & Ferguson, M. J. (2020). Implicit evaluations of moral agents reflect intent and outcome. *Journal of Experimental Social Psychology, 90*, Article 103990.

Kurdi, B., Mann, T. C., & Ferguson, M. J. (2022). Persuading the implicit mind: Changing negative implicit evaluations with an 8-minute podcast. *Social Psychological and Personality Science, 13*(3), 688–697.

Kurdi, B., Melnikoff, D. E., Hannay, J. W., Korkmaz, A., Lee, K. M., Ritchie, E., et al. (2024). Testing the automaticity features of the affect misattribution procedure: The roles of awareness and intentionality. *Behavior Research Methods, 56*(4), 3161–3194.

Kurdi, B., Morehouse, K. N., & Dunham, Y. (2023). How do explicit and implicit evaluations shift? A preregistered meta-analysis of the effects of co-occurrence and relational information. *Journal of Personality and Social Psychology, 124*(6), 1174–1202.

Kurdi, B., Morris, A., & Cushman, F. A. (2022). The role of causal structure in implicit evaluation. *Cognition, 225*, Article 105116.

Lieberman, M. D., Gaunt, R., Gilbert, D. T., & Trope, Y. (2002). Reflexion and reflection: A social cognitive neuroscience approach to attributional inference. In M. P. Zanna (Ed.), *Advances in experimental social psychology*, Vol. 34 (pp. 199–249). Academic Press.

Mann, T. C., Cone, J., Heggeseth, B., & Ferguson, M. J. (2019). Updating implicit impressions: New evidence on intentionality and the affect misattribution procedure. *Journal of Personality and Social Psychology, 116*(3), 349–374.

Mann, T. C., & Ferguson, M. J. (2015). Can we undo our first impressions? The role of reinterpretation in reversing implicit evaluations. *Journal of Personality and Social Psychology, 108*(6), 823–849.

Mann, T. C., & Ferguson, M. J. (2017). Reversing implicit first impressions through reinterpretation after a two-day delay. *Journal of Experimental Social Psychology, 68*, 122–127.

Mann, T. C., Kurdi, B., & Banaji, M. R. (2020). How effectively can implicit evaluations be updated? Using evaluative statements after aversive repeated evaluative pairings. *Journal of Experimental Psychology: General, 149*(6), 1169–1192.

McConnell, A. R., Rydell, R. J., Strain, L. M., & Mackie, D. M. (2008). Forming implicit and explicit attitudes toward individuals: Social group association cues. *Journal of Personality and Social Psychology, 94*(5), 792–807.

Melnikoff, D. E., & Bargh, J. A. (2018). The mythical number two. *Trends in cognitive sciences, 22*(4), 280–293.

Moors, A. (2013). Automaticity. In D. Reisberg (Ed.), *The Oxford handbook of cognitive psychology* (pp. 163–175). Oxford University Press.

Moors, A. (2016). Automaticity: Componential, causal, and mechanistic explanations. *Annual Review of Psychology, 67*, 263–287.

Moran, T., & Bar-Anan, Y. (2013). The effect of object-valence relations on automatic evaluation. *Cognition and Emotion, 27*(4), 743–752.

Moran, T., Bar-Anan, Y., & Nosek, B. A. (2017). The effect of the validity of co-occurrence on automatic and deliberate evaluations. *European Journal of Social Psychology, 47*(6), 708–723.

Nosek, B. A., Hardwicke, T. E., Moshontz, H., Allard, A., Corker, K. S., & Dreber, A. (2022). Replicability, robustness, and reproducibility in psychological science. *Annual Review of Psychology, 73*, 719–748.

Oizumi, M., Tsuchiya, N., & Amari, S. (2016). Unified framework for information integration based on information geometry. *Proceedings of the National Academy of Sciences of the United States of America, 113*(51), 14817–14822.

Paul, L. A. (2014). *Transformative experience*. Oxford University Press.

Payne, B. K., Burkley, M. A., & Stokes, M. B. (2008). Why do implicit and explicit attitude tests diverge? The role of structural fit. *Journal of Personality and Social Psychology, 94*(1), 16–31.

Payne, B. K., Brown-Iannuzzi, J., Burkley, M., Arbuckle, N. L., Cooley, R., Cameron, C. D., et al. (2013). Intention invention and the affect misattribution procedure: Reply to Bar-Anan and Nosek (2012). *Personality and Social Psychology Bulletin, 39*(3), 375–386.

Peters, K. R., & Gawronski, B. (2011). Are we puppets on a string? Comparing the impact of contingency and validity on implicit and explicit evaluations. *Personality and Social Psychology Bulletin, 37*(4), 557–569.

Rydell, R. J., & McConnell, A. R. (2006). Understanding implicit and explicit attitude change: A systems of reasoning analysis. *Journal of Personality and Social Psychology, 91*(6), 995–1008.

Shen, X., & Ferguson, M. J. (2021). How resistant are implicit impressions of facial trustworthiness? When new evidence leads to durable updating. *Journal of Experimental Social Psychology, 97*, Article 104219.

Shen, X., Mann, T. C., & Ferguson, M. J. (2020). Beware a dishonest face? How we update our implicit impressions of untrustworthy faces. *Journal of Experimental Social Psychology, 86*, Article 103888.

Sherman, J. W. (2006). On building a better process model: It's not only how many, but which ones and by which means. *Psychological Inquiry, 17*(3), 173–184.

Sherman, J. W., Gawronski, B., & Trope, Y. (Eds). (2014). *Dual process theories of the social mind.* Guilford Press.

Sherman, J. W., & Rivers, A. M. (2020). Social priming: A dubious term. *Nature, 579*(7797), 29.

Sklar, A. Y., Kardosh, R., & Hassin, R. R. (2021). From non-conscious processing to conscious events: A minimalist approach. *Neuroscience of Consciousness, 2021*(2), niab026.

Sloman, S. A. (1996). The empirical case for two systems of reasoning. *Psychological Bulletin, 119*(1), 3–22.

Smith, E. R., & DeCoster, J. (2000). Dual-process models in social and cognitive psychology: Conceptual integration and links to underlying memory systems. *Personality and Social Psychology Review, 4*(2), 108–131.

Smith, C. T., De Houwer, J., & Nosek, B. A. (2013). Consider the source: Persuasion of implicit evaluations is moderated by source credibility. *Personality and Social Psychology Bulletin, 39*(2), 193–205.

Strack, F., & Deutsch, R. (2004). Reflective and impulsive determinants of social behavior. *Personality and Social Psychological Review, 8*(3), 220–247.

Surdel, N., Bigman, Y. E., Shen, X., Lee, W. Y., Jung, M. F., & Ferguson, M. J. (2024). Judging robot ability: How people form implicit and explicit impressions of robot competence. *Journal of Experimental Psychology: General, 153*(5), 1309–1335.

Surdel, N., & Ferguson, M. J. (2025). *Common ground, divergent evaluations: The impact of pragmatics on competence impressions* [Unpublished manuscript].

Tononi, G., Boly, M., Massimini, M., & Koch, C. (2016). Integrated information theory: From consciousness to its physical substrate. *Nature reviews Neuroscience, 17*(7), 450–461.

Tononi, G., & Koch, C. (2015). Consciousness: Here, there and everywhere? *Philosophical Transactions of the Royal Society B: Biological Sciences, 370*(1668), 20140167.

Tulving, E. (1985). Memory and consciousness. *Canadian Psychology, 26*(1), 1–12.

Ullmann-Margalit, E. (2006). Big decisions: Opting, converting, drifting. *Royal Institute of Philosophy Supplement, 58*, 157–171.

Van Dessel, P., Cummins, J., Hughes, S., Kasran, S., Cathelyn, F., & Moran, T. (2020). Reflecting on 25 years of research using implicit measures: Recommendations for their future use. *Social Cognition, 38*(Suppl), S223–S242.

Van Dessel, P., Ye, Y., & De Houwer, J. (2019). Changing deep-rooted implicit evaluation in the blink of an eye: Negative verbal information shifts automatic liking of Gandhi. *Social Psychological and Personality Science, 10*(2), 266–273.

Wilson, T. D., Lindsey, S., & Schooler, T. Y. (2000). A model of dual attitudes. *Psychological Review, 107*(1), 101–126.

Wyer, N. A. (2016). Easier done than undone . . . by some of the people, some of the time: The role of elaboration in explicit and implicit group preferences. *Journal of Experimental Social Psychology, 63*, 77–85.

CHAPTER 12

From Self-Discontinuity to Meaning through Nostalgia

Constantine Sedikides and Tim Wildschut

In his pioneering book *Yearning for Yesterday: A Sociology of Nostalgia*, Fred Davis (1979) suggested that nostalgia serves to temporally connect disjointed self-aspects: "Nostalgia helps the individual construct continuity of identity by encouraging an appreciative stance toward former selves; excluding unpleasant memories; reinterpreting 'marginal, fugitive, and eccentric facets of earlier selves' in a positive light; and establishing benchmarks in one's biography" (pp. 35–36). The prescient sociologist also suggested that when these temporally disjointed self-aspects become salient or accessible, the individual experiences "fears, discontents, anxieties, or uncertainties" (p. 34). In that case, nostalgia comes to the rescue by restoring the temporal bond among self-aspects: "It is these emotions and cognitive states that pose the threat of identity discontinuity . . . that nostalgia seeks, by marshalling our psychological resources for continuity, to abort or, at the very least, deflect" (pp. 34–35). Davis, then, seemed to opine that self-discontinuity triggers nostalgia, which in turn increases self-continuity. We will elaborate on this idea, adding that self-continuity subsequently raises meaning in life (henceforth, *meaning*). We will envelop our proposal within a conceptual framework, the regulatory model of nostalgia.

DEFINITIONS

We will proceed to define and embellish the relevant concepts: self-discontinuity, self-continuity, nostalgia, and meaning.

Self-Discontinuity and Self-Continuity

Self-discontinuity is the subjective experience of disjuncture between one's past and present selves (Sedikides, Wildschut, Gaertner, Routledge, & Arndt, 2008; Sedikides, Wildschut, Routledge, & Arndt, 2015). Self-discontinuity involves identity confusion and discomfort because one's life patterns or sources of meaning are disrupted (Jiang, Cheng, Wang, & Hou, 2021; Sedikides, Hong, & Wildschut, 2023). More generally, self-discontinuity is a marker of psychological ill-being or psychological illness, including distress (Anderzén & Arnetz, 1999; Habermas & Köber, 2015), loneliness (Zhang, Zhang, & Gao, 2022), ineffective coping (Sadeh & Karniol, 2012), depression, anxiety, schizophrenia, and suicidal ideation (Chandler & Proulx, 2008; Sokol & Eisenheim, 2016; Sokol & Serper, 2019).

Conversely, self-continuity is the subjective experience of connectedness between one's past and present selves (Sedikides et al., 2016). Self-continuity synthesizes one's experiential stream and consolidates one's identity (i.e., feeling like the same person across time; Sedikides et al., 2023), contributing to self-concept clarity (Jiang, Chen, & Sedikides, 2020). Also, self-continuity is associated with psychological adjustment, well-being, and equanimity (Landau, Greenberg, & Solomon, 2008; McAdams, Reynolds, Lewis, Patten, & Bowman, 2001), as well as physical health (Anderzén & Arnetz, 1999).

Nostalgia

According to *The New Oxford Dictionary of English* (Pearsall, 1998, p. 1266), the emotion of nostalgia is "a sentimental longing or wistful affection for the past." Prototype approaches, which explore laypersons' understanding of the construct "nostalgia," concur with the dictionary definition. Laypersons, across cultures, regard nostalgia as bittersweet ("a joy tinged with sadness"; Werman, 1977, p. 393) but predominantly positive, involving contentment, calmness, and warmth, but also yearning for one's past (Hepper, Ritchie, Sedikides, & Wildschut, 2012; Hepper et al. 2014). Also, experimental inductions of nostalgia engender more positive affect than negative affect (Leunissen et al., 2021).

The past to which nostalgia refers is personally valued and meaningful (Sedikides & Wildschut, 2018). It often pertains to momentous occasions with close others (e.g., family members, partners, friends), such as birthday celebrations, graduations, and summer vacations (Wildschut, Sedikides, Arndt, & Routledge, 2006). Nostalgia occurs frequently (i.e., several times a week; Wildschut et al., 2006) and across cultures (Sedikides & Wildschut, 2022) and ages (Hepper, Wildschut, Sedikides, Robertson, & Routledge, 2021).

Meaning

Meaning is the subjective experience that one's life is purposeful or goal oriented, is coherent or comprehensible, and is significant or existentially matters (King & Hicks, 2021). These three components are, respectively, motivational, cognitive, and evaluative (Reker & Wong, 1988). Significance or existentially mattering might be the most critical ingredient of meaning (Costin & Vignoles, 2020). Nevertheless, we take an inclusive approach, focusing on the presence of meaning in one's life (Steger, Frazier, Oishi, & Kaler, 2006).

People seek meaning or engage in meaning making (Frankl, 1946/1984). In turn, meaning is characterized by key correlates or outcomes. Specifically, it is associated with, or predicts, psychological health, psychological functioning (e.g., coping, optimism), and physical health (Czekierda, Banik, Park, & Luszczynska, 2017; Hooker, Masters, & Park, 2018).

THE REGULATORY MODEL OF NOSTALGIA

Nostalgia has coping potential. This potential is explicated by the regulatory model (Wildschut & Sedikides, 2023a, 2023b). In its general form, the model posits that a life event might provoke a certain unsettling psychological state, such as a sense of rapture or self-discontinuity, but it will also trigger nostalgia. The individual will move beyond the here and now and connect with distal events in their life in an attempt to self-regulate (Trope et al., 2021). In turn, nostalgia will assuage that psychological state, such as by reducing self-discontinuity or increasing self-continuity. The emotion of nostalgia, then, constitutes a psychological resource, a balancing feedback mechanism that maintains homeostasis. We will use the regulatory model of nostalgia mainly as a framework to discuss the rather fragmented empirical literature on the links among self-discontinuity, nostalgia, and self-continuity. We will also consider meaning as a correlate and consequence of self-continuity.

Self-Discontinuity Is Associated with, or Triggers, Nostalgia

The first tenet of the regulatory model implies that self-discontinuity is related to, or elicits, nostalgia. Qualitative evidence (i.e., content-analyzed interviews, participant observation) is consistent with this tenet. Faculty members in Turkey (Brown & Humphreys, 2002) and Finland (Ylijoki, 2005) confronted with changes in higher education resorted to nostalgia, as did medical practitioners in the United Kingdom (McDonald, Waring, & Harrison, 2006) facing organizational change. Similarly, U.S. community members relied on nostalgia to cope with news of the closure of a community hub (i.e., coffeeshop; Milligan, 2003).

Correlational evidence is likewise generally consistent with this tenet of the regulatory model (Best & Nelson, 1985). In four surveys of U.S. nationals (conducted in 1968, 1974, 1976, and 1980), respondents who were experiencing self-discontinuity rather than self-continuity rated their past more positively on four items (e.g., "People had it better in the old days"; "In spite of what some people say, the lot of the average man is getting worse, not better"); arguably, favorable perceptions of the past under these circumstances constitute an indirect index of nostalgia. However, out of four indices assessing self-discontinuity (i.e., occupational mobility; geographic mobility; work interruption; deteriorating life circumstances, such as divorce and health problems), this pattern emerged for the last index only. Furthermore, in a cross-sectional study (Sedikides, Wildschut, Routledge, & Arndt, 2015, Study 1), British community members reported their level of self-discontinuity due to both unfavorable life events (e.g., "change in financial situation," "death of a close family member") and favorable life events (e.g., "gaining a new family member," "outstanding personal achievement"; Social Readjustment Rating Scale [Holmes & Rahe, 1967]) occurring in the prior 2 years. Those who experienced self-discontinuity due to unfavorable (but not favorable) events expressed higher nostalgia, measured with the 5-item Southampton Nostalgia Scale (Routledge, Arndt, Sedikides, & Wildschut, 2008), which refers to the experiential frequency (e.g., "How often do you experience nostalgia?") and subjective importance (e.g., "How important is it for you to bring to mind nostalgic experiences?") of the emotion. Additional correlational evidence stems from research on addiction. U.S. (MTurkers) disordered gamblers and drinkers indicated their level of self-discontinuity (i.e., "Gambling has changed who I am"; "The person I was before I started gambling is different from the person I am now"). Self-discontinuity was positively related to nostalgia for the pre-addicted self (Kim & Wohl, 2015). Here, nostalgia was measured with three items ("I sometimes feel nostalgic for the life I had before I started gambling"; "I never miss the life I had before I started gambling" [reverse coded]; "I sometimes long for the life I had before gambling") adapted from Iyer and Jetten (2011).

A longitudinal study also provided support for the first tenet of the regulatory model (Wang et al., 2024). For each of their 4 years at university, Chinese undergraduates indicated their level of self-discontinuity and nostalgia. Self-discontinuity was assessed in terms of the presence of life events ranging in unfavorability (Adolescent Self-Rating Life Events Checklist; Liu, Liu, Yang, & Zhao, 1997). Examples are as follows:

"Being fined," "Conflict with friends or classmates," "Failure in a test," "Unable to be with family," and "Get sick seriously." Nostalgia was assessed with the 5-item Southampton Nostalgia Scale (Routledge et al., 2008). Initial self-discontinuity that accompanied transition to university life predicted higher nostalgia, although the strength of this relation weakened in subsequent years.

More importantly, experimental evidence is consistent with the tenet (Sedikides, Wildschut, Routledge, & Arndt, 2015, Study 2). British undergraduates were randomly assigned to three conditions: negative self-discontinuity, positive self-discontinuity, and self-continuity control. In the negative self-discontinuity condition, they read an essay arguing that the university years break off students from family and friends, prompting students to question their self-beliefs, goals, and values. In the positive self-discontinuity condition, they read an essay arguing that the university years are a time of personal transformation during which students become more independent; explore new opportunities; and consolidate their self-beliefs, goals, and values. Lastly, in the self-continuity control condition, they read an essay arguing that the university years strengthen and specify their role as a student surrounded by a steady group of friends in a familiar setting. Negative self-discontinuity (compared with the other two conditions) increased nostalgia, as assessed with the Nostalgia Inventory (Batcho, 1995). The Nostalgia Inventory includes 18 items that refer to persons or objects from one's past (e.g., "my family," "my friends," "TV shows and movies," "my childhood toys"). Finally, an experiment in the context of addiction supported the tenet (Wohl, Kim, Salmon, Santesso, Wildschut, & Sedikides, 2018). Disordered gamblers (Experiment 1) and drinkers (Experiment 2), all U.S. MTurkers, were informed that addiction leads to loss of self through changes in personality, moods, or behavior (self-discontinuity condition) or does not lead to loss of self (control condition). Self-discontinuity increased nostalgia for the pre-addicted self, with nostalgia being measured as in Kim and Wohl (2015).

Nostalgia Is Associated with, or Increases, Self-Continuity

The second tenet of the regulatory model states that nostalgia is related to, or augments, continuity. We review correlational and experimental evidence for this tenet.

Content Analyses and Correlational Evidence

Content analyses suggest that nostalgia bridges one's past with one's present (Stephan, Sedikides, & Wildschut, 2012). Nostalgia was experimentally manipulated among British undergraduates with the event reflection task (ERT; Sedikides, Wildschut, Routledge, Arndt, et al., 2015; Wildschut & Sedikides, 2024). This is the most frequently used nostalgia induction technique (Fetterman et al., 2024). It entails vivid autobiographical recall, a particularly effective method to elicit emotions where high personal relevance is central to the affective experience (Joseph et al., 2020). As part of the ERT, participants in the nostalgia condition visualize a nostalgic event from their past, whereas participants in the control condition visualize an ordinary (e.g., everyday, regular) event from their past. Next, all participants list a few keywords that capture the gist of the corresponding event, then proceed to narrate the event in writing. A manipulation check (e.g., "I feel nostalgic at the moment") follows. The ensuing narratives were coded (Stephan et al., 2012) for abstractness/concreteness based on the Linguistic Inquiry and Word Count (Pennebaker, Booth, & Francis, 2007) and the linguistic category model (Coenen, Hedebouw, & Semin, 2006). Nostalgic (vs. ordinary) narratives contained more abstract terms and more concrete terms. Interestingly, the concrete terms buttressed the relevance of the nostalgic event for the nostalgizer's present. For instance, concrete terms highlighted a behavior or psychological state in the present ("I smile . . . ") that was prompted by a past event (" . . . when I look at my family photo on my desk"). Another content analysis of event memories written by individuals living with dementia revealed that nostalgic (relative to control) events contained more expressions of self-continuity (Ismail et al., 2022). Furthermore, a content analysis of memoirs suggested that nostalgia strengthened self-continuity among Ukrainian resistance fighters during World War II (Batcho, 2021). Lastly, a content analysis of participants' research journals (i.e., experimenter-guided recording of personal experiences) indicated that nostalgic memories tethered to olfaction (i.e., the aroma of various objects) were associated with self-continuity (Waskul, Vannini, & Wilson, 2009).

Additional research provides support for a link between nostalgia and self-continuity. U.S. sports fans watched a 30-second video clip evoking nostalgia for their team and completed the 4-item Self-Continuity Index ("I feel . . . ": "connected with my past," "connected with who I was in the past," "there is continuity in my life," "important aspects of my personality remain the same across time"). Nostalgia was positively associated with self-continuity (Chang, Schneider, Connaughton, Hager, & Ju, 2019). Malaysian community members who were dispositionally nostalgic (with nostalgia assessed with the 7-item Southampton Nostalgia Scale; Sedikides, Wildschut, Routledge, Arndt, et al., 2015) reported higher levels of self-continuity (assessed with the 4-item Self-Continuity Index; Loh, Gaur, & Lim, 2019).

Nostalgia can also serve as a linchpin that connects repatriates' experiences across cultures (Zou, Wildschut, Cable, & Sedikides, 2018). In a large sample of repatriates from 41 countries, nostalgia for the host culture (controlling for nostalgia for the home culture) was associated with higher self-continuity. Host nostalgia, then, facilitated the integration of experiences across varying cultural contexts.

The relevant literature has broadened the construct of self-continuity and measured it accordingly. Self-continuity was conceptualized as the subjective experience of connection among one's past, present, and future selves (Becker et al., 2018), a construct termed *global self-continuity* (Sedikides et al., 2023). It was measured as follows. Participants listed identities that best represented who they were, then rated whether they considered each identity as continuous ("To what extent does [each identity] make you feel that your past, present, and future are connected?"). The average score across the listed identities represented global self-continuity. In relevant research, nostalgia was positively associated with global self-continuity among Canadian undergraduates (Hong, Sedikides, & Wildschut, 2021, Study 1), Korean undergraduates, U.S. MTurk workers, and British Prolific workers (Hong, Sedikides, & Wildschut, 2022, Studies 1–3).

Experimental Evidence

DIRECT EFFECTS OF NOSTALGIA ON SELF-CONTINUITY. The positive association of nostalgia with self-continuity invites explication. As mentioned previously, nostalgic reflections typically refer to events (e.g., achievements, family customs, cultural rituals) that are steeped in meaning (Routledge et al., 2011; Wildschut et al., 2006; Yin, Jiang, Wildschut, & Sedikides, 2024). These events are personally important and textured, and they often reflect traditions that unite one's past with one's present. The events enshroud and elucidate the person's life trajectory (e.g., how one transitioned "from then to now") and serve as signposts that aid navigation through life. Memories of those events are likely to foster temporal continuity.

A sizeable literature has established the causal influence of nostalgia on self-continuity. Pertinent research has induced nostalgia and assessed self-continuity in multiple ways, following a converging operations approach (Campbell & Fiske, 1959). Nostalgia, induced via the ERT, increased self-continuity, assessed with the 8-item Self-Continuity Index, in U.S. undergraduates (Sedikides, Wildschut, Routledge, & Arndt, 2015, Experiment 3). This index subsumes the 4-item Self-Continuity Index and also includes the following items: "The past and present flow seamlessly together"; "The present is a mere continuation of the past";

"There is continuity between the past and present"; "The past merges nicely into the present." Likewise, nostalgia, induced via the ERT, (1) elevated self-continuity, assessed with the 8-item Self-Continuity Index in Chinese participants recruited from So Jump Survey (a survey platform; Wang, Tian, Sarigöllü, & Xu, 2020), and (2) elevated self-continuity, assessed with 4-item Self-Continuity Index, in U.S. MTurkers (Lasaleta & Loveland, 2019, Study 1) and British undergraduates (Biskas, Juhl, Wildschut, Sedikides, & Saroglou, 2022, Study 3). These findings were replicated in British undergraduates with a variant of the ERT that included not only a neutral memories condition (i.e., ordinary event) but also a positive memories condition (i.e., a positive event; Sedikides, Wildschut, Routledge, & Arndt, 2015, Experiment 4). Moreover, the findings were replicated with the standard ERT in undergraduates from 28 countries and a special administrative region of China (i.e., Hong Kong) across five continents (Hepper et al., 2024).

Other ERT experiments demonstrated the robustness of nostalgia's causal impact on self-continuity, assessed with the 4-item Self-Continuity Index. In particular, nostalgia increased self-continuity in Syrian refugees residing in Saudi Arabia (Wildschut, Sedikides, & Alowidy, 2019) and in British individuals living with Alzheimer disease (Ismail et al., 2018, Experiment 1).

Is the effect of nostalgia on self-continuity independent of other modes of contemplating one's past? Such modes include reflection and brooding. Reflection is an attempt to understand the reasons underlying one's (especially negative) affective states, whereas brooding is a persistent, if not repetitive, focus on the causes of one's (especially negative) affective states (Miranda & Nolen-Hoeksema, 2007; Treynor, Gonzalez, & Nolen-Hoeksema, 2003). An experiment testing both British and Chinese undergraduates addressed this issue (Jiang, Cheung, Wildschut, & Sedikides, 2021). The experiment additionally introduced a novel manipulation of nostalgia and, correspondingly, of reflection and brooding. The nostalgia manipulation relied on analyses of the prototype of the construct across cultures (Hepper et al., 2012, 2014). These analyses revealed the following five highly prototypical features of the construct: "bringing to mind rose-tinted memories," "reflecting on keepsakes," "longing for a time or place from my past," "thinking about my family and friends," and "remembering my childhood" (see also Cheung, Sedikides, & Wildschut, 2017). Based on standardized scales of reflection and brooding (Treynor et al., 2003), the authors (Jiang, Cheung, et al., 2021) abstracted five prototypical features of reflection (i.e., "analyzing the event, trying to understand why it happened"; "going away and reflect on why I feel in certain ways"; "writing down what I was thinking and analyze it"; "analyzing my personality to try to understand why it happened"; "going somewhere along to think about my feelings related to what happened") and five prototypical features of brooding ("wishing things had gone better," "asking why I have problems other people don't have," "asking why I always react this way," "asking what am I doing to deserve this," "asking why can't I handle things better"). An advantage of this manipulation is that it does not include the pertinent terms (i.e., "nostalgia," "reflection," "brooding"), thus reducing potential demand characteristics. Participants were randomly assigned to the nostalgia, reflection, and brooding conditions. They brought to mind an event in their lives that was characterized by the five features corresponding to their mode of contemplating the past and described the event in writing. Nostalgia increased self-continuity (assessed with the 4-item Self-Continuity Index) in both British and Chinese samples, above and beyond reflection and brooding.

All reviewed experiments so far manipulated nostalgia either with the ERT (Hepper et al., 2024; Ismail et al., 2018, Experiment 1; Sedikides, Wildschut, Routledge, & Arndt, 2015, Experiments 3 and 4; Wildschut et al., 2019) or an alternative narrative induction technique (Jiang, Cheung, et al., 2021). Nostalgia has also been manipulated with music among individuals living with Alzheimer disease (Ismail et al., 2018, Experiment 2). Initially, participants submitted three of their favorite nostalgic songs. At a later session, they were randomly assigned to the nostalgia or control condition. A given participant in the nostalgia condition listened to one of three songs (randomly determined) that they had submitted previously. The same song was played to a yoked participant in the control condition. Participants immersed themselves in the song, spent a couple of minutes thinking about how it made them feel, and wrote about a past experience or event associated with the song. Participants in the nostalgia condition reported higher self-continuity (assessed with the 4-item Self-Continuity Scale) than their control-condition counterparts.

Relatedly, nostalgia has been evoked via scents among U.S. undergraduates (Reid, Green, Wildschut, & Sedikides, 2015). A pretest identified 12 appropriate scented oils for later use (out of 33). These included Chanel No. 5 (a perfume), Purrs and Paws (a pet fragrance scented with citrus and fresh flowers), eggnog, apple pie, fresh-cut roses, and cappuccino. In the quasi-experiment that followed, participants were presented with scents in glass test tubes, one at a time and in random order, and continued to smell each scent while completing the dependent measures. In particular, they reported their level of nostalgia ("How nostalgic does this scent make you feel?") and level of self-continuity ("connected with my past," "important aspects of my personality remain the same across time"—both items derived from the Self-Continuity Index). Higher intensity of scent-evoked nostalgia predicted greater self-continuity. Similarly, nostalgia has been manipulated among U.S. MTurkers with scents (i.e., fragrance, sunscreen) that were past focused to elicit nostalgia versus present focused (control). Self-continuity was measured with the 4-item Self-Continuity Index. Nostalgia amplified self-continuity (Ju, Kim, Chang, & Bluck, 2016, Studies 1a and 1b).

In addition, nostalgia has been manipulated behaviorally. Chinese master of business administration (MBA) students who chose cookies from a nostalgia brand (Want Want) versus a non-nostalgic brand (Kraft Foods) reported higher self-continuity, as measured by the 4-item Self-Continuity Index (Xu & Jin, 2020).

As mentioned previously, self-continuity has been conceptualized and measured not just in terms of the perceived connection between one's past and present selves but also in terms of the perceived connection among one's past, present, and future selves (i.e., global self-continuity; Becker et al., 2018). Nostalgia, manipulated with the ERT, elevated global self-continuity in a British Prolific sample (Hong et al., 2021, Study 2).

The influence of nostalgia on self-continuity has also been examined in an intervention (Layous, Kurtz, Wildschut, & Sedikides, 2022). U.S. undergraduates completed the ERT every week for 6 consecutive weeks. Self-continuity was assessed (with the 4-item Self-Continuity Index) immediately after each weekly nostalgia induction. Nostalgia fostered self-continuity throughout the 6-week intervention.

Finally, nostalgia and self-continuity are transmitted intergenerationally (Wildschut, Sedikides, & Robertson, 2018). Participants were younger adults (i.e., British undergraduates). They were presented with one of five nostalgic narratives and one of five ordinary narratives, randomly selected from a large pool of narratives. The 10 narratives were statistically treated as a random variable (Judd, Westfall, & Kenny, 2012) for generalizability purposes. Participants learned that each narrative referred to a genuine event recalled and written by an older adult. Participants took a few minutes to read and reflect on each narrative. Subsequently, they rated their level of nostalgia on three items (e.g., "Right now, I am feeling quite nostalgic"; Wildschut et al., 2006) and their level of self-continuity on the 4-item Self-Continuity Index. Participants who read a nostalgic (vs. ordinary) narrative reported greater nostalgia, which in turn was associated with higher self-continuity.

INDIRECT EFFECTS OF NOSTALGIA ON SELF-CONTINUITY. How might nostalgia increase self-continuity? Social connectedness, the subjective experience of acceptance and belongingness, is a prime candidate. Nostalgia is a social emotion. During nostalgic reverie, "the mind is 'peopled'" (Hertz, 1990, p. 195) as one reestablishes a symbolic bond with close others. Nostalgic events often depict socializing with close others (Abeyta, Routledge, Roylance, Wildschut, & Sedikides, 2015; Wildschut et al., 2006). As a case in point, nostalgic (vs. ordinary) narratives contain a higher proportion of first-person plural pronouns, more social interactions, stronger expressions of companionship (Wildschut et al., 2018), and an increased number of social terms (e.g., *family*, *friend*, *love*, *child*, *people*; Chen, Wildschut, Layous, & Sedikides, 2023). Moreover, manipulated nostalgia galvanizes a sense of attachment to close others (Wildschut et al., 2006; Wildschut, Sedikides, Routledge, Arndt, & Cordaro2010) and ingroups (Abakoumkin, Wildschut, Sedikides, & Bakarou, 2017), and it strengthens perceptions of social support from one's networks (Zhou, Sedikides, Wildschut, & Gao, 2008). In all, nostalgia augments social connectedness (Juhl & Biskas, 2023; Sedikides & Wildschut, 2019).

Nostalgic events often reflect relational or cultural rituals, such as Thanksgiving, festivals, and national holidays (Yin et al., 2024; Yin, Jiang, Thomas, Wildschut, & Sedikides, 2025). These rituals are largely defined by the people surrounding the nostalgizer, and they weave the narrative thread of one's close relationships. For example, nostalgic recollections of a childhood family Thanksgiving may evoke memories of other Thanksgivings and thus constitute a mental storyboard of one's relationships with parents and siblings across the years, thereby contributing to self-continuity.

A series of experiments tested and supported the idea that social connectedness mediates the effect of nostalgia on self-continuity (Sedikides et al., 2016). In all experiments, social connectedness was assessed with the relevant 4-item ("I feel connected to loved ones"; "I feel protected"; "I feel loved"; "I feel I can trust others") subscale of the Nostalgia Functions Scale (Hepper et al., 2012), whereas self-continuity was assessed with the 4-item Self-Continuity Index. In Experiment 1, testing British undergraduates, nostalgia was induced via music (as in Ismail et al., 2018, Experiment 2). In Experiment 2, testing both British and Chinese undergraduates, nostalgia was induced with the ERT. In Experiment 3, testing U.S. MTurk workers, nostalgia was induced with a variation of the ERT, in which control participants brought to mind a positive past event ("[B]ring to mind a lucky event in your life. Specifically, try to think of a positive past event that was brought on by chance rather than through your own actions"; Sedikides et al., 2016, p. 529).

Follow-up research replicated and extended this mediational pattern (Abakoumkin, Hepper, Wildschut, & Sedikides, 2019). Social connectedness and self-continuity were assessed as described previously. In Experiment 1, a three-condition ERT was implemented among Greek undergraduates. One control condition provided general instructions ("[T]hink of an ordinary event in your life"; p. 132), whereas the other gave specific instructions ("[T]hink of a past event that is completely ordinary, common, everyday. For example, an event like taking the city bus to get from one place to another"; p. 133). In Experiment 2, nostalgia was induced via both the standard ERT and a prototype-based manipulation (as in Jiang, Cheung, et al., 2021) among British undergraduates. With the prototype-based manipulation, participants in the nostalgia condition brought to mind an event characterized by central features of nostalgia (e.g., "reminiscence," "keepsakes, "familiar smells," "rose-tinted memories"), whereas participants in the control condition brought to mind an event characterized by peripheral nostalgia features (i.e., "daydreaming," "wishing," "bittersweet," "achievements").

All five experiments that we reviewed (Abakoumkin et al., 2019, Experiments 1 and 2; Sedikides et al., 2016, Experiments 1–3) tested and supported the mediational model—namely, that the impact of nostalgia on self-continuity is transmitted by social connectedness. However, these experiments implemented a measurement-of-mediation design. Such designs have come under criticism for leaving open alternative interpretations (Maxwell & Cole, 2007; O'Laughlin, Martin, & Ferre, 2018). In our case, both the mediator (i.e., social connectedness) and the dependent variable (i.e., self-continuity) were measured, a practice that introduces uncertainty regarding their causal ordering. Yet measurement-of-mediation designs are also informative because they place the hypothesis at risk (Anderson & Bushman, 1997; Fiedler, Schott, & Meiser, 2011), thus increasing its empirical plausibility when supported. Nevertheless, more conclusive evidence would be obtained by using an experimental-causal-chain design (Spencer, Zanna, & Fong, 2005), in which the mediator is manipulated, assessing its causal influence on the dependent measure.

Sedikides et al. (2016, Experiment 4) used such a design among British undergraduates. Social connectedness was operationalized in terms of loneliness (Wildschut et al., 2006; Zhou et al., 2008). High social connectedness was assumed to involve low loneliness, and vice versa. Participants filled out the ostensible "Southampton Loneliness Scale," which consisted of 15 statements derived from the UCLA Loneliness Scale (Russell, Peplau, & Cutrona, 1980). Participants indicated whether they disagreed or agreed with each item. In the high-social-connectedness condition, the items were worded so as to draw out disagreement (e.g., "I always feel that I am 'out of tune' with the people around me"), whereas in the low-social-connectedness condition, the items were worded so as to draw out agreement (e.g., "I sometimes feel that I am 'out of tune' with the people around me"). Next, participants received bogus feedback. Those in the high-social-connectedness condition were told that they were in the 12th percentile of the loneliness score distribution and were thus "very low on loneliness" relative to their peers. Those in the low-social-connectedness condition were told that they were in the 62nd percentile of the loneliness score distribution and were thus "above average on loneliness" relative to their peers. Finally, participants were asked to list reasons why their scores were so low or high. The manipulation of social connectedness was effective. Afterward, participants complete the 4-item Social Continuity Index. Participants with high social connectedness reported greater self-continuity compared with those with low social connectedness. This finding reinforced the status of social connectedness as a mediator of nostalgia's effect on self-continuity.

Self-Continuity Is Associated with, or Augments, Meaning

Self-continuity engenders the perception that one's life is coherent, predictable, or comprehensible (Sedikides et al., 2023). It stands to reason, then, that nostalgia-induced self-continuity would be positively related to meaning, and this hypothesis was supported in several studies (Evans et al., 2021; Hepper et al., 2024; Wildschut et al., 2019). In these studies, self-continuity was measured with the 4-item Self-Continuity Scale, and meaning was measured with the 4-item subscale of the Nostalgia Functions Scale (Hepper et al., 2012). The specific items, preceded by the stem "I feel that . . . ," were as follows: "life is meaningful," "life has a purpose," "there is a greater purpose to life," and "life is worth living."

Further, self-continuity causally affects meaning (Van Tilburg, Sedikides, Wildschut, & Vingerhoets, 2019, Study 1). U.S. MTurkers underwent a self-continuity manipulation (after Sedikides, Wildschut, Routledge, & Arndt, 2015, Study 2). Participants in the high-self-continuity condition were asked to describe an important aspect of their lives that "you believe characterized you in the past, and continues to characterize you in the present," whereas participants in the low-self-continuity condition were asked to describe an important aspect of their life that "you believe characterized you in the past, but no longer characterizes you in the present" (Van Tilburg et al., 2019, p. 523). Afterward, all participants responded to two meaning items ("I feel that life is meaningful"; "I feel that life has a purpose"). Participants in the high-self-continuity condition reported greater meaning than those in the low-self-continuity condition.

A large literature has established not only that nostalgic events are meaningful but also that experimentally manipulated nostalgia increases meaning (Sedikides & Wildschut, 2018, 2024a). More importantly, self-continuity mediates the effect of nostalgia on meaning (Van Tilburg et al., 2019, Study 1). In a sample of Irish community members, nostalgia was induced with the ERT, self-continuity was measured with the 4-item Self-Continuity Scale, and meaning was measured with five items (preceded by the stem "This memory gives me . . ."): "a sense of meaning," "a sense of purpose," "the impression that things make sense," "a sense of value," and "a sense of significance" (after Van Tilburg, Igou, & Sedikides, 2013, Study 6). Nostalgia augmented meaning via self-continuity. This finding was replicated in an ERT experiment in which self-continuity was also measured with the 4-item Self-Continuity Scale, but meaning was measured with the 4-item subscale of the Nostalgia Functions Scale (Biskas et al., 2022, Study 3).

Moreover, this pattern was replicated with a music induction of nostalgia in Dutch community samples. In a within-participants design (Van Tilburg et al., 2019, Study 3), participants listened to a nostalgic song and a happy (control) song. After listening to each song, they completed measures of self-continuity (whether the song made them feel "connected to your past" and "that there is continuity in your life") and of meaning (whether the song made them feel that "life is meaningful" and "life has a purpose"). In a between-participants design (Van Tilburg et al., 2019, Study 4), participants listened either to a nostalgic song or a happy (control) song before completing the same measures of self-continuity and meaning. In both studies, the effect of nostalgia on meaning was transmitted by self-continuity.

CONCLUDING REMARKS

Guided by the regulatory model of nostalgia, we reviewed findings on the interplay of self-discontinuity, nostalgia, self-continuity, and meaning. Self-discontinuity is associated with, or leads to, nostalgia. In turn, nostalgia reestablishes self-continuity, which is a source of meaning. The regulatory model is based on the assumption that people actively create meaning (chapter 1, Fishbach, Fujita, and Liberman, this volume), and we argued that they do so, in part, through nostalgia and self-continuity. Yet the regulatory model could be enriched by addressing various issues.

The Character of the Instigating Events

One set of issues entails the character of the event that sets the regulatory cycle in motion. How disruptive or unfavorable should an event be? A longitudinal study included events ranging in unfavorability, but data analyses collapsed across them (Wang, Wildschut, Sedikides, Wu, & Ca,

2024). A curvilinear relation is plausible: Nostalgia might be instigated by moderately disruptive, rather than trivially or overwhelmingly disruptive, events.

Self-discontinuity can involve temporal or psychological distance from the present; it can also involve social distance, such as when a person was an important part of one's life but no longer has that role (Liberman & Trope, 2014). Is the strength of nostalgia as a regulatory mechanism equally effective for both kinds of distance?

We discussed discontinuity between one's past and present selves. Discontinuity, however, can also pertain to one's present versus future selves (Hershfield, 2023). For example, one may interact virtually with their aged future self (Shen, Nelson, & Oberlin, 2022) or write a letter to their future self that differs on socioeconomic (e.g., social class) variables (Simić, Vardo, & Solaković, 2021). Is the regulatory model equally effective in the case of future self-discontinuity? Preliminary evidence indicates that it is.

Metamotivation

Another set of issues entails metamotivation, the "psychological processes that monitor and modify motivational states" (Fujita, Le, Scholer, & Miele, 2024, p. 2). What is the nature of the association between self-discontinuity and nostalgia? Is this association part of the individual's coping repertoire intended to maintain homeostasis (Sedikides, 2021), or is it formed consciously or metamotivationally? The same questions apply to the association between nostalgia and self-continuity, as well as meaning.

As a potent response to self-discontinuity, nostalgia could be widely implemented as an intervention strategy. Prior attempts, though, have indicated that nostalgia is more effective among individuals who are dispositionally high on nostalgia (Layous et al., 2022; Sedikides & Wildschut, 2024b). It is likely that high nostalgics have better metamotivational insight into the emotion's benefits than low nostalgics. If so, interventions should be tailored differently for low nostalgics, teaching them how to reap the benefits of nostalgic reverie.

Generalizability and Neuronal Underpinnings

Our conceptual framework invites comprehensive testing in cross-sectional, longitudinal, momentary-ecological-assessment, and experimental investigations. Also, it invites examinations of its generalizability across cultures and across ages. For example, some research suggests that Chinese (compared with Canadians of European descent) individuals report higher self-continuity as a result of feeling closer to their past and present selves (Ji et al., 2019). In addition, some research indicates that older (compared with younger) adults experience more nostalgia (Madoglou, Gkinopoulos, Xanthopoulos, & Kalamaras, 2017) and self-continuity (Liao & Bluck, 2023). Might this explain why older adults sometimes report more meaning than younger adults (Morgan & Robinson, 2013; Reker, Peacock, & Wong, 1987)? Finally, future work will do well to examine how the interplay among self-discontinuity, nostalgia, self-continuity, and meaning is reflected in brain processes (Di Domenico et al., 2018; Kang et al., 2019; Yang, Strecher, Kim, & Falk, 2023).

REFERENCES

Abakoumkin, G., Hepper, E. G., Wildschut, T., & Sedikides, C. (2019). From nostalgia through social connectedness to self-continuity: Replication and extension. *Hellenic Journal of Psychology, 16*(2), 127–144.

Abakoumkin, G., Wildschut, T., Sedikides, C., & Bakarou, M. (2017). Nostalgia in response to group-based exclusion: The role of attachment-related avoidance. *European Journal of Social Psychology, 47*(3), 373–381.

Abeyta, A., Routledge, C., Roylance, C., Wildschut, R. T., & Sedikides, C. (2015). Attachment-related avoidance and the social and agentic content of nostalgic memories. *Journal of Social and Personal Relationships, 32*(3), 406–413.

Anderson, C. A., & Bushman, B. J. (1997). External validity of "trivial" experiments: The case of laboratory aggression. *Review of General Psychology, 1*(1), 19–41.

Anderzén, I., & Arnetz, B. B. (1999). Psychophysiological reactions to international adjustment: Results from a controlled, longitudinal study. *Psychotherapy and Psychosomatics, 68*(2), 67–75.

Batcho, K. I. (1995). Nostalgia: A psychological perspective. *Perceptual and Motor Skills, 80*(1), 131–143.

Batcho, K. I. (2021) The role of nostalgia in resistance: A psychological perspective. *Qualitative Research in Psychology, 18*(2), 227–249.

Becker, M., Vignoles, V. L., Owe, E., Easterbrook, M. J., Brown, R., Smith, P. B., et al. (2018). Being oneself through time: Bases of self-continuity across 55 cultures. *Self and Identity, 17*(3), 276–293.

Best, J., & Nelson, E. E. (1985). Nostalgia and discontinuity: A test of the Davis hypothesis. *Sociology and Social Relations, 69*(2), 221–233.

Biskas, M., Juhl, J., Wildschut, T., Sedikides, C., & Saroglou, V. (2022). Nostalgia and spirituality: The roles of self-continuity and meaning in life. *Social Psychology, 53*(3), 152–162.

Brown, A. D., & Humphreys, M. (2002). Nostalgia and the narrativization of identity: A Turkish case study. *British Journal of Management, 13*(2), 141–159.

Campbell, D. T., & Fiske, D. W. (1959). Convergent and discriminant validation by the multitrait-multimethod matrix. *Psychological Bulletin, 56*(2), 81–105.

Chandler, M. J., & Proulx, T. (2008). Personal persistence and persistent people: Continuities in the lives of individuals and whole cultural communities. In F. Sani (Ed.), *Self-continuity: Individual and collective perspectives* (pp. 213–226). Taylor & Francis.

Chang, N. J., Schneider, R. C., Connaughton, D. P., Hager, P. F, & Ju, I. (2019). The effect of nostalgia on self-continuity, pride, and intention to visit a sport team's hometown. *Journal of Sport & Tourism, 23*(2–3), 115–131.

Chen, J., Wildschut, T., Layous, K., & Sedikides, C. (2023). Identifying nostalgia in text: The development and validation of the Nostalgia Dictionary. *Journal of Consumer Psychology, 33*(4), 728–742.

Cheung, W.-Y., Sedikides, C., & Wildschut, T. (2017). Nostalgia and prejudice reduction. *Personality and Individual Differences, 109*, 89–97.

Coenen, L. H. M., Hedebouw, L., & Semin, G. R. (2006). *Measuring language abstraction: The linguistic category model (LCM). www.cratylus.org/resources/uploadedFiles/1151434261594- 8567.pdf*

Costin, V., & Vignoles, V. L. (2020). Meaning is about mattering: Evaluating coherence, purpose, and existential mattering as precursors of meaning in life judgments. *Journal of Personality and Social Psychology, 118*(4), 864–884.

Czekierda, K., Banik, A., Park, C. L., & Luszczynska, A. (2017). Meaning in life and physical health: Systematic review and meta-analysis. *Health Psychology Review, 11*(4), 387–418.

Davis, F. (1979). *Yearning for yesterday: A sociology of nostalgia.* Free Press.

Di Domenico, S. I., Fournier, M. A., Rodrigo, A. H., Dong, M., Ayaz, H., & Ruocco, A. C. (2018). Need fulfillment and the modulation of medial prefrontal activity when judging remembered past, perceived present, and imagined future identities. *Self Identity, 17*(3), 259–275.

Evans, N. D., Reyes, J., Wildschut, T., Sedikides, C., & Fetterman, A. K. (2021). Mental transportation mediates nostalgia's psychological benefits. *Cognition and Emotion, 35*(1), 84–95.

Fetterman, A. K., Evans, N. D., Ravey, E. P., Henderson, P. R., Tran, B. H. L., & Boyd, R. L. (2024). The topics of nostalgic recall: The benefits of nostalgia depend on the topics that one recalls. *Social Psychological and Personality Science, 16*(4), 444–456.

Fiedler, K., Schott, M., & Meiser, T. (2011). What mediation analysis can (not) do. *Journal of Experimental Social Psychology, 47*(6), 1231–1236.

Frankl, V. E. (1984). *Man's search for meaning.* Washington Square Press. (Original work published 1946)

Fujita, K., Le, P. Q., Scholer, A. A., & Miele, D. N. (2024). The metamotivation approach: Insights into the regulation of motivation and beyond. *Social and Personality Psychology Compass, 18*(2), e12937.

Habermas, T., & Köber, C. (2015). Autobiographical reasoning in life narratives buffers the effect of biographical disruptions on the sense of self-continuity. *Memory, 23*(5), 664–674.

Hepper, E. G., Ritchie, T. D., Sedikides, C., & Wildschut, T. (2012). Odyssey's end: Lay conceptions of nostalgia reflect its original Homeric meaning. *Emotion, 12*(1), 102–119.

Hepper, E. G., Sedikides, C., Wildschut, T., Cheung, W.-Y., Abakoumkin, G., Arikan, G., et al. (2024). Pancultural nostalgia in action: Prevalence, triggers, and psychological functions of nostalgia across cultures. *Journal of Experimental Psychology: General, 153*(3), 754–777.

Hepper, E. G., Wildschut, T., Sedikides, C., Ritchie, T. D., Yung, Y.-F., Hansen, N., et al. (2014). Pancultural nostalgia: Prototypical conceptions across cultures. *Emotion, 14*(4), 733–747.

Hepper, E. G., Wildschut, T., Sedikides, C., Robertson, S., & Routledge, C. D. (2021). Time capsule: Nostalgia shields psychological wellbeing from limited time horizons. *Emotion, 21*(3), 644–664.

Hershfield, H. (2023). *Your future self: How to make tomorrow better today.* Hachette.

Hertz, D. G. (1990). Trauma and nostalgia: New aspects of the coping of aging holocaust survivors. *Israeli Journal of Psychiatry and Related Sciences, 27*(4), 189–198.

Holmes, T. H., & Rahe, R. H. (1967). The Social Readjustment Rating Scale. *Journal of Psychosomatic Research, 11*(2), 213–218.

Hong, E. K., Sedikides, C., & Wildschut, T. (2021). Nostalgia strengthens global self-continuity through holistic thinking. *Cognition and Emotion, 35*(4), 730–737.

Hong, E. K., Sedikides, C., & Wildschut, T. (2022). How does nostalgia conduce to global self-continuity? The roles of identity narrative, associative links, and stability. *Personality and Social Psychology Bulletin, 48*(5), 735–749.

Hooker, S. A., Masters, K. S., & Park, C. L. (2018). A meaningful life is a healthy life: A conceptual model linking meaning and meaning salience to health. *Review of General Psychology, 22*(1), 11–24.

Ismail, S., Christopher, G., Dodd, E., Wildschut, T., Sedikides, C., Ingram, T. A., Jones, R. W., Nooman, K. A., Tingley, D., & Cheston, R. (2018). Psychological and mnemonic benefits of nostalgia for people with dementia. *Journal of Alzheimer's Disease, 65*(4), 1327–1344.

Ismail, S., Dodd, E., Christopher, G., Wildschut, T., Sedikides, C., & Cheston, R. (2022). The content and function of nostalgic memories of people living with dementia. *International Journal of Aging and Human Development, 94*(4), 436–459.

Iyer, A., & Jetten, J. (2011). What's left behind: Identity continuity moderates the effect of nostalgia on well-being and life choices. *Journal of Personality and Social Psychology, 101*(1), 94–108.

Ji, L.-J., Hong, E., Guo, T., Zhang, Z., Su, Y., & Li, Y. (2019). Culture, psychological proximity to the past and future, and self-continuity. *European Journal of Social Psychology, 49*(4), 735–747.

Jiang, T., Chen, Z., & Sedikides, C. (2020). Self-concept clarity lays the foundation for self-continuity: The restorative function of autobiographical memory. *Journal of Personality and Social Psychology, 119*(4), 945–959.

Jiang, T., Chen, Z., Wang, S., & Hou, Y. (2021). Ostracism disrupts self-continuity. *Personality and Social Psychology Bulletin, 47*(9), 1390–1400.

Jiang, T., Cheung, W.-Y., Wildschut, T., & Sedikides, C. (2021). Nostalgia, reflection, brooding: Psychological benefits and autobiographical memory functions. *Consciousness and Cognition, 90*, Article 103107.

Joseph, D. L., Chan, M. Y., Heintzelman, S. J., Tay, L., Diener, E., & Scotney, V. S. (2020). The manipulation of affect: A meta-analysis of affect induction procedures. *Psychological Bulletin, 146*(4), 355–375.

Ju, I., Kim, J., Chang, M., J., & Bluck, S. (2016). Nostalgic marketing, perceived self-continuity, and consumer decisions. *Management Decision, 54*(8), 2063–2083.

Judd, C. M., Westfall, J., & Kenny, D. A. (2012). Treating stimuli as a random factor in social psychology: A new and comprehensive solution to a pervasive but largely ignored problem. *Journal of Personality and Social Psychology, 103*(1), 54–69.

Juhl, J., & Biskas, M. (2023). Nostalgia: An impactful social emotion. *Current Opinion in Psychology, 49*, Article 101545.

Kang, Y., Strecher, V. J., Kim, E., & Falk, E. B. (2019). Purpose in life and conflict-related neural responses during health decision-making. *Health Psychology, 38*(6), 545–552.

Kim, H. S., & Wohl, M. J. A. (2015). The bright side of feeling disconnected with the past self: Self-discontinuity (via nostalgia) increases readiness to change unhealthy behaviors. *Social Psychology and Personality Science, 6*(2), 229–237.

King, L. A., & Hicks, J. A. (2021). The science of meaning in life. *Annual Review of Psychology, 72*, 561–584.

Landau, M. J., Greenberg, J., & Solomon, S. (2008). The never-ending story: A terror management perspective on the psychological function of self-continuity. In F. Sani (Ed.), *Self-continuity: Individual and collective perspectives* (pp. 87–100). Taylor & Francis.

Lasaleta, J. D., & Loveland, K. E. (2019). What's new is old again: Nostalgia and retro-styling in response to authenticity threats. *Journal of the Association for Consumer Research, 4*(2), 172–184.

Layous, K., Kurtz, J. L., Wildschut, T., & Sedikides, C. (2022). The effect of a multi-week nostalgia intervention on well-being: Mechanisms and moderation. *Emotion, 22*(8), 1952–1968.

Leunissen, J. M., Wildschut, T., Sedikides, C., & Routledge, C. (2021). The hedonic character of nostalgia: An integrative data analysis. *Emotion Review, 13*(2), 139–156.

Liao, H.-W., & Bluck, S. (2023). Recalling self-disruptive events and maintaining self-continuity in adulthood. *Psychology and Aging, 38*(1), 17–29.

Liberman, N., & Trope, Y. (2014). Traversing psychological distance. *Trends in Cognitive Sciences, 18*(7), 364–369.

Liu, X. C., Liu, L. Q., Yang, J., & Zhao, G. F. (1997). 青少年 生活事件量表的信度效度检验 [Reliability and validity of the Adolescent Self-Rating Life Events Checklist]. 中国临 床心理学杂志/ [*Chinese Journal of Clinical Psychology*], *5*, 34–36.

Loh, H. S., Gaur, S. S., & Lim., R. J.-H. (2019). Childhood brand nostalgia, perceived self-continuity and brand loyalty. *Journal of Emerging Trends in Marketing and Management, 1*(1), 52–62.

Madoglou, A., Gkinopoulos, T., Xanthopoulos, P., & Kalamaras, D. (2017). Representations of autobiographical nostalgic memories: Generational effect, gender, nostalgia proneness and communication of nostalgic experiences. *Journal of Integrated Social Sciences, 7*(1), 60–88.

Maxwell, S. E., & Cole, D. A. (2007). Bias in cross-sectional analyses of longitudinal mediation. *Psychological Methods, 12*(1), 23–44.

McAdams, D., Reynolds, J., Lewis, M., Patten, A., & Bowman, P. (2001). When bad things turn good and good things turn bad: Sequences of redemption and contamination in life narrative, and their relation to psychosocial adaptation in midlife adults and in students. *Personality and Social Psychology Bulletin, 27*(4), 472–83.

McDonald, R., Waring, J., & Harrison, S. (2006). At the cutting edge? Modernization and nostalgia in a hospital operating theatre department. *Sociology, 40*(6), 1097–1115.

Milligan, M. J. (2003). Displacement and identity discontinuity: The role of nostalgia in establishing new identity categories. *Symbolic Interaction, 26*(3), 381–403.

Miranda, R., & Nolen-Hoeksema, S. (2007). Brooding and reflection: Rumination predicts suicidal ideation at 1-year follow-up in a community sample. *Behaviour Research and Therapy, 45*(12), 3088–3095.

Morgan, J., & Robinson, O. (2013). Intrinsic aspirations and personal meaning across adulthood: Conceptual interrelations and age/sex differences. *Developmental Psychology, 49*(5), 999–1010.

O'Laughlin, K. D., Martin, M. J., & Ferrer, E. (2018). Cross-sectional analysis of longitudinal mediation processes. *Multivariate Behavioral Research, 53*(3), 375–402.

Pearsall, J. (Ed.). (1998). Nostalgia. In *The new Oxford dictionary of English.* Oxford University Press.

Pennebaker, J. W., Booth, R. J., & Francis, M. E. (2007). *Linguistic inquiry and word count: LIWC2007. Operator's manual.* LIWC.net

Reid, C. A., Green, J. D., Wildschut, T., & Sedikides, C. (2015). Scent-evoked nostalgia. *Memory, 23*(2), 157–166.

Reker, G. T., Peacock, E. J., & Wong, P. T. (1987). Meaning and purpose in life and well-being: A life-span perspective. *Journal of Gerontology, 42*(1), 44–49.

Reker, G. T., & Wong, P. T. P. (1988). Aging as an individual process: Toward a theory of personal meaning. In J. E. Birren & V. L. Bengtson (Eds.), *Emergent theories of aging* (pp. 214–246). Springer.

Routledge, C., Arndt, J., Sedikides, C., & Wildschut, T. (2008). A blast from the past: The terror management function of nostalgia. *Journal of Experimental Social Psychology, 44*(1), 132–140.

Routledge, C., Arndt, J., Wildschut, T., Sedikides, C., Hart, C. M., Juhl, J., et al. (2011). The past makes the present meaningful: Nostalgia as an existential resource. *Journal of Personality and Social Psychology, 101*(3), 638–652.

Russell, D., Peplau, L. A., & Cutrona, C. E. (1980). The revised UCLA Loneliness Scale: Concurrent and discriminant validity evidence. *Journal of Personality and Social Psychology, 39*(3), 472–480.

Sadeh, N., & Karniol, R. (2012). The sense of self-continuity as a resource in adaptive coping with job loss. *Journal of Vocational Behavior, 80*(1), 93–99.

Sedikides, C. (2021). Self-construction, self-protection, and self-enhancement: A homeostatic model of identity protection. *Psychological Inquiry, 32*(4), 197–221.

Sedikides, C., Hong, E., & Wildschut, T. (2023). Self-continuity. *Annual Review of Psychology, 74*, 333–361.

Sedikides, C., & Wildschut, T. (2018). Finding meaning in nostalgia. *Review of General Psychology, 22*(1), 48–61.

Sedikides, C., & Wildschut, T. (2019). The sociality of personal and collective nostalgia. *European Review of Social Psychology, 30*(1), 123–173.

Sedikides, C., & Wildschut, T. (2022). Nostalgia across cultures. *Journal of Pacific Rim Psychology, 16*, 1–16.

Sedikides, C., & Wildschut, T. (2024a). Nostalgia: The existential value of temporal longing. In K. Vail, D. Van Tongeren, B. Schlegel, J. Greenberg, L. King, & R. Ryan (Eds.), *Handbook of the science of existential psychology* (pp. 200–214). Guilford Press.

Sedikides, C., & Wildschut, T. (2024b). Trait nostalgia. *Personality and Individual Differences, 221*, Article 112554.

Sedikides, C., Wildschut, T., Cheung, W.-Y., Routledge, C., Hepper, E. G., Arndt, J., et al. (2016). Nostalgia fosters self-continuity: Uncovering the mechanism (social connectedness) and the consequence (eudaimonic well-being). *Emotion, 16*(4), 524–539.

Sedikides, C., Wildschut, T., Gaertner, L., Routledge, C., & Arndt, J. (2008). Nostalgia as enabler of self-continuity. In F. Sani (Ed.), *Self-continuity: Individual and collective perspectives* (pp. 227–239). Psychology Press.

Sedikides, C., Wildschut, T., Routledge, C., & Arndt, J. (2015). Nostalgia counteracts self-discontinuity and restores self-continuity. *European Journal of Social Psychology, 45*(1), 52–61.

Sedikides, C., Wildschut, T., Routledge, C., Arndt, J., Hepper, E. G., & Zhou, X. (2015). To nostalgize: Mixing memory with affect and desire. *Advances in Experimental Social Psychology, 51*, 189–273.

Shen, Y. I., Nelson, A. I., & Oberlin, B. J. (2022). Virtual reality intervention effects on future self–continuity and delayed reward preference in substance use disorder recovery: Pilot study results. *Discover Mental Health, 2*(1), 19.

Simić, A., Vardo, E., & Solaković, S. (2021). Future self-continuity increases responsibility during Covid-19 restrictions. *Psihologijske Teme, 30*(2), 205–223.

Sokol, Y., & Eisenheim, E. (2016). The relationship between continuous identity disturbances, negative mood, and suicidal ideation. *Primary Care Companion for CNS Disorders, 18*(1).

Sokol, Y., & Serper, M. (2019). Temporal self, psychopathology, and adaptive functioning deficits: An examination of acute psychiatric patients. *Journal of Nervous and Mental Disease, 207*(2), 76–83.

Spencer, S. J., Zanna, M., & Fong, G. T. (2005). Establishing a causal chain: Why experiments are often more effective than mediational analyses in examining psychological processes. *Journal of Personality and Social Psychology, 89*(6), 845–851.

Steger, M. F., Frazier, P., Oishi, S., & Kaler, M. (2006). The meaning in life questionnaire: Assessing the presence of and search for meaning in life. *Journal of Counseling Psychology, 53*(1), 80–93.

Stephan, E., Sedikides, C., & Wildschut, T. (2012). Mental travel into the past: Differentiating recollections of nostalgic, ordinary, and positive events. *European Journal of Social Psychology, 42*(3), 290–298.

Treynor, W., Gonzalez, R., & Nolen-Hoeksema, S. (2003). Rumination reconsidered: A psychometric analysis. *Cognitive Therapy and Research, 27*(3), 247–259.

Trope, Y., Ledgerwood, A., Liberman, N., & Fujita, K. (2021). Regulatory scope and its mental and social supports. *Perspectives on Psychological Science, 16*(2) 204–224.

Van Tilburg, W. A. P., Igou, E. R., & Sedikides, C. (2013). In search of meaningfulness: Nostalgia as an antidote to boredom. *Emotion, 13*(3), 450–461.

Van Tilburg, W. A. P., Sedikides, C., Wildschut, T., & Vingerhoets, A. J. J. M. (2019). How nostalgia infuses life with meaning: from social connectedness to self-continuity. *European Journal of Social Psychology, 49*(3), 521–532.

Wang, Y., Tian, H., Sarigöllü, E., & Xu, W. (2020). Nostalgia prompts sustainable product disposal. *Journal of Consumer Behaviour, 19*(6), 570–580.

Wang, Y., Wildschut, T., Sedikides, C., Wu, M., & Cai, H. (2024). Trajectory of nostalgia in emerging adulthood. *Personality and Social Psychology Bulletin, 50*(4), 629–644.

Waskul, D. D., Vannini, P., & Wilson, J. (2009). The aroma of recollection: Olfaction, nostalgia, and the shaping of the sensuous self. *The Senses and Society, 4*(1), 5–22.

Werman, D. S. (1977). Normal and pathological nostalgia. *Journal of the American Psychoanalytic Association, 25*(2), 387–398.

Wildschut, T., & Sedikides, C. (2023a). Benefits of nostalgia in vulnerable populations. *European Review of Social Psychology, 34*(1), 44–91.

Wildschut, T., & Sedikides, C. (2023b). Water from the lake of memory: The regulatory model of nostalgia. *Current Directions in Psychological Science, 32*(1), 57–64.

Wildschut, T., & Sedikides, C. (2024). Psychology and nostalgia: A primer on experimental nostalgia inductions. In T. Becker & D. Trigg (Eds.), *The Routledge handbook of nostalgia* (pp. 54–69). Routledge.

Wildschut, T., Sedikides, C., & Alowidy, D. (2019). *Hanin*: Nostalgia among Syrian refugees. *European Journal of Social Psychology, 49*(7), 1368–1384.

Wildschut, T., Sedikides, C., Arndt, J., & Routledge, C. (2006). Nostalgia:

Content, triggers, functions. *Journal of Personality and Social Psychology, 91*(5), 975–993.

Wildschut, T., Sedikides, C., & Robertson, S. (2018). Sociality and intergenerational transfer of older adults' nostalgia. *Memory, 26*(8), 1030–1041.

Wildschut, T., Sedikides, C., Routledge, C., Arndt, J., & Cordaro, P. (2010). Nostalgia as a repository of social connectedness: The role of attachment-related avoidance. *Journal of Personality and Social Psychology, 98*(4), 573–586.

Wohl, M. J. A., Kim, H. S., Salmon, M., Santesso, D., Wildschut, T., & Sedikides, C. (2018). Self-discontinuity-induced nostalgia improves the odds of a self-reported quit attempt among people living with addiction. *Journal of Experimental Social Psychology, 75*, 83–94.

Xu, W., & Jin, X.-T. (2020). Effects of social exclusion and implicit theories of personality on nostalgic consumption. *Social Behavior and Personality: An International Journal, 48*(3), 1–12.

Yin, Y., Jiang, T., Thomas, S., Wildschut, T., & Sedikides, C. (2025). Nostalgia promotes parents' tradition transfer to children: The role of self-child overlap. *Personality and Social Psychology Bulletin, 51*(3), 394–408.

Yin, Y., Jiang, T., Wildschut, T., & Sedikides, C. (2024). Nostalgia, ritual engagement, and meaning in life. *Personality and Social Psychology Bulletin*. Advance online publication. *doi.org/10.1177/01461672241235*7

Ylijoki, O.-H. (2005). Academic nostalgia: A narrative approach to academic work. *Human Relations, 58*(5), 555–576.

Zhang, F., Zhang, S., & Gao, X. (2022). Relationship between socioeconomic status and win-win values: Mediating roles of childhood neglect and self-continuity. *Frontiers in Psychiatry, 13*, Article 882933.

Zhou, X., Sedikides, C., Wildschut, T., & Gao, D. G. (2008). Counteracting loneliness: On the restorative function of nostalgia. *Psychological Science, 19*(10), 1023–1029.

Zou, X., Wildschut, T., Cable, D., & Sedikides, C. (2018). Nostalgia for host culture facilitates repatriation success: The role of self-continuity. *Self and Identity, 17*(3), 327–342.

CHAPTER 13

Continuity in Psychological Space Creates a Sense of Meaning in Life

Nira Liberman

WHAT CREATES A SENSE OF MEANING IN LIFE?

In this chapter, I examine the experience of meaning in life from the perspective of construal-level theory (CLT; Liberman & Trope, 2008; Trope & Liberman, 2010; Trope, Ledgerwood, Liberman, & Fujita, 2020). I propose that three conditions must be met for a person to feel that their life is meaningful. The first condition requires individuals to feel engaged with reality—sensing both their impact on the world and the world's significance to them—and that their self is continuous across the dimensions of that reality, that is, across time, space, social relations, and hypothetical possibilities. In CLT, these are psychological distances that constitute a person's ecology. Second, a person must form a higher-level, abstract concept of their life, such as a narrative or a purpose. This is a mental operation that creates continuity in mental space. Finally, these two—namely, the continuous self in the real world and the abstract mental construct of it—must align such that a person's narrative and sense of purpose will help integrate them into the swaths of time, space, social relations, and possible alternatives that are relevant to their life. In other words, I suggest that the experience of meaningfulness requires the immersion and continuity of the self in its ecology, the continuity of the mental constructs, and their successful mapping on each other. In a nutshell, a sense of meaning emerges from connecting elements, whereas a sense of meaninglessness results from rupture and disconnection between elements. In the case of meaning in life, we are talking about a connection between the self and the environment, between elements within one's mental system, and between the mental system and the environment. The remainder of this chapter elaborates on these concepts and situates them within the existing literature on meaning in life.

The present notion of meaning builds on the three core ideas of CLT. The first is that human ecology—namely, the environment that affects a person's life—consists not only of the places around them and their past and future (i.e., spatial and temporal scope) but also of their social surroundings and counterfactual worlds (i.e., social and hypotheticality scope). The second is that expanding scope—that is, considering more distant places, times, people, and possibilities—introduces the need to take into account more objects that are potentially more different from each other. In other words, expanding scope increases variability. Finally, the third relevant principle of CLT is that abstraction is a tool for finding unity within that variability, a tool that helps one regulate themselves with respect to distal times, places, people, and possibilities (Trope et al., 2020; see also Gilead, Trope, & Liberman, 2020).

The notion of meaning I present here is consistent with two different views on how people come to experience their life as meaningful. According to the first view, meaning is essentially a mental construct akin to "understanding" (Heintzelman & King, 2014b) that emerges when one's life makes sense (e.g., when one has a coherent narrative of one's life). A sense of meaning, in this view, is achieved via operations within one's mind, so in a crisis of meaninglessness, one could, for example, seek help from a psychotherapist, who would help one reach a better understanding of their life. According to the second view, meaning emerges from engagement and immersion in (as opposed to detachment from) one's ecology, and it arises when one is connected to (i.e., acts in, interacts with, affects and is affected by, is a part of) the real outside world that stretches across time, space, social networks, and the realm of possibilities. In this view, in a crisis of meaninglessness, one should seek engagement and oppose detachment (Hayes, 2005; Wilson & Murrell, 2004; Žižek, 2022). The present notion of meaning does not lean toward one of these views but rather embraces both and suggests that they are intertwined, a proposition that will repeatedly surface throughout this chapter. I turn now to elaborate on each of the proposed components of meaning.

MEANING AND CONTINUITY OF THE SELF IN TIME, SPACE, SOCIAL RELATIONS, AND HYPOTHETICAL WORLDS

The study of ecology suggests that an organism's physical environment plays an important role in shaping it and determining its behavior. Psychologists largely adopt this view (Todd & Gigerenzer, 2012) while also emphasizing that the relevant environment, at least in the case of humans, stretches not only across space but also across time, the network of social connections and hypothetical possibilities. People (re) act toward and regulate themselves with respect to objects that can be proximal or distal in these four dimensions of psychological distance: They make decisions about proximal or distal objects and situations, communicate over large or small distances, and understand and react to proximal or distal events. CLT (Liberman & Trope, 2008, 2014; Trope & Liberman, 2010) examines how the way people act and react toward objects depends on the object's psychological distance. For example, it suggests that people would construe "attending a political rally" in more abstract terms (e.g., as "being politically active" as opposed to "standing in a crowd and holding a banner") when the rally is next month rather than tonight (Liberman & Trope, 1998; Nguyen, Grinfeld, Liberman, & Wakslak, 2023; Sanchez, Coleman, & Ledgerwood, 2021), when it is far away rather than nearby (Fujita, Henderson, Eng, Trope, & Liberman, 2006), when it is more rather than less likely to happen (Grinfeld, Wakslak, Trope, & Liberman, 2024; Wakslak, Trope, Liberman, & Alony, 2006), and when advising a friend rather than deciding whether to attend the rally themselves (Danziger, Montal, & Barkan, 2012). The notion of regulatory scope (Trope et al., 2020) emphasizes that people have to regulate with respect to both proximal and distal objects (e.g., that they often have to plan to attend both proximal and distal rallies, that they might seek to motivate both close friends and total strangers to attend a rally), and that they use abstraction strategically to achieve that goal. I propose that expanding scope while maintaining continuity and successfully using abstraction to accommodate expansive yet continuous scope is not only adaptive but also creates a sense of meaning.

A recent study examined the relationship between meaning in life and dispositional regulatory scope (DRS; Sverdlik, Kalkstein, Levit, Trope, & Liberman, 2025). People with an expansive scope tend to make more distal plans, take into account more distal considerations when making decisions, and consider more distal outcomes of their actions across all four dimensions of scope. Sverdlik and her colleagues administered to participants a newly developed self-report measure of DRS, the Meaning in Life Questionnaire (MLQ; Steger, Frazier, Oishi, & Kaler, 2006), and a subjective well-being scale (Diener et al., 1985). As in previous studies (Li, Dou, & Liang, 2021), subjective well-being was positively correlated with having meaning in life but not with searching for it. In contrast, DRS was positively correlated with both having and searching for meaning, and this correlation remained positive even after controlling for well-being. These results are presented in Table 13.1.

TABLE 13.1. Multiple Regression Analyses Predicting the Two Components of Meaning in Life (MIL) from Dispositional Regulatory Scope (DRS) and Subjective Wellbeing

	Presence of MIL			Search for MIL		
Predictors	B	T	P	β	T	p
Subjective Wellbeing	.48	6.34	<.001	–.087	–1.01	.315
DRS	.17	2.19	.030	.24	2.74	.007

Note. β values are the standardized regression coefficients. Significant effects are marked in bold.

Going beyond the association between scope and meaning, I propose that meaning requires that the self is experienced as continuous. When the continuity of the self is ruptured, or when the scope expands but one does not "find themselves" in that expanded scope (in other words, when one cannot expand the self to encompass the expanded scope), a sense of meaninglessness ensues. For example, a person might experience meaninglessness upon realizing that they are very different from their past self (e.g., because they lost religious faith and are no longer the believer they used to be), upon being removed from their social and physical environment (e.g., because they immigrated to a new country), or upon losing their social role (e.g., because they were the breadwinner of the family and lost their job).

Typically, discontinuity results from negative events, and much of the literature on loss of meaning has examined how people cope with hardship, loss, and disaster. But neutral or even positive events can also engender meaninglessness if they create discontinuity in scope or expand it beyond what the self can accommodate. For example, people might experience meaninglessness when they find themselves in a social world that is far larger than what they were used to (e.g., a child who learns about other cultures or religions, a high school graduate who goes to college away from home), when they transition to a new social role (e.g., become parents), or when they consider stretches of scope beyond what they used to know (e.g., a person learns that life on earth dates back 4 billion years, rather than only 6,000 years). In fact, existential mattering, which is an important component of meaning in life (King & Hicks, 2021) and a precursor of a sense of meaning (Costin & Vignoles, 2020), has been operationalized as agreement with such statements as "Even considering how big the universe is, I can say that my life matters," and "Given the vastness of the universe, my life does not matter" (reverse scored; Costin & Vignoles, 2020). These statements reflect, in the present terminology, a successful accommodation of the self in a very expansive scope.

A loss of meaning due to expansion or rupture in scope often instigates a process of meaning making, which might involve adjusting to the expansion or mending of the rupture (Park, 2010). For example, when a young person leaves their family and local community to go to college, they expand both spatial and social scope. If these new experiences remain disconnected from the self, a loss of meaning ensues. However, once the person "finds their place" and accommodates to the expanded scope, they will experience personal growth and a reinstated sense of meaning. In this way, ruptures in and expansions of scope both challenge the sense of meaning and strengthen it. This is how coping systems typically work: Challenges to the sense of meaning may enhance it, just like an intense physical effort both challenges and builds muscles, and viral diseases both challenge the immune system and bolster it.

I now turn to examine experiences of continuity versus discontinuity in each dimension of scope: time, space, social relations, and the realm of hypothetical possibilities. Subsequently, I discuss the interrelations between these dimensions and how they apply to continuity.

Continuity in Time

One day, Gregor Samsa, a traveling salesman in Franz Kafka's *The Metamorphosis*, wakes up to find himself transformed into a giant insect. Initially, he struggles to adjust to his new body and tries to continue with his daily routine, but these efforts fail. He experiences loss of meaning. Gregor's presence becomes a burden to his family, and they decide that Gregor must be removed from their lives. In his final moments, Gregor is left alone and neglected (Kafka, 1912/1996).

Most personal transitions are less extreme: Adolescence, pregnancy, parenthood, retirement, and physical changes due to illness and accidents all threaten the continuity of the self in time and may create a sense of loss of meaning. More generally, discontinuity in time occurs when one feels that they are no longer the person that they used to be. The chapter by Sedikides and Wildschut in this volume presents a regulatory model of nostalgia, according to which discontinuity of the self across (past) time threatens the sense of meaning and instigates nostalgia, which signals the need to restore meaning and is followed by (oftentimes successful) attempts to do that (see also Routledge et al., 2011). For example, Sedikides, Wildschut, Routledge, and Arndt (2015, Experiment 3) induced nostalgia in participants by making them visualize a nostalgic event (vs. an ordinary event in the control condition) and found that it increased a sense of self-continuity (measured by items like "I feel connected with my past," and "The past and present flow seamlessly together.")

Theoretically, temporal discontinuity can emerge not only with the past self but also with the future self, for example, in anticipation of both adverse and more neutral changes (e.g., "when I get dementia," "when I become less of a workaholic"). I am not aware, however, of research on the effects of such anticipated future discontinuity on the sense of meaning.

Why is discontinuity of the self across time experienced as a problem? Why does it create a sense of meaninglessness? Is it a problem for the mind because it robs the self of its clarity and makes the self difficult to comprehend? Because it requires the person to simultaneously hold two inconsistent, "dissonant" beliefs about their self? Or does it pose a problem for functioning in the world? It is worth emphasizing that continuity of the self over time matters a lot in the real world: We always reap the fruits of our past self's labor and seed the life of our future self. Other people and social institutions also assume that we are continuous across time by assigning to our current and future selves legal and moral responsibility over past actions and expecting us to hold on to our interpersonal relationships and social roles. If our past and future selves are not "us," such a stance would undermine much of the value of our actions and decisions and would have the potential to untie social bonds, roles, and institutions. Hence, a self that lacks continuity in time is not only a "mental challenge" but also a problem for one's functioning in the real world.

CONTINUITY OF SOCIAL NETWORKS

Loss of social ties and social isolation are a potent cause of a sense of meaninglessness. Durkheim's (1897/1951) classic essay, which identified social disintegration as a major cause of suicide, is perhaps the earliest of a long line of studies on the adverse effects of social isolation. Studies that examined the sense of meaninglessness more directly found that it can be elicited by social rejection and ostracism (e.g., Williams, 2012). In contrast, close relationships and social support enhance a sense of meaning (Costin & Vignoles, 2020; Hicks & King, 2009, Hicks, Schlegel, & King, 2010), and people often explicitly report that social relationships make their lives meaningful (Lambert et al., 2010). In the lab, enhancing feelings of belongingness was found to increase the belief that one's life is meaningful (Lambert et al., 2013).

Ruptures in social ties often ensue from adverse events, such as the death of a close friend or family member, divorce, incarceration, or loss of a job. But they can also result from normal and even positive life transitions, such as attending a new high school or college, marriage, parenthood, and retirement. Both positive and negative transitions may rupture social connections and thereby engender a sense of meaninglessness (Park, 2010).

Of particular interest here is the literature on self-affirmation (Cohen & Sherman, 2014; Steele, 1988; Sherman, 2013), which looks at the transition to college/high school in individuals who, because of their socioeconomic background, tend to feel that they do not belong to the new environment.

Viewed from the current theoretical perspective, studies on self-affirmation propose that a person might experience distress and loss of meaning if they belong to two social networks that are disconnected from or inconsistent with each other. These studies suggest that such discontinuity can be mended by self-affirmation—a process through which a person connects to and reaffirms their core values, which presumably remain constant across the two "inconsistent" social environments. Imagine, for example, a person who is the first in their family to go to college. Regardless of how well they are doing, they might be distressed by thoughts such as "My parents would have looked lost and ridiculous here," and "None of my high-school friends would understand, let alone appreciate, what I am doing here." A self-affirmation manipulation might get that person thinking, for example, "Honesty and hard work are important to me, and these virtues are valued both here, in college, and back at home." This thought is soothing because by connecting to a deeper and more abstract facet of the self, it helps to bridge the gap between the seemingly incompatible social groups to which the person belongs. In other words, it mends the rupture in the social world by means of abstraction. Consistent with this idea, research has shown that successful self-affirmation is accompanied by adopting a more abstract way of thinking (Wakslak & Trope, 2009).

Is discontinuity in one's social world a psychological or, rather, a realistic problem? This is a classic controversy in social psychology. Heider's (1958) balance theory suggested that "imbalanced relations," whereby I like person A and person B, but A and B dislike each other, are problematic because they represent a "mental inconsistency" akin to a "bad Gestalt." Abelson (1983), however, illuminated a different, realistic aspect of imbalance, having to do with the difficulty of, for example, having A and B stay together at my place. The same logic applies to many examples of social discontinuity, including the aforementioned example of trying to excel in a college environment that one's family and old friends do not value or understand.

CONTINUITY IN SPACE

Immigration, even under the best circumstances, is a very stressful life event (Eggerth & Flynn, 2020). Even a milder change in spatial environment, such as moving to a new place within one's country, is relatively high on the list of life stressors (Wallace, Cooper, Sel, & Russo, 2023). Relocating to a new environment can disrupt established routines, social connections, and familiar surroundings, leading to feelings of disorientation, alienation, and meaninglessness.

The present framework suggests that relocation would be particularly prone to inducing a sense of meaninglessness if it introduces discontinuity—that is, if the new place is very different from the place of origin, if returning to the place of origin is impossible, and/or if the place of origin has undergone a major transformation after one's leaving. For example, a refugee who thinks that they will return to rebuild their home country would experience less meaninglessness than a refugee whose country will never be the same and/or who thinks that they will not be able to go back in the foreseeable future.

As with expansions across other dimensions of scope, mild expansions of spatial scope could promote a sense of meaningfulness rather than undermine it. For example, perhaps leisure travel broadens spatial scope but challenges the sense of meaning only mildly, ensuring a successful process of making meaning (see, for example, Chen and Petrick [2013] for findings that are generally consistent with this idea). Also related to this notion is a study by Waytz, Hershfield, and Tamir (2015) in which participants who wrote about being in a different location (compared with participants who wrote about their current location) reported more meaning in lives.

CONTINUITY IN THE REALM OF HYPOTHETICAL POSSIBILITIES

In a series of studies, Kray, George, Liljenquist, Galinsky, Tetlock, and Roese (2010, Studies 3 and 4) asked participants to write about a turning point in their lives: "Turning points are not very common moments or episodes in a person's life in which rapid, intense, and clear change occurs, such that the person and his or her life are never the same again"; participants in the counterfactual condition then described "how your life would be now if the turning point incident had never occurred" (pp. 109–110). In terms of the present framework, participants in the counterfactual condition expanded scope in the hypotheticality dimension. Moreover, because a turning point was defined as a major change, the counterfactual condition produced discontinuity of the self across hypothetical alternatives to reality.

Kray and her colleagues (2010) found that participants in the counterfactual condition reported more meaning in life compared with participants who wrote factual descriptions of the turning point and compared with participants who contemplated the meaning of the turning point, the two control conditions in the study. They also found that counterfactual reflection increased perceptions of fate, which mediated its effect on meaning. Banerjee and Bloom (2014) likewise found that even nonreligious participants tended to think that significant life events were not arbitrary but rather "happened for a reason." Along the same lines, Heintzelman, Christopher, Trent, and King (2013) found that counterfactual thinking about one's birth enhanced reported meaning in life.

Kray and colleagues (2010) note, "Although it might seem that counterfactual reflections could just as easily highlight life's arbitrariness, we propose an ironic relationship between the perceived mutability of life events and the sense that those events were destined and thus infused with underlying meaning" (p. 106). This reasoning, as well as the results of the studies described previously, is consistent with the current framework. An awareness of life's arbitrariness is akin to a sense of meaninglessness, and believing in faith may be seen as counteracting it by suggesting that events are connected to each other as well as to a greater sense of purpose. Just as nostalgia restores meaning that is threatened by discontinuity of the self in time, a belief in fate restores meaning that is threatened by discontinuity of the self in the realm of hypothetical possibilities.

THE INTERCHANGEABILITY OF DISTANCES

Distances are related to each other in many ways. For one, they tend to covary in reality (e.g., it takes longer to go to a place that is farther away; one needs to sample larger swaths of time, space, and population to come across an event that is rarer; Fiedler, 2020; Fiedler, Jung, Wänke, & Alexopoulos, 2012; Fiedler, Jung, Wänke, Alexopoulos, & de Molière, 2014). Distances are also associated with each other in people's minds and in cultures (e.g., people tend to complete "a long time ago, in a ________ land" with "faraway" rather than "nearby"; Bar Anan, Liberman, Trope, & Algom, 2007; Stephan, Liberman, & Trope, 2010). Finally, the dimensions of distance have similar psychological effects (e.g., objects that are farther away from us on any dimension of distance are represented more abstractly and have a less potent effect on us; Trope & Liberman, 2010).

Continuity and discontinuity follow the same logic, in that (dis) continuity in one distance often involves (dis)continuity in another. For example, immigration, although it originates from and is most easily described as a discontinuity in space, would typically involve a rupture in social ties, in time (before vs. after immigration), and in the realm of counterfactual possibilities (one's counterfactual life would have been very different had they not immigrated).

An interesting question is whether reestablishing continuity in one dimension may help heal a rupture in another. In their chapter on nostalgia in this volume, Sedikides and Wildschut describe how reinstatement of social connections heals the pain that is associated with discontinuity in time, which is nostalgia. Can this also happen over other distances? Consistent with this possibility is the finding that some of the adverse effects of immigration, including increased risk for anxiety, depression, and psychosis, are mitigated when immigrants live in communities of people who share their culture of origin and identify with that culture (Brance, Chatzimpyros, & Bentall, 2023). To use the terms of the current framework, social continuity may mitigate discontinuity in space.

As another example, consider the idea that travel may present a minor and easy-to-overcome challenge to self-continuity in space. Would travel, because it is likely to reinstate continuity, help heal discontinuity in time (i.e., or nostalgia)? Can it help mend rupture in social connections? Consider the finding that contemplating how your life could have taken a completely different turn makes life seem meaningful, guided by purpose and destiny. Would it also alleviate the pain of nostalgia? Would it help cope with ruptured social networks?

MEANING AND ABSTRACTION

In his book *Meaning of Life*, Roy Baumeister (1991) suggests that "a rough definition [of meaning] would be that meaning is shared mental representations of possible relationships among things, events, and relationships. Thus, meaning connects things" (p. 15). I agree. To make meaning is to abstract, and any act of abstraction, according to CLT, creates a meaningful connection between elements. More precisely, Gilead et al. (2020) suggest that abstraction occurs when two subjectively distinct objects are deemed equivalent for a purpose. For example, when we represent "reading a book" and "attending class" as "studying," we gloss over the many differences between these activities (e.g., that one involves being around people, whereas the other does not) and deem them equivalent (e.g., their potential contribution to knowledge). Any act of abstraction is a decision about what is more important (this is the dimension of equivalence; in the previous example, "the activity contributes to exam-relevant knowledge" is one dimension of equivalence) and what is less important (this is the dimension of difference; in the previous example, "involves being around people" is one dimension of difference). Of course, many abstractions of the same objects are possible, and each involves a different decision about what is and what is not important. For example, abstracting "attending class" as "socializing" would group it together with "partying" and would render the social aspect primary and "gaining exam-relevant knowledge" secondary or incidental.

Abstraction and the creation of meaning, in this view, stand in contrast to representing haphazard, disjoint elements. When an act of abstraction fails, that is, when one attends to a number of objects and fails to find an important aspect that connects them, they are left with, to use a famous quote, "a heap of broken images" (Eliot, 1922/2001, p. 5) and a sense of meaninglessness.

Two types of abstraction stand out as being particularly important for (research on) meaning making: coherent narratives (in contrast to representing a disjoint, disconnected series of events) and sense of purpose (in contrast to futile, disorganized, senseless action). In fact, recent theories conceptualize coherence and sense of purpose as two of the three primary components of meaning in life (King & Hicks, 2021; Heintzelman & King, 2014a; George & Park, 2017; Krause & Hayward, 2014). (The third component, "existential mattering," which King and Hicks [2021] define as "the belief that one's existence will continue to influence others across time and space" (p. 567), is more related to expansion across social, temporal, and spatial scope, which I discussed earlier.)

Coherent Personal Narratives

The coherence of a narrative is typically defined as the extent to which it conveys the content and meaning of the described events in a structurally and thematically consistent manner. For example, one popular operationalization codes a narrative as coherent to the extent that (1) the context of the described event is defined, consisting of specific time and place indications; (2) the event is structured in a logical and chronological order using time indication words (e.g., *thereafter*, *next*); and (3) the event is elaborated on not merely factually but also emotionally and includes a resolution, closure, and a link to other important events or to the self (Reese et al., 2011).

Much research has examined the coherence of traumatic or negative memories (e.g., Booker et al., 2020; Vanaken, Bijttebier, Fivush, & Hermans, 2021; Tuval-Mashiach et al., 2004; Waters & Fivush, 2015) and found that it was associated with better emotional outcomes and well-being. Research also suggests that coherent life narratives are associated with both satisfaction with and experiencing meaning in life (George & Park, 2016). Consistent with these findings, the first step in narrative therapy, termed *personal narrative construction*, involves assisting the patient in authoring a coherent life story (White & Epston, 1990).

All abstractions, including the construction of coherent narratives, are mental acts that organize objects in the mind rather than in the real world. But that does not mean that their effects are confined to mental outcomes, such as facilitating understanding and acceptance of traumatic events. Rather, narratives (like other abstractions) determine how one relates to and acts in the real world and are especially useful for expanding psychological scope and for mending ruptures in scope. For example, coherence of narratives has been found to serve a social function. Studies by Vanaken and colleagues (2021; Vanaken, Bijttebier, & Hermans, 2020) show that listeners react more positively to more coherent narratives, granting the narrator more social support. A study also found that perceived social support partly mediated the effect of narrative coherence on enhancing the sense of meaning (Vanaken, Bijttebier, Fivush, & Hermans, 2021). This line of research demonstrates that the construction of coherent narratives helps in creating continuity in one's scope of social relations.

Let me also reiterate the obvious: Narratives, by their very definition, help create continuity in time (and mend discontinuity in time), which, as noted earlier, contributes to a sense of meaning (and offsets the sense of meaninglessness; Sedikides et al., 2025). A successful narrative can help connect one's current self to an otherwise potentially disconnected past self. Moreover, by virtue of being logical and offering resolution and closure, a successful narrative makes the events it narrates seem nonarbitrary and thus creates continuity in the realm of counterfactual possibilities.

Sense of Purpose

Goals form hierarchies in which more concrete means are subordinated to more abstract ends (Carver & Scheier, 2002). For example, "organizing a party" may be subordinate to (i.e., be the means to achieve) the goal of "socializing," and it may be superordinate to (i.e., be fulfilled by means of) "baking a cake." To go up a level in this hierarchy, one asks the question of why an action is done, and to go down a level, one asks the question of how it is done (Vallacher & Wegner, 1987). At the lowest level of this hierarchy are motor actions: Repeated "how" questions will eventually lead to physical actions such as "moving my mouth," for which "how" questions can no longer be answered. At the highest level of the goal hierarchy are abstract "being goals," such as "to be a good person" (Carver & Scheier, 2002). The goals at the top of the hierarchy are relatively stable, encompass many subgoals, and tend to have no definite end points. For example, "helping my grandmother move into her new place" is a concrete goal with a clear end point, but the more abstract goal of "being a helpful person" does not have an end point—any activity that is performed within this goal instantiates it but does not close it. Values, defined as "broad goals that apply across contexts and time" (Bardi & Schwartz, 2003, p. 1208), can be conceptualized as goals at the top of the goal hierarchy. Purpose-of-life goals, which "often represent abstract, long term, intrinsically valuable goals" (King & Hicks, 2021, p. 567), are obviously at the top of the goal hierarchy, and their relation to abstraction is self-evident.

Some theories conceptualize the sense of purpose as a component of well-being (Ryff & Keyes, 1995; King & Hicks, 2021). Others have treated it as an independent construct but nevertheless emphasized its theoretical and empirical relation to well-being, meaningfulness, and mental health (McKnight & Kashdan, 2009). Both approaches are consistent with theories of goal hierarchies and with the present notion that meaning in life comes from using abstract constructs that help extend one's scope. This consistency is, admittedly, somewhat superficial because theories of goal hierarchy typically assume that all goals of all people are organized into hierarchies, and theories of values assume that all people have values, whereas theories of purpose in life imply that some people have more of a sense of purpose in life compared with others.[1] Theories of goal hierarchies thus cannot easily explain variations in meaning in life between people.

Is there a meaningful interpersonal and situational variation in the tendency to think about one's actions in terms of values and superordinate, "being" goals? And does doing so promote a sense of meaning?

[1]A cynical view could have noted that measures of purpose in life, which often gauge agreement with items like "My life has clear purpose," simply reflect general satisfaction with oneself and one's life rather than anything related more specifically to goal hierarchies. This problem does not detract from the importance of findings showing that self-reports of purpose predict physical health, mortality rates, resilience in the face of adverse situations, and health-related behaviors (see review in King & Hicks, 2021). It only renders these findings uninformative with respect to the question of whether abstract construal of actions has anything to do with these outcomes.

The Behavior Identification Form (Vallacher & Wegner, 1989), constructed within action identification theory, measures people's tendency to identify actions in terms of abstract goals versus concrete means, but even the abstract identifications in this questionnaire remain fairly concrete (e.g., the high-level, "why" identification of "reading a book" is "gaining knowledge," which is still fairly far from values and overall life goals). I am not aware of any finding on the relationship between this questionnaire and a sense of meaning in life. Although the theory developed in this chapter might suggest a positive correlation, the relative concreteness of high-level identifications in this questionnaire might mitigate this prediction (in addition, the authors of action identification theory proposed a more complex relation between the level of action identification and sense of meaning than the one I discuss here; Michael, Parkin, & Vallacher, 2013).

I am not aware of studies that examined how identification of actions in value-relevant terms relates to experiencing life as meaningful. Researchers did, however, examine value fulfillment, which was measured by asking participants about the extent to which they have acted in accordance with their values. For example, participants were provided a short definition of *hedonism* and were asked, "How much do you feel you have acted in accordance with the value of Hedonism during the day?" They found that fulfilling one's values predicted well-being (Hanel, Tunç, Bhasin, Litzellachner, & Maio, 2024; Oppenheim-Weller, Roccas, & Kurman, 2018). I am not aware, however, of studies that used meaning in life as the dependent measure using this paradigm. More importantly, although value fulfillment, as measured in these studies, could reflect *construal* of actions in value-related terms, it could also reflect *successful instantiation* of the value (Schwartz & Sortheix, 2018).

Recently, Fujita, Trope, and Liberman (2025) proposed another approach to how action hierarchies may play out differently between people and between situations. They noted that sometimes, the outcomes of actions are dependent on other actions and on circumstances beyond the immediate, such that the utility of an action when considered in isolation might be quite different from its utility when considered in the broader context of other actions that span across time, space, social perspectives, and hypothetical outcomes. These authors defined successful self-control as considering an action's expansive rather than only contractive utility. For example, in the classic self-control problem of dieting, the contractive utility of eating a high-calorie dessert is high, but an expansive perspective would take into account the utility that comes from relevant superordinate goals, as well as the value of more distant future outcomes (e.g., how it will affect my weight and looks), value that comes from other social perspectives (e.g., what would my partner say?), and value from considering hypothetical worlds (e.g., what if tomorrow I see an even more tempting dessert?). This is somewhat similar, the authors argue, to how in institutions, some actions (e.g., admitting a minority student with below-threshold grades) might have a different value when viewed in isolation than when considered within a policy (e.g., affirmative action in view of historic injustice). A policy, in this view, may be defined as an expansive, system-level (rather than a contractive, case-level) view of utility.

Extending this reasoning to a sense of purpose in life, I suggest that a person would experience life as purposeful when they evaluate a current action in view of their highest-level goals. Purpose in life, according to this view, would be an extension of self-control, in the sense that it stems from evaluating action based on a policy rather than in isolation, except that in this case, the relevant policy is, so to speak, "life's grand policy." For example, if one of my highest-level goals is to preserve the environment, then I would experience my actions as meaningful to the extent that I see how they help preserve the environment or fit into a goal hierarchy that subserves that goal (e.g., I study engineering in order to develop a technology to combat ocean pollution, a goal of which I'm aware during my studies). A sense of purpose in life, according to this view, stands in contrast to disorganized action that wastes energy instead of optimizing actions by coordinating them in view of the higher-level goal. Therefore, reminders of one's limited resources, most notably of one's limited time on earth, should sensitize people to their ultimate goals and to utilities that derive from those goals. It is perhaps for that reason that mortality salience increases adherence to values and the importance of meaningful social relations (Plusnin, Pepping, & Kashima, 2018; Mikulincer & Florian, 2000; Florian, Mikulincer, & Hirschberger, 2002; Yaakobi, Mikulincer, & Shaver, 2014).

Why does thinking in terms of high-level rather than low-level goals and in terms of policies rather than isolated action contribute to a sense of meaning in life? Is it by fostering mental balance, clarity, and structure or, rather, by better embedding one in the ecology—namely, via building effective bridges over time, social networks, and hypothetical possibilities? As with personal narratives, I would like to propose that the answer is "both."

SUCCESSFULLY MAPPING ONE'S NARRATIVE AND SENSE OF PURPOSE ONTO SCOPE

According to some Jewish traditions, Abraham, one of the founding fathers of Judaism, grew up among idolaters and, to use the language of the present chapter, was fully integrated within his extended family, which, in that time and place, formed most of one's social network. His family's business, the tradition goes, was manufacturing and trading statues of local deities. Abraham was already a mature person when he started to question the powers of the human-made idols and arrived at a belief in a single, invisible, almighty God, the original cause of everything (Ginzberg, 1909, pp. 209–217). We might say, using the language of the present chapter, that he developed a coherent narrative and sense of purpose that did not match those of his social, spatial, and temporal environment. I would like to suggest, furthermore, that this situation is likely to cause a sense of meaninglessness, which would persist until the "misfit" is fixed by changing one's narrative, the narrative of the community, or the community itself. In the case of Abraham, the "misfit" was fixed by founding a new religion and a new community in a new place after experiencing a major socio-spatial discontinuity upon following God's instruction to "go from your country and your kindred and your father's house to the land that I will show you" (Genesis 12:1).

More generally, when a person's beliefs, values, and plans are coherent and purposeful yet do not fit with the social, cultural, ideological, or epistemic environment, a sense of meaninglessness may arise. This can happen if a person arrives at a worldview or a narrative that is not shared by their social group and therefore does not serve to integrate the person into their environment but rather to set them apart from it. Take, for example, a person who came to view their own gender as a category that was wrongly imposed on them by society. If they live in a society in which gender plays a major role in people's narratives and sense of purpose, they might experience meaninglessness, unless they join a new community of similarly minded individuals and either cut connections to the old social environment, change its narrative, or develop a narrative that mends the social rupture.

There might be, of course, other examples of personal narratives that come to clash with those of the spatial and social environment of their time, in which they might be otherwise perfectly integrated. People who developed new, revolutionary theories and artists who establish new schools come to mind. But perhaps less dramatic examples are all around us: People who, without being part of a social or a political movement, come to view the "dominant narrative" of their society as misguided might feel estranged and experience meaninglessness even if they develop an alternative coherent narrative of their own.

SUMMARY AND OPEN QUESTIONS

Using CLT, I suggested a framework for understanding how people come to experience a sense of meaning in life. I suggested that a sense of meaning in life requires (1) continuity of the self in the physical world, in the relevant scope of time, space, social relationships, and possible alternatives; (2) a narrative and a sense of purpose, which are abstractions that introduce continuity in one's mental constructs; and (3) an alignment of the mental and the real, such that a person's narrative and sense of purpose help integrate them into their scope of time, space, social network, and possibilities.

It would be interesting to examine whether the principles of meaning in life suggested here and the way they operate vary across cultures. For example, are some cultures more tolerant of intertemporal or cross-situational inconsistencies of the self? Do some cultures supply their members with better, more readily available means to mend such inconsistencies by way of abstraction? Possibly, the present framework can offer an interesting lens for looking at cross-cultural differences.

Finally, this chapter subscribes to CLT's notion that expansion into scope and mending of ruptures in scope are afforded by abstraction. It would be interesting to explore whether concrete mental representations, because they serve to highlight discontinuity across scope, can be used strategically to induce mental pain (à la nostalgia) or a sense of meaninglessness or, conversely, to instigate a process of meaning making. It is also interesting to consider what happens when concrete details rather than abstract constructs are used as bridges over scope. Wisława Szymborska's poem "Teenager" describes a visit by her adolescent self. She does not feel connected to the visitor, to her poems, and to her entire attitude. "Only when she vanishes, / leaving her scarf in her haste. //A scarf of genuine wool, / in colored stripes / crocheted for her / by our mother. // I've still got it" (Szymborska, 2009, lines 39–45.) Why is it that only the most concrete detail—the colored, striped wool scarf—finally creates the connection to her distant past self? The present chapter, as well as other theories of self and meaning, would expect more abstract constructs to do the job better. The striped wool scarf, these theories would say, is a flimsy bridge over the vast sea of time. Perhaps the poet wants us to appreciate the flimsiness of that bridge? Or to linger in the pain of the discontinued self rather than venturing to heal the sting of nostalgia? Or maybe the present chapter misses something important about what gives life a sense of meaning.

REFERENCES

Abelson, R. P. (1983). Whatever became of consistency theory? *Personality and Social Psychology Bulletin*, *9*(1), 37–54.

Banerjee, K., & Bloom, P. (2014). Why did this happen to me? Religious believers' and non-believers' teleological reasoning about life events. *Cognition, 133*(1), 277–303.

Bar-Anan, Y., Liberman, N., Trope, Y., & Algom, D. (2007). Automatic processing of psychological distance: Evidence from a Stroop task. *Journal of Experimental Psychology: General, 136*(4), 610–622.

Bardi, A., & Schwartz, S. H. (2003). Values and behavior: Strength and structure of relations. *Personality and Social Psychology Bulletin, 29*(10), 1207–1220.

Baumeister, R. F. (1991). *Meanings of life*. Guilford Press.

Booker, J. A., Fivush, R., Graci, M. E., Heitz, H., & Hudak, L. A., Jovanovic, T., et al. (2020). Longitudinal changes in trauma narratives over the first year and associations with coping and mental health. *Journal of Affective Disorders, 272*, 116–124.

Brance, K., Chatzimpyros, V., & Bentall, R. P. (2023). Increased social identification is linked with lower depressive and anxiety symptoms among ethnic minorities and migrants: A systematic review and meta-analysis. *Clinical Psychology Review, 99*, 102216.

Carver, C. S., & Scheier, M. F. (2002). Control processes and self-organization as complementary principles underlying behavior. *Personality and Social Psychology Review, 6*(4), 304–315.

Chen, C. C., & Petrick, J. (2013). Health and wellness benefits of travel experiences: A literature review. *Journal of Travel Research, 52*(6), 709–719.

Cohen, G. L., & Sherman, D. K. (2014). The psychology of change: Self-affirmation and social psychological intervention. *Annual Review of Psychology, 65*(1), 333–371.

Costin, V., & Vignoles, V. L. (2020). Meaning is about mattering: Evaluating coherence, purpose, and existential mattering as precursors of meaning in life judgments. *Journal of Personality and Social Psychology, 118*(4), 4864–4884.

Danziger, S., Montal, R., & Barkan, R. (2012). Idealistic advice and pragmatic choice: A psychological distance account. *Journal of Personality and Social Psychology, 102*(6), 1105–1117.

Diener, E., Emmons, R. A., Larsen, R. J., & Griffin, S. (1985). The Satisfaction With Life Scale. *Journal of Personality Assessment, 49*(1), 71–75.

Durkheim, E. (1951). *Suicide. A study in sociology* (J. Spaulding & G. Simpson, Trans.). Free Press. (Original work published 1897)

Eggerth, D. E., & Flynn, M. A. (2020). Immigration and stress. In T. Ringeisen, P. Genkova, & F. T. L. Leong (Eds.), *Handbuch stress und kultur* (pp. 1–19). Springer.

Eliot, T. S. (2001). *The waste land* (M. North, Ed.). W. W. Norton. (Original work published 1922)

Fiedler, K. (2020). Cognitive representations and the predictive brain depend heavily on the environment. *Behavioral and Brain Sciences, 43*, e121.

Fiedler, K., Jung, J., Wänke, M., & Alexopoulos, T. (2012). On the relations between distinct aspects of psychological distance: An ecological basis of construal-level theory. *Journal of Experimental Social Psychology, 48*(5), 1014–1021.

Fiedler, K., Jung, J., Wänke, M., Alexopoulos, T., & de Molière, L. (2014). Toward a deeper understanding of the ecological origins of distance construal. *Journal of Experimental Social Psychology, 57*, 78–86.

Florian, V., Mikulincer, M., & Hirschberger, G. (2002). The anxiety-buffering function of close relationships: Evidence that relationship commitment acts as a terror management mechanism. *Journal of Personality and Social Psychology, 82*(4), 527–542.

Fujita, K., Trope, Y., & Liberman, N. (2025). Understanding self-control as a problem of regulatory scope. *Psychological Review, 132*(1), 50–75.

Fujita, K. F., Henderson, M. D., Eng, J., Trope, Y., & Liberman, N. (2006). Spatial distance and mental construal of social events. *Psychological Science, 17*(4), 278–282.

George, L. S., & Park, C. L. (2016). Meaning in life as comprehension, purpose, and mattering: Toward integration and new research questions. *Review of General Psychology, 20*(3), 205–220.

George, L. S., & Park, C. L. (2017). The multidimensional existential meaning scale: A tripartite approach to measuring meaning in life. *Journal of Positive Psychology, 12*(6), 613–627.

Gilead, M., Trope, Y., & Liberman, N. (2020). Above and beyond the concrete: The diverse representational substrates of the predictive brain. *Behavioral and Brain Sciences, 43*, Article e121.

Ginzberg, L. (1909). *The legends of the Jews* (Vol. 1). Jewish Publication Society of America.

Grinfeld, G., Wakslak, C., Trope, Y., & Liberman, N. (2024). Construing hypotheticals: How hypotheticality affects level of abstraction. *Journal of Experimental Social Psychology, 110*, Article 104543.

Hanel, P. H., Tunç, H., Bhasin, D., Litzellachner, L. F., & Maio, G. R. (2024). Value fulfillment and well-being: Clarifying directions over time. *Journal of Personality, 92*(4), 1037–1049.

Hayes, S. C. (2005). *Get out of your mind and into your life*. New Harbinger.

Heider, F. (1958). *The psychology of interpersonal relations*. Wiley.

Heintzelman, S. J., Christopher, J., Trent, J., & King, L. A. (2013). Counterfactual thinking about one's birth enhances well-being judgments. *Journal of Positive Psychology, 8*(1), 44–49.

Heintzelman, S. J., & King, L. A. (2014a). Life is pretty meaningful. *American Psychologist, 69*(6), 561–574.

Heintzelman, S. J., & King, L. A. (2014b). (The feeling of) meaning-as-information. *Personality and Social Psychology Review, 18*(2), 153–167.

Hicks, J. A., & King, L. A. (2009). Positive mood and social relatedness as information about meaning in life. *Journal of Positive Psychology, 4*(6), 6471–6482.

Hicks, J. A., Schlegel, R. J., & King, L. A. (2010). Social threats, happiness, and the dynamics of meaning in life judgments. *Personality and Social Psychology Bulletin, 36*(10), 1305–1317.

Kafka, F. (1996). *The metamorphosis and other stories* (S. Appelbaum, Trans.). Dover Publications. (Original work published 1912)

King, L. A., & Hicks, J. A. (2021). The science of meaning in life. *Annual Review of Psychology, 72*(1), 561–584.

Krause, N., & Hayward, R. D. (2014). Assessing stability and change in a second-order confirmatory factor model of meaning in life. *Journal of Happiness Studies, 15*(2), 2237–2253.

Kray, L. J., George, L. G., Liljenquist, K. A., Galinsky, A. D., Tetlock, P. E., & Roese, N. J. (2010). From what *might* have been to what *must* have been: Counterfactual thinking creates meaning. *Journal of Personality and Social Psychology, 98*(1), 106–118.

Lambert, N. M., Stillman, T. F., Baumeister, R. F., Fincham, F. D., Hicks, J. A., & Graham, S. M. (2010). Family as a salient source of meaning in young adulthood. *Journal of Positive Psychology, 5*(5), 5367–5376.

Lambert, N. M., Stillman, T. F., Hicks, J. A., Kamble, S., Baumeister, R. F., & Fincham, F. D. (2013). To belong is to matter: Sense of belonging enhances meaning in life. *Personality and Social Psychology Bulletin, 39*(11), 1418–1427.

Li, J.-B., Dou, K., & Liang, Y. (2021). The relationship between presence of meaning, search for meaning, and subjective well-being: A three-level meta-analysis based on the Meaning in Life Questionnaire. *Journal of Happiness Studies, 22*(1), 467–489.

Liberman, N., & Trope, Y. (1998). The role of feasibility and desirability considerations in near and distant future decisions: A test of temporal construal theory. *Journal of Personality and Social Psychology, 75*(1), 5–18.

Liberman, N., & Trope, Y. (2008). The psychology of traversing the here and now. *Science, 322*(5905), 1201–1205.

Liberman, N., & Trope, Y. (2014). Traversing psychological distance. *Trends in Cognitive Sciences, 18*(7), 364–369.

McKnight, P. E., & Kashdan, T. B. (2009). Purpose in life as a system that creates and sustains health and well-being: An integrative, testable theory. *Review of General Psychology, 13*(3), 242–251.

Michaels, J. L., Parkin, S. S., Vallacher, R. R. (2013). Destiny is in the details: Action identification in the construction and destruction of meaning. In J. Hicks & C. Routledge (Eds.), *The experience of meaning in life* (pp. 103–115). Springer.

Mikulincer, M., & Florian, V. (2000). Exploring individual differences in reactions to mortality salience: Does attachment style regulate terror management mechanisms? *Journal of Personality and Social Psychology, 79*(2), 260–273.

Nguyen, T., Grinfeld, G., Liberman, N., & Wakslak, C. J. (2023). Effects of temporal distance on a dynamic measure of action identification. *Journal of Experimental Social Psychology, 108*, Article 104493.

Oppenheim-Weller, S., Roccas, S., & Kurman, J. (2018). Subjective value fulfillment: A new way to study personal values and their consequences. *Journal of Research in Personality, 76*, 38–49.

Park, C. L. (2010). Making sense of the meaning literature: An integrative review of meaning making and its effects on adjustment to stressful life events. *Psychological Bulletin, 136*(2), 257–301.

Plusnin, N., Pepping, C. A., & Kashima, E. S. (2018). The role of close relationships in terror management: A systematic review and research agenda. *Personality and Social Psychology Review, 22*(4), 307–346.

Reese, E., Haden, C. A., Baker-Ward, L., Bauer, P., Fivush, R., & Ornstein, P. A. (2011). Coherence of personal narratives across the lifespan: A multidimensional model and coding method. *Journal of Cognition and Development, 12*(4), 424–462.

Routledge C., Arndt, J., Wildschut, T., Sedikides, C., Hart, C. M., Juhl, J., et al. (2011). The past makes the present meaningful: Nostalgia as an existential resource. *Journal of Personality and Social Psychology, 101*(3), 638–652.

Ryff, C. D., & Keyes, C. L. M. (1995). The structure of psychological well-being revisited. *Journal of Personality and Social Psychology, 69*(4), 719–727.

Sanchez, A. M., Coleman, C. W., & Ledgerwood, A. (2021). Does temporal distance influence abstraction? A large pre-registered experiment. *Social Cognition, 39*(3), 352–365.

Schwartz, S. H., & Sortheix, F. (2018). Values and subjective well-being. In E. Diener, S. Oishi, & L. Tay (Eds.), *Handbook of well-being* (pp. 871–885). DEF Publishers.

Sedikides, C., Wildschut, T., Routledge, C., & Arndt, J. (2015). Nostalgia counteracts self-discontinuity and restores self-continuity. *European Journal of Social Psychology, 45*(1), 52–61.

Sherman, D. K. (2013). Self-affirmation: Understanding the effects. *Social and Personality Psychology Compass, 7*(11), 834–845.

Steele, C. M. (1988). The psychology of self-affirmation: Sustaining the integrity of the self. In L. Berkowitz (Ed.), *Advances in experimental social psychology, Vol. 21. Social psychological studies of the self: Perspectives and programs* (pp. 261–302). Academic Press.

Steger, M. F., Frazier, P., Oishi, S., & Kaler, M. (2006). The meaning in life questionnaire: Assessing the presence of and search for meaning in life. *Journal of Counseling Psychology, 53*(1), 80–93.

Stephan, E., Liberman, N., & Trope, Y. (2010). Politeness and psychological distance: A construal level perspective. *Journal of Personality and Social Psychology, 98*(2), 268–280.

Sverdlik, N., Kalkstein, D., Levit, O., Trope, Y., Liberman, N. (2025). *The dispositional lantern: Individual differences in regulatory scope* [Manuscript in preparation].

Szymborska, W. (2010). *Here* (C. Cavanagh & S. Baranczak, Trans.). Houghton Mifflin Harcourt.

Todd, P. M., & Gigerenzer, G. (Eds.). (2012). *Ecological rationality: Intelligence in the world.* Oxford University Press.

Trope, Y., Ledgerwood, A., Liberman, N., & Fujita, K. (2020). Regulatory scope and its mental and social supports. *Perspectives on Psychological Science, 16*(2), 204–224.

Trope, Y., & Liberman, N. (2010). Construal-level theory of psychological distance. *Psychological Review, 117*(2), 440–463.

Tuval-Mashiach, R., Freedman, S., Bargai, N., Boker, R., Hadar, H., & Shalev, A. Y., (2004). Coping with trauma: Narrative and cognitive perspectives. *Psychiatry, 67*(3), 280–293.

Vallacher, R. R., & Wegner, D. M. (1987). What do people think they're doing? Action identification and human behavior. *Psychological Review, 94*(1), 3–15.

Vallacher, R. R., & Wegner, D. M. (1989). Levels of personal agency: Individual variation in action identification. *Journal of Personality and Social Psychology, 57*(4), 660–671.

Vanaken, L., Bijttebier, P., Fivush, R., & Hermans, D. (2021). Narrative coherence predicts emotional well-being during the COVID-19 pandemic: A two-year longitudinal study. *Cognition and Emotion, 36*(1), 70–81.

Vanaken, L., Bijttebier, P., & Hermans, D. (2020). I like you better when you are coherent. Narrating autobiographical memories in a coherent manner has a positive impact on listeners' social evaluations. *PLOS ONE, 15*(4), Article e0232214.

Wakslak, C. J., & Trope, Y. (2009). Cognitive consequences of affirming the self: The relationship between self-affirmation and object construal. *Journal of Experimental Social Psychology, 45*(4), 927–932.

Wakslak, C. J., Trope, Y., Liberman, N., & Alony, R. (2006). Seeing the forest when entry is unlikely: Probability and the mental representation of events. *Journal of Experimental Psychology: General, 135*(4), 641–653.

Wallace, D., Cooper, N. R., Sel, A., & Russo, R. (2023). The Social Readjustment Rating Scale: Updated and modernised. *PLOS ONE, 18*(12), Article e0295943.

Waters, T. E., & Fivush, R. (2015). Relations between narrative coherence, identity, and psychological well-being in emerging adulthood. *Journal of Personality, 83*(4), 441–451.

Waytz, A., Hershfield, H. E., & Tamir, D. I. (2015). Mental simulation and meaning in life. *Journal of Personality and Social Psychology, 108*(2), 336–355.

White, M., & Epston, D. (1990). *Narrative means to therapeutic ends.* W. W. Norton & Company.

Williams, K. D. (2012). Ostracism: The impact of being rendered meaningless. In M. Mikulincer & P. Shaver (Eds.), *Meaning, mortality, and choice: The social psychology of existential concerns* (pp. 309–324). American Psychological Association.

Wilson, K. G., & Murrell, A. R. (2004). Values work in acceptance and commitment therapy: Setting a course for behavioral treatment. In S. C. Hayes,

V. M. Follette, & M. M. Linehan (Eds.), *Mindfulness and acceptance: Expanding the cognitive-behavioral tradition* (pp. 120–151). Guilford Press.

Yaakobi, E., Mikulincer, M., & Shaver, P. R. (2014). Parenthood as a terror management mechanism: The moderating role of attachment orientations. *Personality and Social Psychology Bulletin, 40*(6), 762–774.

Žižek, S. (2022). *Surplus enjoyment: A guide for the non-perplexed.* Bloomsbury.

CHAPTER 14

Significance-Questing or Awe-Stricken

On Two Paradigms of Meaning

Sophia Moskalenko and Arie W. Kruglanski

The dichotomy between self-focus and self-transcendence has inspired the religious traditions that shaped our civilization. From Jesus telling his followers to "give to the Caesar what's Caesar's and to God what's God's" to the Buddha's transition from a rich prince to ascetic monk before finding "the middle way," major religious teachings emerged from attempts to reconcile these alternative systems of meaning. We are proposing a psychological view on this dichotomy, building on the well-researched psychologies of significance-questing and awe.

The self-focused manner of relating to the world highlights one's sense of significance and social worth, the degree to which one feels that one's existence is imbued with value and that one matters to members of one's ingroup (Kruglanski et al., 2022). The self-transcendent mode highlights awe (Keltner & Haidt, 2003): the diminishment of self in response to the vast and incomprehensible, such as God, beauty, starry skies, grand music, and mathematical equations of supreme elegance, or threatening stimuli such as death, pain, Hitler, the atomic bomb, or natural disasters (Gordon et al., 2017).

Thus far, the phenomena of significance and awe have been addressed within their respective research programs and in relative isolation from each other. Yet there are ways in which they are intricately intertwined. Here, we propose that both significance and awe represent basic human needs that individuals strive to satisfy and that cause suffering when these needs are not met. Second, we propose that these two needs, for significance and awe, exist in a state of unstable equilibrium: The pursuit of each entails psychological costs, which accumulate and prompt a switch to the alternative. Third, we propose that individuals, as well as large collectives such as nations, ethnic groups, or cultures, may consistently prioritize one need above the other, and the result of this emphasis creates respective *awe-centric* or *significance-centric* tendencies to imbue events and situations with divergent meanings.

SIGNIFICANCE AND AWE AS NEEDS

Questing Significance

The *need for significance* is a need to feel as though one matters, is important, and is respected by others. It is the motivation at the heart of a variety of pursuits: academic achievement, romantic relationships, career strivings—but also crime, violence, and terrorism, depending on the kind of values (narratives) one's reference group (network) holds in high regard (Kruglanski, Bélanger, & Gunaratna, 2019; Kruglanski, Fernandez, Factor, & Szumowska, 2019). The quest for significance involves competition with others––the insatiable *unidirectional drive upward* (Festinger, 1954), and is laced with fear of failure and social anxiety.

One of the fundamental human motivations, the desire for significance gain (and fear of significance loss) permeates human affairs from individual psychology to national and international policies. When whole classes of people feel downtrodden and discriminated against, they may coalesce into social movements (e.g., the civil rights movement, Black Lives Matter) that fight for their members' rights to a dignified existence. Major revolutions that shaped world history (e.g., the French Revolution, the American Revolution, the Russian Revolution) emanated from the sense of humiliation that a class of people felt and rose against (Kruglanski et al., 2022).

Activating the Significance Quest

As with any motivational state, the need for significance can be activated through priming by semantic terms, events, or memories associated with this particular striving (Bargh, 1990) but also through significance deprivation or incentivization. Humiliation and feelings of significance loss activate the significance quest through significance deprivation. In contrast, incentivization consists of the opportunity to attain "greatness" through accumulating wealth, conquest, and dominance over competitors or adversaries. Hitler's ambition to dominate the world, which launched World War II, and Vladimir Putin's dreams of glory that motivated the Russian 2022 invasion of Ukraine were explicitly in the service of the significance these acts were hoped to bestow upon their respective nations and their leaders.

The pursuit of significance and social worth has been implicit in varied psychological analyses, like those emphasizing the need for competence and autonomy (Deci & Ryan, 2000), self-esteem (Tesser, 2000), social identity (Tajfel & Turner, 2004), self-enhancement (Fiske, 2010), and others. It is the common core of the semantic space inhabited by these terms. But the question is whether the self-focused pursuit of social worth and recognition, however prevalent, is the exclusive mode of relating to oneself and the world. Recent research on the awe phenomenon identifies an important alternative to significance-questing. We consider it next.

Needing Awe

According to Keltner (2024, p. xvi): "We have a basic need for awe wired into our brains and bodies." There is indeed evidence that the experience of awe is universal and, hence, that it is a basic aspect of human nature. Furthermore, there is evidence that it is indeed a need that human societies attempt to meet in various forms, including through religion and art.

All known human societies have some form of religion (Glazier & Ember, 2018), and although the content of religions varies a great deal, one commonality they all share is the concept of "mystical power"—different from and greater than physical and social forces (Child & Child, 1993; Glazier, 1999). William James describes the mysticism common to all religious and spiritual traditions as an opening of a window through which the soul "looks out upon a more extensive and inclusive world" (James, 2002, p. 335). James's description of religious mysticism closely echoes psychologists' definitions of awe (vastness and a change of perspective; Keltner & Haidt, 2003). That every known human society in history has offered an outlet in the form of religion for the need to experience something vast and incomprehensible—something awe-inspiring—speaks to the universality of the human need for awe.

In parallel to the pervasiveness of religion, every known human society has incorporated art whose utility is not fully captured by metrics of evolutionary fitness, such as status, survival, or procreation (Dissanayake, 2015). A philosopher of art, Dennis Dutton, claimed that there is an inborn "instinct" for art and art appreciation, divorced from acculturation (Dutton, 2009). As evidenced by Spain's 40,800-year-old El Castillo cave paintings (Than, 2012) and the limestone Leang Tedongnge cave painting from 45,500 years ago in Sulawesi, Indonesia (Brumm et al., 2021), the presence of art in even the earliest human collectives suggests a universal need that art and beauty satisfy. Research on political refugees and displaced peoples shows that even in conditions of extreme scarcity and insecurity, people still invest time and resources in beautifying their living environments (Acker, 2023; Neumark, 2013), implying the profound importance of the awe of beauty even amid most dire living circumstances.

Theorists of emotion (e.g., Frijda, 1986; Higgins, 1996) have viewed it as a psychological experience inseparable from motivational states where unfulfilled needs induce negative feelings (of frustration, deficit, and want), whereas fulfilled needs induce positive feelings (of satisfaction, relief, pride, etc.). Accordingly, different emotional states were found to be induced in positive and negative states of awe. Exposure to threatening, vast, and uncontrollable stimuli, including powerful tyrants and natural disasters (Gordon et al., 2017), was found to induce negative affect (Gordon et al., 2017; Piff, Dietze, Feinberg, Stancato, & Keltner, 2015), whereas positive awe stimuli were found to elicit positive affect (Shiota, Keltner, & John, 2006). Whether positively or negatively valenced, the awe experience makes a person feel small and insignificant (Bai et al., 2017), and the positive affect occasioned by fulfillment of one's need for awe may be overridden by the threatening aspects of the experience (as can be occasioned by watching horror films, for example). The fact that the awe experience is aligned with affect attests to its motivational roots.

Activating Awe

Awe can be activated by exposure to a variety of stimuli (starry skies, videos of extraordinary heroism or generosity, beauty, nature, or certain kinds of music; Shiota Campos, & Keltner, 2003; Shiota et al., 2006; Yaden et al., 2019; Stellar et al., 2018). As with other motivational states, awe can also be activated by incentivization. The latter is evidenced in the multibillion-dollar tourism industry, where advertisements tempt customers with nature's grand spectacles. Traveling to experience the world's natural and artistic treasures is a major incentive for retirement. According to the 19th Annual Transamerica Retirement Survey, 67% of American workers dream of traveling once they retire (Lake, 2024). The countless travel books, travel blogs, and guides extol the appeal of witnessing the world's wonders away from the competitive pressures of the workplace, awakening people's wanderlust and the quest for awe. Especially when it comes to traveling to natural marvels such as the Grand Canyon, the Aurora lights, Niagara Falls, or the Alaskan wilderness, a desire to experience the awe they inspire, rather than mere curiosity, is likely the primary motivation behind such sightseeing tourism.

Just as with significance and mattering, then, the awe experience appears to constitute a fundamental need to which human societies have responded through their engagement in religion, art, and tourism. Fulfillment of one's need for awe is pleasurable, of course, as is the fulfillment of any need or desire, but qualitatively, it is experienced very differently than the pleasure one feels on winning a tennis game or on satisfying one's hunger--each need is associated with a different emotional state that accompanies its pursuit and its satisfaction.

Physiological Markers of Significance and Awe

Physiologically, awe can manifest as aesthetic chills, shivers, and tingles (Bannister, 2019). Awe can also manifest in *frisson*—a sensation people can experience when listening to particular kinds of music, contemplating a thrilling idea, or witnessing a breathtaking sunset—which includes physiological reactions such as tears, a lump in the throat, and muscle tension or relaxation (Harrison & Loui, 2014). The neurophysiology of frisson is related to the release of the hormone oxytocin (Casto & Edwards, 2016; Sapolsky, 1998; Suay et al., 1999; Wein, 2015), which supports affiliative bonding (Feldman, 2012) and relaxation (Uvnäs-Moberg, 1997). Consistent with this, experiencing awe while contemplating morally courageous and kind acts is associated with increased oxytocin release (Thomson & Siegel, 2017). More generally, awe experiences correspond with reduced activation of the sympathetic nervous system, indicating lowered stress (Chirico et al., 2017) and lower inflammation (Stellar et al., 2018). Awe, then, is associated with increased oxytocin release, reduced stress, and reduced inflammation.

The physiology of significance-questing is less well studied. However, because significance-questing is closely related to status seeking and competition and to significance attainment upon winning, it is reasonable to assume that hormones related to those behaviors would correspond to high levels of significance seeking. Status concerns and status-seeking behaviors are related to changes in testosterone (Mazur & Lamb, 1980; Sapolsky, 1998), a hormone that also mediates aggression and violence (Book, Starzyk, & Quinsey, 2001). An increase in testosterone has been consistently demonstrated (in both men and women) to biologically mark victory in competitions, including in physically demanding sports such as soccer; games of skill that do not require physical exertion, such as chess; and economic games, such as hawk–dove games (Carré, 2006; Hasegawa, Toda, & Morimoto, 2008; Mehta, Lawless DesJardins, van Vugt, & Josephs, 2017; Oliveira, Gouveia, & Oliveira, 2009; Zilioli & Watson, 2012). This rise in testosterone in response to success in competition is observed even when the participant does not personally compete but is instead rooting for a sports team that wins and even when it is the participant's dog who is the winner in an agility competition (Bernhardt, Dabbs, Fielden, & Lutter, 1998; Mehta, Jones, & Josephs, 2008). In other words, testosterone seems to both fuel competitive behavior (significance seeking) and surge in response to success in competition (significance attainment), including in cases where significance is attained by association (e.g., with a winning team or one's champion dog). Another hormonal correlate of competition is cortisol (Casto & Edwards, 2016; Edwards & Casto, 2013), a biomarker for stress (Hellhammer, Wüst, & Kudielka, 2009). High levels of cortisol undermine and weaken the immune system (Padgett & Glaser, 2003). In competitive settings, winning corresponds to a reduction in cortisol, and losing corresponds to an increase in cortisol—in parallel with the opposite dynamic in testosterone, a relationship that gave rise to the "dual-hormone hypothesis," which states that, together, testosterone and cortisol fuel and demarcate competition and attainment or the loss of significance that results from it (Grebe, Sarafin, Strenth, & Zilioli, 2019). Jointly, testosterone and cortisol also regulate dominance (Mehta & Josephs, 2010), which is closely related to significance (Kruglanski et al., 2023).

In short, whereas awe is related to an increase in oxytocin, reduced stress, and enhanced immune function, significance-questing, as represented in competitiveness and status attainment, is related to an increase in testosterone, increased stress, and decreased immune function.

Developmental Origins of Significance and Awe Strivings

Almost as soon as a child can explore the world outside of the caregiver's arms, their actions fall into two distinct patterns, one seemingly foreshadowing future significance quests and the other foreshadowing future quests for awe. One of these patterns identified by developmental psychologists is the development of skilled action in infancy (Bruner, 1968, 1973), where a child's activities help them to understand action and intentionality (Kalnins & Bruner, 1973). The *attainment of competence* in infants consists of three themes: intention, feedback, and the patterns of action that mediate between them (Bruner, 1973). We believe this early need to develop control, competence, and mastery over one's environment, with caretakers' feedback acting as an integral component, begets a sense of significance, endowing the self with agency and a sense of achievement that characterizes significance pursuits throughout the lifespan.

The second characteristic pattern of early development is the child's exploration of the environment. Researchers have emphasized the contrast between familiarity and novelty as playing an important role in the child's ventures into new territory (Rheingold & Eckerman, 1969; Ross, 1974). Independent of attachment to the caregiver or mastery of competence or skills, research has highlighted the infant's urge to explore new territory on their own initiative, propelled by a need to learn about the world (Rheingold & Eckerman, 1969; Rheingold, 1985). This developmental pattern, we believe, is an early manifestation of a need and capacity for awe, where the vastness, unpredictability, and incomprehensibility of the world invite infants as young as 9 months to explore it, to pause, and to take it in (Scherer, Zentner, & Stern, 2004).

It is important to emphasize, as does the developmental research discussed earlier, the irrelevance of social praise in this exploratory behavior, suggesting that the need to explore and experience the unfamiliar is an intrinsic motivation independent of significance concerns that are satisfied at this early age by the praise of caretakers. Indeed, the need for exploration can often get children in trouble with caretakers, yet despite these social costs, they tend to persist, attesting to this need's importance.

Introduction of the child to society begins in the preschool years, when they discover the norms, rules, and standards by which their self-worth is measured (Rakoczy & Schmidt, 2013; Schmidt & Tomasello, 2012). They discover that to be appreciated requires behaving in specific ways and obtaining certain outcomes--or inviting the risk of being neglected or rejected. In Western culture, the significance modality tends to dominate people's adult years, manifested in concerns about professional status, sexual attractiveness, and legacy (Kruglanski et al., 2022). Indeed, "adulting" entails taking responsibility; following norms and rules; and managing emotions, money, and time commitments (Golden et al., 2020; Stalp & Hill, 2019), which leaves little capacity for idle contemplation or appreciation of the vast and the incomprehensible—in short, more time pursuing significance and less time for awe.

In older adults, significance quests decline in parallel with the declining ability to compete (Mayr, Wozniak, Davidson, Kuhns, & Harbaugh, 2012). At the same time, exposure to awe-inducing experiences likely increases because of increased exposure to uncontrollable events, such as illness or death, as well as to grandchildren one can enjoy in awe rather than as a significance quest of parenthood. Consistent with this, research finds a greater capacity to experience awe among older adults than among both middle-aged and young adults (Ebert, Patrick, Huggins, Yadava, & Collett, 2021). Notably, a closely corresponding temporal dynamic can be observed in changes in testosterone levels over the lifespan (Handelsman, Sikaris, & Ly, 2016), which begin to rise in pre-adolescence (in parallel to a rise in significance orientation), peak in young and middle adulthood, and decline in older adults (in concert with a decline in significance concerns). This pattern is consistent in both men and women.

Developmentally, then, the needs for significance and awe seem to emerge simultaneously in early infancy as a need to master and a need to explore. Preparation for adult life in Western culture and its demands later in life emphasize and hone significance seeking over awe seeking, a pattern that reverses in older adults when they retire, which reduces their competitiveness, and face the inevitability, incomprehensibility, and vastness of mortality, as well as encounter sources of awe in leisure time spent in nature, creative pursuits, or grandparenting.

Evolutionary Functionality of the Significance–Awe Balance

If significance and awe are indeed basic human motives, the question, then, is why they evolved and what vital functions they have served. The evolutionary function of significance and status has to do with the resources and credit that high-significance individuals are accorded in a group in exchange for performing activities that the group values (Willer, 2009). Significance needs thus appraise opportunities to advance one's status and stature and enhance one's reproductive fitness. By contrast, awe needs seek occasions to note one's limits, to acknowledge the forces far exceeding one's capacities, to recognize and embrace one's humble place in the world and among people.

If significance is a *go* signal, a green light to carve out and cultivate one's unique space under the sun, then awe is a *stop* signal, a yellow or red light alerting the individual to pause, reappraise, and reconnect with others. In evolutionary terms, significance seeking would fuel early human interpersonal and intergroup competition, with status concerns promoting aggression and violence (Buss & Shackelford, 1997; Kruglanski et al., 2023) but also such socially beneficial by-products of competition as agriculture (Thrall, Bever, & Burdon, 2010), technology (Basalla, 1988), and culture (Winegard, Winegard, & Geary, 2018). Significance striving would help individuals accumulate resources and mates, increasing their chances of procreation and survival and enhancing individuals' evolutionary fitness (van Vugt & Tybur, 2014; von Rueden, Gurven, & Kaplan, 2010). At the same time, the human capacity to contemplate the future and the past, our own mortality, and the vastness of the world beyond our immediate surroundings results in the humbling realization that there are forces that even the strongest cannot conquer, powers that no amount of wealth can insulate from (Stellar et al., 2018). This realization of one's insignificance inspires awe, the feeling of smallness, vulnerability, and lack of control over the vast and the incomprehensible. This, in turn, leads to affiliation and altruism.

Although the reason behind the relationship between awe and affiliative tendencies is a question best answered through empirical exploration, one possibility is that "safety in numbers" offers an escape from the feeling of vulnerability elicited by awe; alternatively, awe may highlight one's shared humanity (as opposed to one's unique competitive advantage, which is highlighted in competition and significance seeking), and this leads to a desire to affiliate. Whatever the underlying psychology may be, awe leads to stronger intragroup bonding, altruistic action, and cohesive collective action in the face of dangers (Bai et al., 2017; Graziosi & Yaden, 2021; Guan, Chen, Chen, Liu, & Zha, 2019; Luo, Zou, Yang, & Yuan, 2023; Piff et al., 2015; Song, Klebl, & Bastian, 2023; Takano & Nomura, 2023; Yang & Hu, 2021)-- benefitting the evolutionary (inclusive) fitness of a group as a whole as opposed to the individual (Hamilton, 1964; Silk & House, 2011).

One's significance is affected both by one's *individual* attainments and attributes and those of the *social group or category* to which one belongs. Attempts by the individual to enhance the status of one's group (e.g., by leading a social movement to enhance one's group standing in society) promise to boost this actor's significance through both sources: the group source whose significance would be enhanced and the individual source by the actor gaining appreciation from fellow group members for efforts on their behalf.

Although both significance and awe-inspired behaviors can be prosocial, awe-inspired behaviors can incur significance costs. The Dutch painter Vincent van Gogh cultivating his own unique style despite a continual lack of its appreciation; Chinese multimillionaire Liu Jingchong giving up his money and lifestyle to pursue spiritual growth in an isolated hut in the woods (Sumitra, 2015); Polish Catholic priest Josef Kowalski suffering repeated beatings, ridicule, and humiliation and ultimately drowning in excrement at the hands of Nazis guards at Auschwitz for refusing to renounce his ministry (Rodrigues, 2014)—these are examples of awe-inspired behaviors that carried significance costs. And significance can be pursued at the expense of awe, as exemplified by Herostratus, the 4th-century B.C. Greek arsonist who destroyed the Temple of Artemis, one of the seven wonders of the world, to become famous (Smith, 1867), as well as by the modern-day fame-seeking vandal attackers of Da Vinci's *Mona Lisa* painting in the Louvre (Nayeri, 2022).

Another possible evolutionary function of awe and significance needs is in their reciprocal and mutually mediating relationship. Significance striving, including competition, conflict, and aggression, is taxing; the testosterone and cortisol that regulate these behaviors tend to strain the cardiac and circulatory systems and weaken the immune function (Casto & Edwards, 2016; Sapolsky, 1998; Suay et al., 1999; Wein, 2015). There is no respite from the rat race for success: When John D. Rockefeller, the first billionaire and then the richest man on earth, was asked how much money is enough, he famously answered, "Just a little bit more" (Rastogi, 2021, para. 2). Significance seeking is relentless. And sooner or later, even the most successful individuals may face defeat and the ensuing loss of significance, which can be psychologically devastating (Hobfoll, 1991). Awe offers a reprieve from significance seeking, an escape from the costs of competition, and comfort in defeat. On the other hand, awe and the feelings of vulnerability that it elicits can be difficult to sustain without suffering adverse psychological effects stemming from the experiences of smallness and childlike helplessness; the suffering these induce invites switching to significance striving to relieve the burdens of awe. Thus, in combination, significance and awe enhance individual and collective fitness by mitigating their respective costs and increasing the capacity to respond adaptively to the challenges of the environment.

It merits an empirical investigation, but we hypothesize that rather than being on opposite ends of a continuum where lost significance elicits awe, and vice versa, awe and significance are two independent needs that can overshadow one another when in dominant focus. In this sense, we predict that loss of significance can occur without an experience of awe—if the person dwells on their low significance. Failure itself is not yet awe. However, once significance is left behind (involuntarily or by choice), this opens the possibility to experience awe by focusing, for example, on the transience of achievement in the context of greater things, such as God, nature, beauty, and so forth.

The Complementarity of Awe and Significance

We propose that the relationship between awe and significance is conditionally reciprocal, such that pursuing one temporarily closes off the possibility of pursuing the other.

Developmentally

In early childhood, significance is pursued through acquiring competencies for which one is praised by caregivers, and awe is pursued by initiating exploration independent of caregivers' feedback. Juxtaposing these two pursuits as extrinsic versus intrinsic motivation, an early study by Lepper, Greene, and Nisbett (1973) had preschool children engage in a drawing activity for either an expected reward ("Good Player" certificate) or for no reward. There was also an unexpected-reward condition, in which the children engaged in the activity without mention of a reward but unexpectedly received a reward after they had finished with the activity. Two weeks later, the target activity (drawing) was made available for children for several days to gauge their intrinsic interest in the activity. It was found that children in the expected-reward condition showed a significant decrease in interest in the activity (compared with baseline) compared with children in the remaining two conditions. Several studies have confirmed that the children who were paid money or rewarded with tokens for playing were significantly less likely to subsequently select the same activity; when explicitly queried by the experimenters, they also reported less interest in this activity (Deci, Koestner, & Ryan, 1999). The original study focused on the role of extrinsic rewards in reducing intrinsic motivation; however, a slightly different interpretation of this result is that self-initiated exploration (awe) can be turned into a significance pursuit by an extrinsic reward.

Awe can be intrinsically motivated, but that does not mean that every intrinsically motivated activity is necessarily awe related. According to the means–ends fusion of intrinsic motivation (Kruglanski et al., 2018), any activity can be experienced as intrinsically motivated if its association with its goal is sufficiently strengthened. Awe relates to a special type of self-transcendent goal, focused on the vastness and incomprehensibility of the world outside. Children in the classic Lepper et al. (1973) study were arguably experiencing awe when engaged in their drawing activity, lost in its pursuit and transcending their egos in the process.

Physiologically

As noted earlier, significance attainment is related to testosterone, whereas awe attainment is related to oxytocin. Interestingly, these two hormones were observed to change jointly and inversely in an experimental study that induced empathy by exposing participants to a video of a sick child (Procyshyn, Watson, & Crespi, 2020), such that an increase in oxytocin corresponded to a decrease in testosterone. In general, testosterone and oxytocin seem to covary reciprocally across domains, including social cognition (Crespi, 2016), mood disorders (Dai et al., 2017), parenting, and pair bonding (Grebe et al., 2019), with a reduction in one corresponding to an increase in the other, and vice versa.

Psychologically

Inducing awe tends to decrease the need for significance. For example, one study induced awe experimentally (by having participants watch a 5-min film of aerial shots of avalanches, waterfalls, mountains, oceans, and forests) or naturalistically (the researchers intercepted people at awe-inspiring places in nature) and measured self-focused attention with items such as "In general, I feel insignificant" (Bai et al., 2017)—which directly assesses significance concerns. There was an inverse relationship between awe and significance, such that participants high on awe reported less significance concerns than those low on awe.

Awe and significance were found to exert opposite effects on aggressive tendencies. Thus, one study compared the effects of awe on aggression with those of a neutral condition or with the effects of another positive emotion on aggression (Yang, Yang, Bao, Liu, & Passmore, 2016) and found that awe reduced participants' aggression motivation and aggressive behavior. In contrast, aggression is positively related to significance-questing (Kruglanski et al., 2023). In other words, whereas awe predicts lower aggression, significance predicts higher aggression.

A similar disparity between awe and significance was observed with respect to *social dominance orientation* (Pratto, Sidanius, Stallworth, & Malle, 1994): a preference for social hierarchy and inequality based on group membership. Awe is negatively related to a social dominance orientation (Zhao, Zhang, Xu, Lu, & He, 2018), whereas significance-questing is positively related to a social dominance orientation (Kruglanski et al., 2016; Troian et al., 2019).

Similarly, opposing effects of significance and awe can be observed in their respective effects on attitudes toward money. Specifically, accumulation of wealth and riches is positively related to significance-questing (Milyavsky, Kruglanski, Gelfand, Chernikova, Ellenberg, & Pierro, 2022). By contrast, awe weakens people's desire for money (Jiang, Yin, Mei, Zhu, & Zhou, 2018) and makes them more willing to give away money to others (Guan et al., 2019).

Awe and significance are also differentially related to the *need for cognitive closure*—an individual difference in desire for predictability, preference for order and structure, discomfort with ambiguity, decisiveness, and close-mindedness (Webster & Kruglanski, 1994). Thus, awe is negatively correlated with the need for closure (Shiota, Keltner, & Mossman, 2007), but the need for significance is positively correlated with the need for closure (Kruglanski, Molinaro, & Sensales, 2021).

In short, not only does an increase in awe reduce significance concerns, but also, across a wide range of attitudinal and behavioral variables—including aggression, prejudice, attitudes toward money and wealth, social dominance, and need for closure––awe and significance were shown to exert opposite effects.

UNSTABLE EQUILIBRIUM

Because the needs for significance and awe are so central to the evolutionary fitness of both the individual and the larger collective, and because their pursuits are mutually exclusive, we propose that these two psychological orientations exist in an unstable equilibrium, where the pursuit of one need is intermittently interrupted by concerns of the other, raising the possibility of switching from self-focused concerns of significance to self-transcendent concerns of awe. Thus, successful athletes whose careers revolve around practice, mastery, and competitions—hence professional significance seeking—are known to pray for performance enhancement and victory (Aicinena, 2018). Appeals to a religious power were found to reduce anxiety, especially in high-profile competitions, and increase well-being (Shahdan, Noh, & Adnan, 2022). Even elite athletes who have achieved extraordinary significance feel the need for awe and derive psychological benefits from fulfilling this need through religious rituals. Relatedly, research suggests that successful business professionals with high job authority and high incomes (who presumably have achieved high professional significance) may be especially vulnerable to feelings of meaninglessness and emptiness (Barnard, 2008; Pudrovska & Karraker, 2014; Walton, 2015), possibly stemming from awe deficit. Jim Carrey, whose humble beginnings included living in a van with his homeless family before he became a world-famous actor, commanding tens of millions in movie contracts, said, "I think everybody should get rich and famous and do everything they ever dreamed of so they can see that it's not the answer" (Brown, 2016, Quote 15). In short, even individuals who are immensely successful in pursuing significance still seem to need awe, suffer without it, and benefit from it.

It is worth pointing out that awe is not simply "nonselfish" goals, for example, altruistic or ideological goals (for freedom, democracy, king and country, etc.). The pursuit of ideological goals can be for the sake of significance, as in the case of a terrorist who expects to become a hero or a martyr for their group—or they can be for the sake of awe, as in the case of someone sacrificing their own needs without an expectation to be recognized or compensated for it. The motivation and expectations at the time of the decision, as opposed to actual consequences, are what determine whether an action stems from significance or awe. Apropos, if one buys a treadmill, the motivation is to use it for running or walking. Later, the treadmill may become a clothes rack—but that eventuality does not change the original motivation behind the decision to purchase it. So, too, with a selfless action that is carried out without an expectation of significance rewards—whether or not such reward is granted at a later time does not change the motivational roots of the action.

A nonselfish action can be seen as driven by awe and not significance when it either does not enhance one's significance (e.g., "when you give to the needy, do not let your left hand know what your right hand is doing"; anonymous donations; random acts of kindness) or detracts from it (e.g., "turning the other cheek," accepting humiliation and not seeking justice against wrongdoers). On the other hand, significance and not awe can be seen as motivating an action when behavior aimed at acquiring riches or status is carried out without any concern for self-transcendent ideals such as honor, loyalty, morality, or virtue. Awe can sometimes override significance concerns, for instance, in contemplating death, the epitome of negative awe, which dwarves and trivializes significance pursuits. On the other hand, focusing on significance can help override the ill effects of dark awe elicited by thoughts of death: People who have a greater fear of death and who prefer to avoid thoughts of mortality are more likely to endorse death-related status consumption (desire to spend lavishly on death-related expenses such as funerals for self and loved ones) than people with less fear or avoidance of death-related thoughts (Cengiz & Cacciatore, 2024).

The ill effects of too much awe are not circumscribed to contemplating death. Even the most successful artists whose awe-inducing visions of beauty have moved countless others feel vulnerable against the vastness of awe that inspires them. The famous French impressionist Claude Monet said, "I'm never finished with my paintings; the further I get, the more I seek the impossible and the more powerless I feel" (Neuendorf, 2016, p. 114). The notion of a *tortured artist*—someone perpetually trying and failing to faithfully represent their inspirations (awe) as well as to earn recognition and income from them (significance)—is a cultural stereotype and an empirical reality among creative individuals (Alacovska & Kärreman, 2023; Ceci & Kumar, 2016).

Hallowed religious texts affirm that those pursuing divine awe are no more immune from wavering into significance concerns than are artists. Moses decried the children of Israel's "murmuring" and doubting him even as he faithfully followed God's instruction to lead them out of Egypt: a messenger of awe, yearning for significance. Jesus, on the night before his arrest, chastised the disciples for not offering him enough significance when they fell asleep instead of praying with him.

Thus, even at the pinnacle of significance, whether from wealth, fame, or professional achievement, lurks the humility of awe, and even at the height of awe of artistic or religious pursuits, the need for significance beckons. Rich people are often anxious to be loved (to elicit awe) for who they are rather than for what they have (Keller, 2011; Liu, Zhang, & Hao, 2017). Successful professionals often suffer from impostor syndrome, doubting that they deserve the significance they have achieved (Bravata et al., 2020). A scientist may be in awe of a theory they develop, but then they want the theory to be viewed as significant. An author may be inspired to write a book (awe), but then they want the book to sell (significance). The balance between awe and significance is ever rocky, tipping from one side to the other.

SIGNIFICANCE- VERSUS AWE-CENTRIC CULTURES

Cultures differ in the extent to which they emphasize significance versus awe. The 19th-century Romantic movement's use of old religious notions of innocence, fall, and redemption demarcates the difference between the Western cultural narratives focused on utilitarianism and significance and awe-directed narratives, including those centered on the Russian soul, the Aryan race, State Shinto, and fundamentalist Islam (Buruma & Margalit, 2005).

Consistent with our notion of an unstable balance between awe and significance, Buruma and Margalit (2005, p. 101) observe that the lines between the two are never so clear: "Islam sometimes becomes a form of Arab chauvinism: State Shinto extolled the Japanese as a divine race." Nonetheless, the differences between significance- and awe-oriented cultures can be striking, as we show next in comparing the cultures of the United States and Russia.

Significance-Centric Culture: USA

The USA's market-driven capitalist economy inspires the accumulation of wealth and pursuit of the *American Dream*, the idea of an individual rising from rags to riches and thus achieving social status and significance (Dallmann, Boesenberg, & Klepper, 2016). Even in childhood, when awe-inspiring exploration of the world is an integral part of normal development, in the decades since the 1980s, the USA has increasingly introduced competition and striving through structured extracurricular activities heavy on competition and achievement focus, greatly reducing children's exposure to nature, play, and self-initiated art and the awe these inspire (Haidt, 2024).

American adults (compared with those from collectivist cultures such as Japan or Puerto Rico) place more value on self-reliance, competition, and subordination of ingroup goals to personal goals (Triandis,

Bontempo, Villareal, Asai, & Lucca, 1988), preferring to advance individual significance even at a cost to the larger collective. Even among athletes who dwell in a significance-oriented domain of competition, achievement, and status hierarchy, Americans demonstrate greater competitiveness on psychological measures than, for example, Japanese athletes (Hayashi & Weiss, 1994). Advancement of individual significance, therefore, is a guiding principle that is culturally imprinted on individuals from childhood onward, resulting in greater value placed on individual achievement, competitiveness, and materialistic attainment. Even in religion, American significance culture has given rise to a Protestant belief equating wealth and status acquisition with evidence of God's favor (Stark, 2005), quite a departure from the original Christian gospel's proclamation that it is "easier for a camel to go through the eye of a needle than for a rich man to enter the kingdom of Heaven."

American poet Mary Oliver described her significance-seeking homeland as follows: "We will be known as a culture that feared death and adored power, that tried to vanquish insecurity for the few and cared little for the penury of the many. We will be known as a culture that taught and rewarded the amassing of things. . . . All the world, in our eyes, they will say, was a commodity" (Oliver, 2008, p. 46).

Awe-Centric Culture: Russia

The Russian culture cultivates tolerance and acceptance of awe in the kind of fatalism that gave rise to the game of Russian roulette and the notion of *avos'*—a complete reliance on luck, God, or some higher power often used in place of making efforts to personally advance the goal one cares about (Murray, 2012). Russian superstitiousness and fatalism, represented in popular culture through linguistic phrasing and folklore (Kuzmina, 2012), present everything through the prism of humility, uncertainty, and ultimate lack of control over outcomes.

Russian cultural discourse continually examines the differences between Russia and the West, often finding the latter shallow and materialistic in contrast to Russian passion and spirituality. This comparison permeates Dostoyevsky's novels and is embodied, for example, in *The Brothers Karamazov*'s characters of Dmitrij Karamazov, a typical Russian (passionate, unpredictable, and selfless), and Smerdyakov, a Westerner at heart (calculating, cold-blooded, and self-serving). Accordingly, Russian public opinion juxtaposes what it sees as *Western values* of individualism and materialism and *Russian values* of collectivism and spirituality. Sociological surveys find that Russians feel disdain toward the Western worship of wealth and Western soullessness (Ionova, 2008). Of 1,600 Russians surveyed, 26% said they consider Western values destructive, and an additional 33% said that Western values were inappropriate for Russia (Russian Public Opinion Research Center, 2022). Among its own values that Russia juxtaposes to those of the West are patriotism, service to the country, high moral ideals, priority of the spiritual over the material, collectivism, mutual help, historical memory, and intergenerational continuity (Timofeev, 2021). The prevailing narrative in Russian public discourse often claims that the West hates Russia because of Russia's superior values, such as spirituality, faith, and high morals (Lepekhin, 2016).

Consistent with the low regard for individual significance, individual humiliation is frequent in Russia: It is routine among school students as well as between teachers and students (Gorbatkova, 2017); it is practiced as a management style in corporate situations (Korotov, 2022) and is routine in Russian prisons (Mukhamedzhanov, 2016) and in the Russian military (Kulikov, 2022). Humiliation is common not only in Russian daily life but also on widely watched Russian television shows, with no legal consequences against perpetrators (Smolin, 2011), instilling a broad social norm of acceptance for both humiliation and impunity for those who inflict it. Echoing the low priority of individual significance in Russia are findings that individual life is also not nearly as valued there as it is in the West. *Forbes* reports that the relative price of a human life, as measured by either court decisions to compensate for loss or payments for soldiers who died in service, is significantly lower in Russia than in the European Union or North America (Zubets, 2018). A recent video of newly recruited Russian soldiers about to be sent off to fight in Ukraine shows their commander's speech to them: "All of you will die. But you must know that Mother Russia will remember us" (The Racecar Driver, 2024). In the same spirit of valuing awe over significance, recent catastrophic flooding in Russia was addressed not with efforts to evacuate people but with Orthodox priests being flown over the flooded region in a helicopter to pray (AFP, 2024). Some political observers claim that Russia has a "cult of death" (Motyl, 2023), glorifying suffering and death as the highest aspirations, an awe to strive for.

This is not to say that Russians are insensitive to significance needs or material rewards. Far from it. Russian oligarchs are notorious for grabbing as much money and power as they can (Shinar, 2015), and Russian soldiers loot everything, including toilets and washing machines, from the Ukrainian homes they invade (Ong, 2022). When a basic need is suppressed by cultural norms, its fulfillment can take on extreme and destructive forms. Just as extreme hunger can lead a person to eat tree bark or extreme thirst can lead one to drink seawater, a motivational imbalance in awe or significance needs can result in extremism (Kruglanski, Szumowska, Kopetz, Vallerand, & Pierro,, 2021).

Deprivation of significance needs in Russia's case can lead to extreme greed for money and power; deprivation of awe needs in the USA may lead to the rise of belief in conspiracy theories like QAnon (Bloom & Moskalenko, 2021).

Of importance, here we hypothesize about a difference between Russia and the United States in awe versus significance approach at the level of cultural norms. As with other cultural norms, exposure to extreme situations, including imminent threats to one's life, is known to weaken cultural norms (Appleby-Arnold, Brockdorff, Jakovljev, & Zdravković, 2021; Hennekam & Shymko, 2020). We therefore predict a greater difference between these two cultures in adherence to the hypothesized awe-significance cultural default in normative contexts than in extreme contexts, a prediction that merits empirical exploration.

With approaches to daily routine and disasters, life and death, war and peace as vastly divergent as those of the United States and Russia, understanding the other side's motives and ultimate goals can be challenging—especially when the two sides' interests are at odds, one striving for significance and the other aiming for awe. The following case exemplifies such a conflict.

AWE, SIGNIFICANCE, AND MEANING IN THE ISRAEL–HAMAS CONFLICT

The war in Gaza, begun in 2023, is but the latest move in the tragic dance between Israelis and Palestinians, at least since the establishment of the Israeli state in 1948. Typically, the Israeli–Palestinian conflict is perceived as a "realistic" one over a concrete scarce resource: the territory of Palestine. We submit, however, that land is a proxy, of symbolic rather than literal value, and the real issue at hand is the *self-meaning* that possession of the land represents. It derives from two separate meaning systems to which actors in the conflict subscribe: the significance and awe systems that, in an intermingled way, affect the players' attitudes and ultimately drive their actions.

Significance

In the early 20th century, both European Jews and Palestinian Arabs were waking up to a new opportunity to enhance their significance, which had been wanting for centuries. The nationalist spirit that had been shaping the international order throughout the 19th century beckoned to both parties, which, for different reasons, felt downtrodden and humiliated. Nationhood required a home, a territory, a land to call one's own. For both Jews and Arabs, the path to significance led to the sovereignty of the land of Palestine. Those who had sovereignty had significance and could proudly claim their equal place among the world's nations. Those who did not were stateless, devoid of standing in the international arena.

Awe

The awe system sacralizes the ideological cause and portrays its promotion and defense as a supreme imperative that overrides other considerations (Moskalenko & McCauley, 2019). In the context of the Israel–Hamas conflict, the awe system is represented by the religious nationalism of Hamas on the Palestinian side and the messianic mindset of the settlers on the Israeli side.

Kahn, Klar, and Roccas (2017) proposed a distinction between transgenerational (TG) and intragenerational (IG) views of groups that echoes the distinction between the awe and significance paradigms. Perceiving the group as IG implies focusing mainly on the current cohort of group members, whereas perceiving it as TG implies thinking of the group as extending beyond the current generation, stretching across past, present, and future—in short, viewing the group as an eternal entity. Kahn et al. (2017) find that a tendency to perceive the group as TG is related to the willingness to endure ingroup suffering and sacrifice current members, including oneself, for the group. This relationship is mediated by the degree to which the interest of the group as a whole is given primacy over the interest of the group as a collection of group members. Similarly, research by Atran and colleagues (e.g., Atran, 2016) suggests that when people act as "devoted actors," they are deontic (i.e., duty-based) agents who mobilize for collective action in a way that is divorced from instrumental rationality in resisting material compromises. Devoted actors are willing to advance sacred values through costly sacrifice and extreme actions; they are ready to kill and die in the promotion or protection of those values.

It is true that people may be willing to die and kill for their sense of significance as well, especially when this is tied to their social identity, such as when in danger of being humiliated by an external enemy (Kruglanski, Fernandez, et al., 2019). Unlike when in the awe state of mind, however, when acting on behalf of their personal significance, people can still be swayed to consider alternative routes to that end (Kruglanski et al., 2002, 2023), including individualistic paths unrelated to the collective ideal. When in the awe state of mind, in contrast, such significance-affording alternatives hold no appeal because the only thing that matters is the idealized cause. In other words, the significance-oriented attitude admits substitute paths to significance, ones that include material compromise (e.g., the proposed two-state solution between Israel and Palestine). It represents the strategy of satisficing, in contrast to the maximizing approach of the awe-oriented mindset.

When in an awe state of mind, personal lives do not matter, whether of the enemy or of one's own group's members. In 2005, Yuval Bitton, head of the intelligence division of the Israel Prison Service, interviewed Yahya Sinwar, a chief architect of the October 7, 2023, massacre of 1,200 Israelis by Hamas. He asked Sinwar, "Is it worth it for 10,000 innocent Gazans to die, in order to free 100 prisoners?" The reply was, "Even 100,000 is worth it" (Shani, 2024, para. 17).

There is a qualitative difference in attitudes to the Israeli–Palestinian conflict between the Palestinian Fatah organization and Hamas. Whereas Fatah has viewed the Israeli–Palestinian feud from a significance perspective, Hamas is largely driven by the awe paradigm. As Yuval Bitton reports, "Fatah talked about the 1967 borders, about the occupation, about the Palestinian people. To me, the Hamas inmates would say, 'There's neither 1967 nor 1948. There are no borders and there is nothing to talk about. You are on Waqf land, Muslim sacred ground, and you have no place here'" (Shani, 2024, para, 22).

The distinction between significance-focused and awe-focused modes of thought is represented among the Israelis as well. A survey conducted by the Israel Democracy Institute between November 27 and 30, 2023, found that the religious/national Haredi group is the only one in which only a minority expressed support for a hostage deal that would involve a ceasefire with Hamas. The highest level of support was found among secular respondents. A breakdown by age (Jewish sample) shows that the older the respondents, the stronger their support for the deal, seemingly because older age groups in Israel are generally more secular and identify more strongly as on the Left (Hermann & Anabi, 2023).

In some extremist sections of Israel and the diaspora, the extremist mode of religious thinking, which sees God as a God of holy wars and vengeance and demands that Jews act violently in his name, has been gaining ground for more than half a century. But since the October 7 attacks, it has evolved into a more coherent worldview, a political theology that licenses and even commands collective punishment and dismisses efforts to return the Israeli hostages (Manekin, 2024). Sacralization of the Israel–Palestine conflict on both sides of the divide has moved the prospects of peace between the parties ever further from reach. Again, we distinguish religious ideology as a means to significance (i.e., being a "good" Christian, Muslim, or Jew) from the awe a religious person feels in contemplating the Almighty, which can inspire the kind of mystical experience that prompts an instantaneous conversion and embracement of a faith (James, 1902/2002).

CONCLUSION

In this chapter, we proposed a new psychological theory to capture the dichotomy that has inspired the major religious movements and systems of meaning that have shaped Western civilization: self-focused pursuit of significance and self-transcendent pursuit of awe. Existing research on these two phenomena suggests their intertwined evolutionary and developmental origins, as well as a reciprocal relationship between them, with an increase in significance or its correlates corresponding to a decrease in awe or its correlates, and vice versa. We proposed that the relationship between awe and significance is in a state of unstable equilibrium, tipping continually back and forth between significance and awe concerns, enabling fulfillment of needs for each.

At the same time, it is possible to prioritize one over the other, and some cultures seem to consistently do so, developing a significance- or awe-centric cultural default of imbuing events and situations with meaning. The United States, we suggest, is an example of a significance-centric culture; Russia is an example of an awe-centric culture. Because significance concerns can lead to dramatically different values and pursuits than awe concerns, understanding the cultural (or individual) default is important for navigating conflicts, such as that between Israel and Hamas. Concern for human life and its quality, irrelevant to the awe-centric, is paramount to the significance-centric; offering financial concessions, a valid currency for the significance-centric, can be insulting to the awe-centric. What is lost in translation can result in tragic and historic consequences. A fluency in these two psychological paradigms would allow us to seek a common ground or, in the words of the Buddha, "a middle way" in conflicts between awe and significance concerns that can otherwise be intractable.

REFERENCES

Acker, S. (2023). Beauty and beautification in refugees' lives and their implications for refugee policy. *Refuge: Canada's Journal on Refugees, 39*(1), 1–46.

AFP. (2024, April 12). Russian priests fight river flooding with prayer from above. *The Moscow Times. www.themoscowtimes.com/2024/04/12/russian-priests-fight-river-flooding-with-prayer-from-above-a84821*

Aicinena, S. (2018). Implicit religion and the use of prayer in sport. *American Journal of Sociological Research, 7*(1), 56–65.

Alacovska, A., & Kärreman, D. (2023). Tormented selves: The social imaginary of the tortured artist and the identity work of creative workers. *Organization Studies, 44*(6), 961–985.

Appleby-Arnold, S., Brockdorff, N., Jakovljev, I., & Zdravkovi?, S. (2021). Disaster preparedness and cultural factors: A comparative study in Romania and Malta. *Disasters, 45*(3), 664–690.

Atran, S. (2016). The devoted actor: Unconditional commitment and intractable conflict across cultures. *Current Anthropology, 57*(S13), S192–S203.

Bai, Y., Maruskin, L. A., Chen, S., Gordon, A. M., Stellar, J. E., McNeil, G. D., Peng, K., & Keltner, D. (2017). Awe, the diminished self, and collective engagement: Universals and cultural variations in the small self. *Journal of Personality and Social Psychology, 113*(2), 185–209.

Bannister, S. (2019). Distinct varieties of aesthetic chills in response to multimedia. *PLOS One, 14*(11), e0224974.

Bargh, J. A. (1990). Auto-motives: Preconscious determinants of social interaction. In E. T. Higgins & R. M. Sorrentino (Eds.), *Handbook of motivation and cognition* (Vol. 2, pp. 93–130). New York: Guilford Press.

Barnard, J. W. (2008). *Narcissism, over-optimism, fear, anger, and depression: The interior lives of corporate leaders* (SSRN Scholarly Paper 1136888). SSRN. *papers.ssrn.com/sol3/papers.cfm?abstract_id=1136888*

Basalla, G. (1988). *The evolution of technology*. Cambridge University Press.

Bernhardt, P. C., Dabbs Jr, J. M., Fielden, J. A., & Lutter, C. D. (1998). Testosterone changes during vicarious experiences of winning and losing among fans at sporting events. *Physiology & Behavior, 65*(1), 59–62.

Bloom, M., & Moskalenko, S. (2021). *Pastels and pedophiles: Inside the mind of QAnon*. Stanford University Press.

Book, A. S., Starzyk, K. B., & Quinsey, V. L. (2001). The relationship between testosterone and aggression: A meta-analysis. *Aggression and Violent Behavior, 6*(6), 579–599.

Bravata, D. M., Watts, S. A., Keefer, A. L., Madhusudhan, D. K., Taylor, K. T., Clark, D. M., et al. (2020). Prevalence, predictors, and treatment of impostor syndrome: A systematic review. *Journal of General Internal Medicine, 35*(4), 1252–1275.

Brown, J. (2016, February 20). *27 inspirational Jim Carrey quotes*. Addicted 2 Success. *addicted2success.com/quotes/27-inspirational-jim-carrey-quotes/*

Brumm, A., Oktaviana, A. A., Burhan, B., Hakim, B., Lebe, R., Zhao, J., et al. (2021). Oldest cave art found in Sulawesi. *Science Advances, 7*(3), Article eabd4648.

Bruner, J. S. (1968). *The course of cognitive growth: Thinking and reasoning*. Penguin.

Bruner, J. S. (1973). Organization of early skilled action. *Child Development, 44*(1), 1–11.

Buruma, I., & Margalit, A. (2005). *Occidentalism: The West in the eyes of its enemies*. Penguin.

Buss, D. M., & Shackelford, T. K. (1997). Human aggression in evolutionary psychological perspective. *Clinical Psychology Review, 17*(6), 605–619.

Carré, J. M. (2006). *Salivary testosterone and cortisol: Role of athletic setting, game outcome, and game* [Doctoral dissertation, Brock University].

Casto, K. V., & Edwards, D. A. (2016). Testosterone, cortisol, and human competition. *Hormones and Behavior, 82*, 21–37.

Ceci, M. W., & Kumar, V. K. (2016). A correlational study of creativity, happiness, motivation, and stress from creative pursuits. *Journal of Happiness Studies, 17*(2), 609–626.

Cengiz, H., & Cacciatore, J. (2024). Status consumption as coping with fear of death: The mediating role of death avoidance and the moderating role of materialism. *Psychological Reports*, 00332941241251458.

Child, A. B., & Child, I. L. (1993). *Religion and magic in the life of traditional peoples*. Prentice Hall.

Chirico, A., Cipresso, P., Yaden, D. B., Biassoni, F., Riva, G., & Gaggioli, A. (2017). Effectiveness of immersive videos in inducing awe: An experimental study. *Scientific Reports, 7*(1), 1218.

Crespi, B. J. (2016). Oxytocin, testosterone, and human social cognition. *Biological Reviews, 91*(2), 390–408.

Dai, D., Li, Q.-C., Zhu, Q.-B., Hu, S.-H., Balesar, R., Swaab, D., et al. (2017). Direct involvement of androgen receptor in oxytocin gene expression: Possible relevance for mood disorders. *Neuropsychopharmacology, 42*(10), Article 10.

Dallmann, A., Boesenberg, E., & Klepper, M. (2016). *Approaches to American cultural studies*. Routledge.

Deci, E. L., Koestner, R., & Ryan, R. M. (1999). A meta-analytic review of experiments examining the effects of extrinsic rewards on intrinsic motivation. *Psychological Bulletin, 125*(6), 627.

Deci, E. L., & Ryan, R. M. (2000). The "what" and" why" of goal pursuits: Human needs and the self-determination of behavior. *Psychological Inquiry, 11*(4), 227–268.

Dissanayake, E. (2015). *What is art for?* University of Washington Press.

Dutton, D. (2009). *The art instinct: Beauty, pleasure, & human evolution*. Oxford University Press.

Ebert, A., Patrick, J. H., Huggins, M., Yadava, A., & Collett, S. (2021). Age differences in awe among young, middle-aged, and older adults: Extensions of socioemotional selectivity theory. *Innovation in Aging, 5*(Suppl. 1), 766–767.

Edwards, D. A., & Casto, K. V. (2013). Women's intercollegiate athletic competition: Cortisol, testosterone, and the dual-hormone hypothesis as it relates to status among teammates. *Hormones and Behavior, 64*(1), 153–160.

Feldman, R. (2012). Oxytocin and social affiliation in humans. *Hormones and Behavior, 61*(3), 380–391.

Festinger, L. (1954). A theory of social comparison processes. *Human Relations, 7*(2): 117–140.

Fiske, S. T. (2010). Interpersonal stratification: Status, power, and subordination.

In S. T. Fiske, D. T. Gilbert, & G. Lindzey (Eds.), *Handbook of social psychology* (5th ed., pp. 941–982). Wiley.

Frijda, N. H. (1986). *The emotions*. Cambridge University Press.

Glazier, S. D. (1999). *Anthropology of religion: A handbook* (2nd ed.). Praeger.

Glazier, S. D., & Ember, C. R. (2018). Religion. In C. R. Ember (Ed.), *Explaining human culture*. New Haven: Human Relations Area Files. *hraf.yale.edu/teach-ehraf/religion-explaining-human-culture/*

Golden, L., Moser, J., Vella-Riplee, A., MacPhee, J., Schwartz, V., Levin, L., et al. (2020). Adulting is hard: Understanding the college-to-career transition and supporting young adults' emotional wellbeing. *Psychiatry Information in Brief, 17*(21).

Gorbatkova, O. I. (2017). Проблема насилия в школах в зеркале современных российских медиа. *Media Education*, 2, 189–205.

Gordon, A. M., Stellar, J. E., Anderson, C. L., McNeil, G. D., Loew, D., & Keltner, D. (2017). The dark side of the sublime: Distinguishing a threat-based variant of awe. *Journal of Personality and Social Psychology, 113*(2), 310–328.

Graziosi, M., & Yaden, D. (2021). Interpersonal awe: Exploring the social domain of awe elicitors. *Journal of Positive Psychology, 16*(2), 263–271.

Grebe, N. M., Sarafin, R. E., Strenth, C. R., & Zilioli, S. (2019). Pair-bonding, fatherhood, and the role of testosterone: A meta-analytic review. *Neuroscience & Biobehavioral Reviews, 98*, 221–233.

Guan, F., Chen, J., Chen, O., Liu, L., & Zha, Y. (2019). Awe and prosocial tendency. *Current Psychology, 38*(4), 1033–1041.

Haidt, J. (2024). *The anxious generation*. Penguin.

Hamilton, W. D. (1964). The genetical evolution of social behaviour. I. *Journal of Theoretical Biology,* 7(1): 1–16.

Handelsman, D. J., Sikaris, K., & Ly, L. P. (2016). Estimating age-specific trends in circulating testosterone and sex hormone-binding globulin in males and females across the lifespan. *Annals of Clinical Biochemistry, 53*(3), 377–384.

Harrison, L., & Loui, P. (2014). Thrills, chills, frissons, and skin orgasms: Toward an integrative model of transcendent psychophysiological experiences in music. *Frontiers in Psychology, 5*, Article 790.

Hasegawa, M., Toda, M., & Morimoto, K. (2008). Changes in salivary physiological stress markers associated with winning and losing. *Biomedical Research, 29*(1), 43–46.

Hayashi, C. T., & Weiss, M. R. (1994). A cross-cultural analysis of achievement motivation in Anglo-American and Japanese marathon runners. *International Journal of Sport Psychology, 25*(2), 187–202.

Hellhammer, D. H., Wüst, S., & Kudielka, B. M. (2009). Salivary cortisol as a biomarker in stress research. *Psychoneuroendocrinology, 34*(2), 163–171.

Hennekam, S., & Shymko, Y. (2020). Coping with the COVID-19 crisis: Force majeure and gender performativity. *Gender, Work & Organization, 27*(5), 788–803.

Hermann, T., & Anabi, O. (2023, May). *Israelis sharply divided on the question of a two-state solution in return for US assistance*. Israel Democracy Institute. *en.idi.org.il/articles/51746*

Higgins, E. T. (1996). Emotional experiences: The pains and pleasures of distinct regulatory systems. In R. D. Kavanaugh, B. Zimmerberg, & S. Fein (Eds.), *Emotion: Interdisciplinary Perspectives*, 203–241. Erlbaum.

Hobfoll, S. E. (1991). Traumatic stress: A theory based on rapid loss of resources. *Anxiety Research, 4*(3), 187–197.

Ionova, E. V. (2008). Отношение населения России к ценностям западной культуры (по материалам г. Астрахани). *https://cyberleninka.ru/article/n/otnoshenie-naseleniya-rossii-k-tsennostyam-zapadnoy-kultury-po-materialam-g-astrahani/viewer*

James, W. (2002). *The varieties of religious experience: A study in human nature* (2nd ed.). Routledge. (Original work published 1902)

Jiang, L., Yin, J., Mei, D., Zhu, H., & Zhou, X. (2018). Awe weakens the desire for money. *Journal of Pacific Rim Psychology, 12*, Article e4.

Kahn, D. T., Klar, Y., & Roccas, S. (2017). For the sake of the eternal group: Perceiving the group as trans-generational and endurance of ingroup suffering. *Personality and Social Psychology Bulletin, 43*(2), 272–283.

Kalnins, I. V., & Bruner, J. S. (1973). The coordination of visual observation and instrumental behavior in early infancy. *Perception, 2*(3), 307–314.

Keller, T. (2011). *Counterfeit gods: The empty promises of money, sex, and power, and the only hope that matters*. Penguin.

Keltner, D. (2024). *Awe: The new science of everyday wonder and how it can transform your life*. Penguin.

Keltner, D., & Haidt, J. (2003). Approaching awe, a moral, spiritual, and aesthetic emotion. *Cognition & Emotion, 17*(2), 297–314.

Kruglanski, A. W., Bélanger, J. J., & Gunaratna, R. (2019). *The three pillars of radicalization: Needs, narratives, and networks*. Oxford University Press.

Kruglanski, A. W., Ellenberg, M., Szumowska, E., Molinario, E., Speckhard, A., Leander, N. P., et al. (2023). Frustration–aggression hypothesis reconsidered: The role of significance quest. *Aggressive Behavior, 49*(5), 445–468.

Kruglanski, A. W., Fernandez, J. R., Factor, A. R., & Szumowska, E. (2019). Cognitive mechanisms in violent extremism. *Cognition, 188*, 116–123.

Kruglanski, A. W., Fishbach, A., Woolley, K., Bélanger, J. J., Chernikova, M., Molinario, E., & Pierro, A. (2018). A structural model of intrinsic motivation: On the psychology of means-ends fusion. *Psychological Review, 125*(2), 165.

Kruglanski, A. W., Gelfand, M. J., Sheveland, A., Babush, M., Hetiarachchi, M., Ng Bonto, M., et al. (2016). What a difference two years make: Patterns of radicalization in a Philippine jail. *Dynamics of Asymmetric Conflict, 9*(1–3), 13–36.

Kruglanski, A. W., Molinario, E., Jasko, K., Webber, D., Leander, N. P., & Pierro, A. (2022). Significance-quest theory. *Perspectives on Psychological Science, 17*(4), 1050–1071.

Kruglanski, A. W., Molinaro, E., & Sensales, G. (2021). Why populism attracts. On the allure of certainty and dignity. In J. P. Forgas, W. D. Crano, & K. Fiedler (Eds.), *The psychology of populism: The tribal challenge to liberal democracy* (pp. 97–115). Routledge.

Kruglanski, A. W., Szumowska, E., Kopetz, C. H., Vallerand, R. J., & Pierro,

A. (2021). On the psychology of extremism: How motivational imbalance breeds intemperance. *Psychological Review, 128*(2), 264–289.

Kulikov, A. (2022, November 23). Смерти, унижение и насилие очень распространены в российской армии, и их военным это кажется нормой—Романцова. Громадське радіо. *https://hromadske.radio/ru/podcasts/voynf-ynformatsyonn-y-marafon/smerty-unyzhenye-nasylye-ochen-rasprostranen-v-rossyyskoy-armyy-y-ykh-voenn-m-to-kazhetsia-normoy-romantsova*Lake, R. (2024). *How to plan for travel in retirement.* Investopedia. *www.investopedia.com/retirement/how-plan-travel-retirement/*

Kuzmina, E. O. (2012). Метафизическая сущность «авось», «небось» и «как-нибудь» как средство выражения ментальности русского народа (на материале сказки С. Кржижановского «Когда рак свистнет»). [The metaphysical essence of "maybe," "perhaps," and "somehow," as a means of expressing the mentality of the Russian people (based on S. Krzhizhanovsky's fairy tale "When the Crab Whistles").] «Молодой. *https://moluch.ru/conf/phil/archive/27/2334/*

Lepekhin, V. (2016). Запад видит в России врага, потому что у неё "неправильные" ценности. [The West see Russia as an enemy because it has "wrong" values.] РИА Новости. *https://ria.ru/20160317/1391628897.html*

Lepper, M. R., Greene, D., & Nisbett, R. E. (1973). Undermining children's intrinsic interest with extrinsic rewards: A test of the "overjustification" hypothesis. *Journal of Personality and Social Psychology, 28*(1), 129–137.

Liu, C.-J., Zhang, Y., & Hao, F. (2017). An implicit stereotype of the rich and its relation to psychological connectedness. *Journal of Pacific Rim Psychology, 11*, Article e7.

Luo, L., Zou, R., Yang, D., & Yuan, J. (2023). Awe experience triggered by fighting against COVID-19 promotes prosociality through increased feeling of connectedness and empathy. *Journal of Positive Psychology, 18*(6), 866–882.

Manekin, M. (2024, May 7). In Israel, Jewish extremists worshipping a God of holy war are getting stronger. *Haaretz: www.haaretz.com/opinion/2024-05-07/ty-article-opinion/.premium/in-israel-jewish-extremists-worshipping-a-god-of-holy-war-are-getting-stronger/0000018f-496c-d17f-adcf-f9ef43630000*

Mayr, U., Wozniak, D., Davidson, C., Kuhns, D., & Harbaugh, W. T. (2012). Competitiveness across the life span: The feisty fifties. *Psychology and Aging, 27*(2), 278–285.

Mazur, A., & Lamb, T. A. (1980). Testosterone, status, and mood in human males. *Hormones and Behavior, 14*(3), 236–246.

Mehta, P. H., Jones, A. C., & Josephs, R. A. (2008). The social endocrinology of dominance: Basal testosterone predicts cortisol changes and behavior following victory and defeat. *Journal of Personality and Social Psychology, 94*(6), 1078–1093.

Mehta, P. H., & Josephs, R. A. (2010). Testosterone and cortisol jointly regulate dominance: Evidence for a dual-hormone hypothesis. *Hormones and Behavior, 58*(5), 898–906.

Mehta, P. H., Lawless DesJardins, N. M., van Vugt, M., & Josephs, R. A. (2017). Hormonal underpinnings of status conflict: Testosterone and cortisol are related to decisions and satisfaction in the hawk-dove game. *Hormones and Behavior, 92*, 141–154.

Milyavsky, M., Kruglanski, A. W., Gelfand, M., Chernikova, M., Ellenberg, M., & Pierro, A. (2022). People who need people (and some who think they don't): On compensatory personal and social means of goal pursuit. *Psychological Inquiry, 33*(1), 1–22.

Moskalenko, S., & McCauley, C. (2019). *The marvel of martyrdom: The power of self-sacrifice in a selfish world*. Oxford University Press.

Motyl, O. C. (2023, February 21). Russia's cult of death. *The Hill. thehill.com/opinion/international/3864092-russias-cult-of-death/*

Mukhamedzhanov, B. (2016). "Мочить в сортире"—Тюремная политика России. openDemocracy. *www.opendemocracy.net/ru/mochit-v-sortire/*

Murray, M. (2012, July 30). You shouldn't count on Russian avos for success. *The Moscow Times. www.themoscowtimes.com/2012/07/30/you-shouldnt-count-on-russian-avos-for-success-a16641*

Nayeri, F. (2022, November 3). There is a long history of vandalizing art for a cause. But is it effective? *Artnet News. https://news.artnet.com/art-world-archives/vandals-with-a-cause-op-ed-2203145*

Neuendorf, H. (2016, November 14). *9 brilliant quotes by Claude Monet on his birthday*. Artnet News. *news.artnet.com/art-world/quotes-claude-monet-birthday-747290*

Neumark, D. (2013). Drawn to beauty: The practice of house-beautification as homemaking amongst the forcibly displaced. *Housing, Theory and Society, 30*(3), 237–261.

Oliveira, T., Gouveia, M. J., & Oliveira, R. F. (2009). Testosterone responsiveness to winning and losing experiences in female soccer players. *Psychoneuroendocrinology, 34*(7), 1056–1064.

Oliver, M. (2008). *Red bird: Poems*. Beacon Press.

Ong, D. (2022, April 11). Russians stole wine, washing machine, sofa from abandoned Ukraine homes. *International Business Times. www.ibtimes.com/russian-soldiers-allegedly-stole-wine-washing-machine-sofa-abandoned-ukraine-homes-3470531*

Padgett, D. A., & Glaser, R. (2003). How stress influences the immune response. *Trends in Immunology, 24*(8), 444–448.

Piff, P. K., Dietze, P., Feinberg, M., Stancato, D. M., & Keltner, D. (2015). Awe, the small self, and prosocial behavior. *Journal of Personality and Social Psychology, 108*(6), 883–899.

Pratto, F., Sidanius, J., Stallworth, L. M., & Malle, B. F. (1994). Social dominance orientation: A personality variable predicting social and political attitudes. *Journal of Personality and Social Psychology, 67*(4), 741–763.

Procyshyn, T. L., Watson, N. V., & Crespi, B. J. (2020). Experimental empathy induction promotes oxytocin increases and testosterone decreases. *Hormones and Behavior, 117*, Article 104607.

Pudrovska, T., & Karraker, A. (2014). Gender, job authority, and depression. *Journal of Health and Social Behavior, 55*(4), 424–441.

The Racecar Driver. (2024, May 5). *"All of you will die" Russian commander tells his soldiers* [Video]. YouTube. *www.youtube.com/watch?v=b6JxDvOQx-4*

Rakoczy, H., & Schmidt, M. F. H. (2013). The early ontogeny of social norms. *Child Development Perspectives, 7*(1), 17–21.

Rastogi, S. (2021, April 2). *How much money is enough? Just a little bit more.* CNBCTV18. *www.cnbctv18.com/views/how-much-money-is-enough-just-a-little-bit-more-8800361.html*

Rheingold, H. L. (1985). Development as the acquisition of familiarity. *Annual Review of Psychology, 36*(1), 1–18.

Rheingold, H. L., & Eckerman, C. O. (1969). The infant's free entry into a new environment. *Journal of Experimental Child Psychology, 8*(2), 271–283.

Rodrigues, V. (2014). *Joseph (Józef) Kowalski. Priest and martyr.* Scribd. *www.scribd.com/document/223387833/Jozef-Joseph-Kowalski-by-Victor-Rodrigues*

Ross, H. S. (1974). The influence of novelty and complexity on exploratory behavior in 12-month-old infants. *Journal of Experimental Child Psychology, 17*(3), 436–451.

Russian Public Opinion Research Center. (2022). *Каждый четвертый россиянин назвал западные ценности разрушительными* [Every fourth Russian called Western values destructive]. Lenta RU.

Sapolsky, R. M. (1998). *The trouble with testosterone: And other essays on the biology of the human predicament.* Simon and Schuster.

Scherer, K. R., Zentner, M. R., & Stern, D. (2004). Beyond surprise: The puzzle of infants' expressive reactions to expectancy violation. *Emotion, 4*(4), 389–402.

Schmidt, M. F. H., & Tomasello, M. (2012). Young children enforce social norms. *Current Directions in Psychological Science, 21*(4), 232–236.

Shahdan, S., Noh, Y., & Adnan, Y. (2022). The role of religious faith in sport-related anxiety among elite athletes: An exploratory study. *Jurnal Sains Sukan & Pendidikan Jasmani, 11*(1), Article 1.

Shani, A. (2024, April 12). I Asked Sinwar, Is It Worth 10,000 Innocent Gazans Dying? He Said, Even 100,000 Is Worth It. *Haaretz. archive.is/EDGPY*

Shinar, C. (2015). The Russian oligarchs, from Yeltsin to Putin. *European Review, 23*(4), 583–596.

Shiota, M. N., Campos, B., & Keltner, D. (2003). The faces of positive emotion: Prototype displays of awe, amusement, and pride. *Annals of the New York Academy of Sciences, 1000*(1), 296–299.

Shiota, M. N., Keltner, D., & John, O. P. (2006). Positive emotion dispositions differentially associated with Big Five personality and attachment style. *Journal of Positive Psychology, 1*(2), 61–71.

Shiota, M. N., Keltner, D., & Mossman, A. (2007). The nature of awe: Elicitors, appraisals, and effects on self-concept. *Cognition and Emotion, 21*(5), 944–963.

Silk, J. B., & House, B. R. (2011). Evolutionary foundations of human prosocial sentiments. *Proceedings of the National Academy of Sciences, 108*(Suppl. 2), 10910–10917.

Smith, W. (Ed.). (1867). Herostratus. In *Dictionary of Greek and Roman biography and mythology* (Vol. II). Little, Brown.

Smolin, A. (2011, February 3). Общество унижения. [Society of humiliation.] РАПСИ. *https://rapsinews.ru/incident_publication/20110203/251775031.html*

Song, J. Y., Klebl, C., & Bastian, B. (2023). Awe promotes moral expansiveness via the small-self. *Frontiers in Psychology, 14.*

Stalp, M. C., & Hill, S. (2019). The expectations of adulting: Developing soft skills through active learning classrooms. *Journal of Learning Spaces, 8*(2), Article 2.

Stark, R. (2005). *The victory of reason: How Christianity led to freedom, capitalism, and Western success.* Random House.

Stellar, J. E., Gordon, A., Anderson, C. L., Piff, P. K., McNeil, G. D., & Keltner, D. (2018). Awe and humility. *Journal of Personality and Social Psychology, 114*(2), 258–269.

Suay, F., Salvador, A., González-Bono, E., Sanchís, C., Martínez, M., Martínez-Sanchis, S., et al. (1999). Effects of competition and its outcome on serum testosterone, cortisol and prolactin. *Psychoneuroendocrinology, 24*(5), 551–566.

Sumitra. (2015, August 12). Chinese millionaire gives up fortune, lives in isolation for two years to become Buddhist monk. *Oddity Central. www.odditycentral.com/news/chinese-millionaire-gives-up-fortune-lives-in-isolation-for-two-years-to-become-buddhist-monk.html*

Tajfel, H., & Turner, J. C. (2004). The social identity theory of intergroup behavior. In J. T. Jost & J. Sidanius (Eds.), *Political psychology* (pp. 276–293). Psychology Press.

Takano, R., & Nomura, M. (2023). Strengthened social ties in disasters: Threat-awe encourages interdependent worldviews via powerlessness. *PLOS One, 18*(4), Article e0285049.

Tesser, A. (2000). On the confluence of self-esteem maintenance mechanisms. *Personality and Social Psychology Review, 4*(4), 290–299.

Than, K. (2012, June 14). *World's oldest cave art found—made by Neanderthals?* Adventure. *www.nationalgeographic.com/adventure/article/120614-neanderthal-cave-paintings-spain-science-pike*

Thomson, A. L., & Siegel, J. T. (2017). Elevation: A review of scholarship on a moral and other-praising emotion. *Journal of Positive Psychology, 12*(6), 628–638.

Thrall, P. H., Bever, J. D., & Burdon, J. J. (2010). Evolutionary change in agriculture: The past, present and future. *Evolutionary Applications, 3*(5–6), 405–408.

Timofeev, I. (2021). Аналитика. Клуб «Валдай». [Analytics. Valdai Club.] *https://ru.valdaiclub.com/a/highlights/rossiya-i-zapad-problema-v-tsennostyakh/*

Triandis, H. C., Bontempo, R., Villareal, M. J., Asai, M., & Lucca, N. (1988). Individualism and collectivism: Cross-cultural perspectives on self-ingroup relationships. *Journal of Personality and Social Psychology, 54*(2), 323–338.

Troian, J., Baidada, O., Arciszewski, T., Apostolidis, T., Celebi, E., & Yurtbakan, T. (2019). Evidence for indirect loss of significance effects on violent extremism: The potential mediating role of anomia. *Aggressive Behavior, 45*(6), 691–703.

Uvnäs-Moberg, K. (1997). Oxytocin linked antistress effects—The relaxation and growth response. *Acta Physiologica Scandinavica Supplementum, 640*, 38–42.

van Vugt, M., & Tybur, J. M. (2014). The evolutionary foundations of status hierarchy. In D. Buss (Ed.), *The handbook of evolutionary psychology* (2nd ed., pp. 788–809). Wiley.

von Rueden, C., Gurven, M., & Kaplan, H. (2010). Why do men seek status? Fitness payoffs to dominance and prestige. *Proceedings of the Royal Society B: Biological Sciences, 278*(1715), 2223–2232.

Walton, A. G. (2015). Why the super-successful get depressed. *Forbes*. *www.forbes.com/sites/alicegwalton/2015/01/26/why-the-super-successful-get-depressed/*

Webster, D. M., & Kruglanski, A. W. (1994). Individual differences in need for cognitive closure. *Journal of Personality and Social Psychology, 67*(6), 1049–1062.

Wein, H. (2015, May 22). *The benefits of being a beta male*. National Institutes of Health. *www.nih.gov/news-events/nih-research-matters/benefits-being-beta-male*

Willer, R. (2009). Groups reward individual sacrifice: The status solution to the collective action problem. *American Sociological Review, 74*(1), 23–43.

Winegard, B., Winegard, B., & Geary, D. C. (2018). The status competition model of cultural production. *Evolutionary Psychological Science, 4*(4), 351–371.

Yaden, D. B., Kaufman, S. B., Hyde, E., Chirico, A., Gaggioli, A., Zhang, J. W., & Keltner, D. (2019). The development of the Awe Experience Scale (AWE-S): A multifactorial measure for a complex emotion. *The Journal of Positive Psychology, 14*(4), 474–488.

Yang, Y., & Hu, J. (2021). Self-diminishing effects of awe on consumer forgiveness in service encounters. *Journal of Retailing and Consumer Services, 60*, Article 102491.

Yang, Y., Yang, Z., Bao, T., Liu, Y., & Passmore, H.-A. (2016). Elicited awe decreases aggression. *Journal of Pacific Rim Psychology, 10*, e11.

Zhao, H., Zhang, H., Xu, Y., Lu, J., & He, W. (2018). Relation between awe and environmentalism: The role of social dominance orientation. *Frontiers in Psychology, 9*, Article 2367.

Zilioli, S., & Watson, N. V. (2012). The hidden dimensions of the competition effect: Basal cortisol and basal testosterone jointly predict changes in salivary testosterone after social victory in men. *Psychoneuroendocrinology, 37*(11), 1855–1865.

Zubets, A. (2018, April 26). Скидка на страну. Сколько стоит человеческая жизнь в России. Forbes.ru. *www.forbes.ru/finansy-i-investicii/360649-skidka-na-stranu-skolko-stoit-chelovecheskaya-zhizn v rossii*

PART IV

CLOSING REMARKS

CHAPTER 15

Meaning Making in the Mind and Society

Yaacov Trope

The first two verses of the Hebrew Bible state:

> In the beginning God created the heaven and the earth. And the earth was without form, and void; and darkness was upon the face of the deep.

The first two verses of Hesiod's *Works and Days* (700 B.C.E.), the oldest source of Greek mythology, state:

> In the beginning there was Chaos, a yawning nothingness. Out of the void emerged Gaia (the Earth) and other divine beings—Eros (love), the Abyss (part of the underworld), and the Erebus (the unknowable place where death dwells).

The origins of the two stories of creation couldn't be more different from each other. The biblical story is rooted in monotheistic religions, whereas the Greek mythology story is rooted in polytheistic religions. Nevertheless, both stories construe creation as a process that transforms a formless, empty, and chaotic world into a world that is constitutive of distinct, enduring, and interrelated entities. The entities in the two stories of creation are different—heaven and earth, day and night, land and seas, man and woman in the Bible, and gods giving birth to titans, who then create humans, in Greek mythology. Despite these differences, both the Bible and Greek mythology construe creation as making a meaningful world out of a meaningless pre-creation world.

Thousands of years after the Bible and Greek myths were written, Heider and Simmel (1944) conducted their classic animation experiment to explore meaning making on a more modest human scale. Participants were presented with a cartoon-like animation in which two triangles and a disk moved haphazardly in and around a rectangular shape and were asked to describe what they saw. Heider and Simmel found that the vast majority of their participants did the same—they saw characters with intentions, emotions, and agendas engaging in goal-directed interactions. Remarkably, even when the cartoon was played backward, from end to beginning, to a group of 44 participants, all but 2 construed it in terms of human actions and motives.

The ancient stories of creation and the more recent stories of Heider and Simmel's participants point to entropy reduction as a core aspect of meaning making. In information theory, entropy is a measure of the degree of disorder in a system (Shannon & Weaver, 1949). It reflects the randomness, unpredictability, and chaos in the system. At maximal entropy, all states of the system are equiprobable and the expected information gained by the actualization of one of the states is high. Meaning making transforms an initial high-entropic system into a low-entropic, structured, and predictable system. The cosmic transformation in the creation stories is miraculous because it starts with a maximally entropic, meaningless world and ends with a low-entropic, meaningful world. Although mundane in comparison, the stories told by Heider and Simmel's participants are nevertheless remarkable because almost all of them create a coherent, psychologically meaningful narrative that goes far beyond the erratic movements of the geometric figures in the cartoon. Notably, the notion of entropy applies to both the environment and the construal of the environment. It applies, for example, to both the entropic cartoon featuring geometric figures and to the less entropic construal of the cartoon by participants, to both the origin of the universe and to the biblical or Greek mythological construal of its origin.

In this chapter, meaning making is viewed as a process that reduces the entropy of a system by connecting its disparate elements and integrating them within a coherent structure. The elements in such a structure are interdependent, with a change in one element leading to predictable changes in the other elements. The elements may constitute different levels of abstraction, with discriminable elements on one level being aggregated or treated as equivalent on a higher level of abstraction. For example, constituting a low level of abstraction, a range of unique spatiotemporal configurations of the geometric figures in Heider and Simmel's cartoon are chunked together on the higher level of behavior identifications (e.g., chasing, pushing), which in turn are treated as equivalent on the still higher levels of inferred anthropomorphic mental states (e.g., angry) or traits (e.g., aggressive). At the core of the present perspective is the assumption that the meaning of an object resides in its connections to other objects comprising a structured system rather than in some inherent properties of the object itself (Heider, 1958; Lewin, 1936; Mead, 1934). It is further assumed that meaning making is a domain-general psychosocial process that manifests in the beliefs, preferences, and actions of both individuals and social collectives.

The following sections examine meaning making across different areas of social psychology. Specifically, the first section examines meaning making in two key areas of social cognition, person perception and cognitive consistency. The second section extends the notion of meaning making to constructing preferences, goals, and plans. The third section introduces the idea that meaning making is for expanding the scope of considerations people bring to bear on their current expectations, preferences, and actions. The fourth section examines meaning making at the level of social collectives and its role in expanding the scope of collectives. The chapter concludes with the implications of the current perspective on meaning making for the interface between individuals and society.

I. COGNITIVE MEANING MAKING

Person Perception

Research on person perception provides many examples of meaning making. People have been shown to go beyond surface-level, often noisy, behavioral cues to draw inferences about its more structured underlying causes (e.g., Heider, 1958; Jones & Davis, 1965; Kelley, 1967; Trope, 1986). Guided by people's lay theories of the determinants of behavior (Trope & Gaunt, 2000), these inferences use behavioral cues and the context in which they occur as evidence for the mental states—emotions, preferences, and attitudes—that might have given rise to the behavior (e.g., Aviezer, Trope, & Todorov, 2012; Freeman & Ambady, 2011; Nisbett & Valins, 1971; Speer et al., this volume; Trope, 1974a, 1989a; Trope & Burnstein, 1975). The inferences often proceed from mental states to more abstract personality traits that organize a range of behavioral cues and mental states across a variety of contexts (e.g., Gilbert & Malone, 1995; Jones, 1979; Trope, 1986, 1989a; Winter & Uleman, 1984). There is also ample evidence showing that people read such traits from the face and into the face (Hassin & Trope, 2000; Todorov, 2017).

When the behavioral cues are fallible because they are, for example, retrieved from one's memory (Trope, 1978) or reported by unreliable sources (Trope & Burnstein, 1979), people nevertheless continue to construe them in terms of others' general dispositions. Even when the behavioral cues are perceptually ambiguous, people use their prior knowledge and contextual cues to disambiguate the behavioral cues and draw inferences from them about others' personal dispositions as if the behavioral cues are perceptually unambiguous (Trope, 1986).

Moreover, when given the opportunity to seek information about others' behavior, people do so in a manner that is diagnostic of others' dispositions (Trope & Bassok, 1982, 1983; Trope, Bassok, & Alon, 1984; Trope & Mackie, 1987), and once behavioral information is obtained, they update their prior beliefs about others' dispositions in line with Bayesian inductive inference (Trope, 1974a; Trope & Burnstein, 1975). Notably, when information about others' group membership is available, inferences about their dispositions are based not only on their observed behavior but also, and often mainly, on stereotypes about the groups they belong to (e.g., Cameron & Trope, 2004; Fiske, 1998; Hamilton, Hartter, & Saito, 2015; Trope, 1986, 1989b; Trope & Thompson, 1997).

Further evidence for meaning making through connecting observed "behavioral cues to underlying dispositions comes from research on perceived freedom. One common approach assumes that behavior is perceived as free and meaningful when it is *unexpected* (e.g., Dennet, 2003; Sartre, 1943; Steiner, 1970). However, research has shown that people impute free will to others to the extent that their choices are *expected given* their personal dispositions (Kruglanski & Cohen, 1973; Trope, 1978; Trope & Burnstein, 1977). Consistent with the present framework, these findings suggest that perceiving others' choices as predictable *given* their personal dispositions and thus less entropic can lead to imputing free will to them. In other words, what matters for perceiving a behavior as freely chosen is not the behavior in isolation but rather its connection to the actor's dispositions.

Related meaning-making phenomena have also been found in research on self-assessment. People use their task performance to assess their own general abilities and, accordingly, select tasks in which success and failure are diagnostic of those abilities (e.g., Trope, 1975; Trope & Brickman, 1975; Trope & Ben-Yair, 1982). They undertake hard tasks and exert little effort to make success diagnostic of high ability (because high ability is necessary for success under such circumstances); they undertake easy tasks and exert great effort to make failure diagnostic of low ability (because low ability is necessary for failure under these circumstances); and they undertake intermediate-difficulty tasks and exert moderate effort to make both success and failure moderately diagnostic of high or low ability (Trope, 1975, 1979, 1983). In information theoretic terms, self-assessment renders performance outcomes meaningful by enhancing the transmission of information from the outcomes to one's knowledge about one's abilities and thus reducing its entropy (Trope, 1974b, pp. 113–114).

Finally, a large amount of research has shown that people often underutilize statistical information when making a judgment about a specific person, suggesting that they fail to see the relevance of statistical information to judgments about an individual (Tversky & Kahneman, 1974). However, research suggests that this depends on how the statistical information is construed. When the statistical information is construed as reflecting a meaningful underlying causal factor (e.g., a low base rate of success on a test reflecting the test's difficulty), people readily integrate statistical information into their judgment about an individual (e.g., the likelihood that this individual will succeed in the exam), even in the presence of individuating information (Ajzen, 1977; see also Ginossar & Trope, 1987).

These lines of research demonstrate that people imbue specific behaviors with meaning by connecting them to increasingly more abstract characteristics ranging from mental states to general traits. Importantly, these construals do not end with a compilation of disparate characteristics. Inspired by Asch's (1946) pioneering work on impression formation, person perception research has shown that people integrate their knowledge about others' traits within low-entropic structured representations (e.g., Hastie et al., 1980; Kunda & Thaggard, 1996; Passini & Norman, 1966; Read & Urada, 2003). Specifically, the component traits that comprise these representations are organized around a few dimensions—for example, competence and trustworthiness—that capture people's implicit personality theory (Oosterhoff & Todorov, 2008; Rosenberg & Sedlak, 1972; Schneider, 1973; Thornton & Tamir, 2021). Furthermore, the overall impressions people form about others show Gestalt properties; that is, the inferred traits interact and modify each other, with changes in one trait changing the connotations of the other traits (Asch, 1946). Individual trait inferences are thus imbued with meaning by being construed as parts of a low-entropic whole, with the overall impression reflecting a configural integration of the component traits rather than their additive aggregation.

Cognitive Consistency

Research on cognitive consistency further attests to the ubiquity of meaning making. This research shows that holding incongruous beliefs prompts people to resolve the incongruity and form more coherently structured (or low-entropic) belief systems (Abelson et al., 1968; Gawronski & Strack, 2012). A striking example is Asch and Zukier's (1984) study showing that people can readily make meaning of information about others even when the information is contradictory. Specifically, they show that people are adept at resolving contradictions between others' traits (e.g., a person being both *cheerful and gloomy*, *brilliant and foolish*, *sociable and lonely*). One of the resolution modes construes two opposite traits as having a common source. For example, participants reconciled the two contradictory traits *cheerful* and *gloomy* by construing the person as *moody*. Another mode of resolution assigned each of the contradictory traits to different domains. For example, participants reconciled the two traits *brilliant* and *foolish* by construing the person as *brilliant* intellectually but *foolish* in practical, commonsense matters.

Cognitive consistency research has demonstrated that similar forms of meaning making structure interpersonal relations (e.g., Cartwright & Harary, 1956; Heider, 1958; Newcomb, 1959). This research has shown that people are attuned to imbalanced interpersonal relations (e.g., "I like someone who dislikes a person I like") and attempt to restore cognitive balance by changing their own opinion or their perception of the opinions of the other people involved. Of note, entitativity—the perception of a collection of people as a unified group—evinces similar processes to those that underlie the perception of a person as a unified whole (Hamilton & Sherman, 1996). These processes include construing group actions as reflecting the group's enduring characteristics, interconnecting different group characteristics, organizing the individual characteristics within a coherent structure, and resolving inconsistencies among them. The greater the entitativity of a group, the more similar are the processes of making meaning of the group to the processes of making meaning of an individual. This raises the question of whether group polarization—a pervasive social phenomenon first identified in research on group decision making (e.g., Moscovici & Zavalloni, 1969; Vinokur & Burnstein, 1974; Vinokur, Trope, & Burnstein, 1975)—might reflect an entitative construal of group members and their opinions.

Although consistent construals tend to be more stable than inconsistent construals (e.g., Abelson, 1986), people and their social environment are rarely static. With the social world becoming increasingly dynamic and diverse, people often need to adopt new behavior patterns and change their relationships with others. These changes may introduce entropy into people's social knowledge, threaten to fragment it, and consequently prompt meaning making to restore the integrity of people's knowledge about themselves and their social environment (Frankl, 1946/1962). The challenge posed by change might be particularly acute for making meaning of the self. People tend to construe changes in their behavior as flexible attempts to meet the changing demands of their environment (e.g., Eibach, Libby, & Gilovich, 2003). However, the accumulation of contextualized and disconnected self-construals may reach a level that threatens the sense of an integrated self and the meaning of one's life (e.g., King & Hicks, 2021; Sedikides, Hong, & Wildschu, 2023). The life narratives people sometimes construct can be seen as attempts to restore self-consistency and integrate the diverse self-construals into a unified and stable view of one's selfhood (Gergen & Gergen, 1988).

In general, when a set of beliefs is isolated from other beliefs, it is vulnerable to haphazard influences that can fragment those beliefs and increase their entropy. Embedding the same set of beliefs within a broader interconnected belief system can buffer against and constrain the potential perturbances in those beliefs. For example, when one's beliefs about eating meat are unrelated to one's broader beliefs, they might be influenced by specific and incidental experiences of eating meat or plant-based food. In contrast, when embedded in a broader belief system—comprising, for example, beliefs about climate change, health, or animal welfare—changes in beliefs about eating meat are likely to be constrained by the broader belief systems. And when such changes do occur, they are likely to be predictable rather than erratic reactions to incidental influences.

Consistent, Inconsistent, and Irrelevant Cognitions

Although establishing cognitive consistency can be viewed as a form of meaning making, the two are not the same. Cognitive consistency theories distinguish between consistent and inconsistent relations between cognitions and view irrelevant cognitions as playing no role in cognitive consistency. Cognitive dissonance theory specifically states that the magnitude of dissonance depends on the proportion of dissonant-to-consonant cognitions and is unaffected by irrelevant cognitions (Festinger, 1957). For example, being on a diet is consonant with eating low-calorie food, dissonant with eating high-calorie food; and irrelevant to doing laundry, wearing boots, playing chess, and so forth. However, although irrelevant elements may not affect cognitive dissonance, their disconnectedness can undermine meaningfulness. From the present perspective, a cognitive system consisting of many elements that are irrelevant to each other is highly entropic and devoid of meaning. When being on a diet is an element in a random collection of mutually unrelated cognitions, like doing laundry, wearing boots, or playing chess, the collection has little meaning. When thinking of one's past as a random assortment of unrelated events, one's past has little or no meaning. In fact, knowledge that consists of two conflicting sets of cognitive elements may be more meaningful than knowledge that consists of a hodgepodge of disconnected elements. For example, an ambiguous facial expression—for instance, a smiling face, which can be construed as friendly or sarcastic—can be more meaningful than a degraded image of a face. The ambiguous face allows two conflicting construals that, akin to the figure–ground vase and binocular rivalry, can be readily disambiguated by contextual cues such as shaking someone's hand (Aviezer, Hassin, Bentin, & Trope, 2008; Trope, 1986; Trope & Cohen, 1989). In contrast, the degraded face allows any number of potential construals, none of which is evinced in the face and therefore unlikely to be supported by contextual cues. That is, the degraded information may not even afford an identification of the conflict it might entail. In short, entropic information is meaningless without necessarily being inconsistent. Conversely, although structuring unrelated pieces of information reduces entropy and makes the information more meaningful, it might reveal disagreements among those pieces of information and thus undermine cognitive consistency.

II. CONATIVE MEANING MAKING

Meaning making is not confined to cognition—to what people believe is true; it also applies to conation—to what people want, plan, and do. These psychological functions, reflecting the personal *significance* of one's beliefs (Moskalenko & Kruglanski, this volume), can be characterized in terms of their meaningfulness—namely, the extent to which they are coherently structured. In some cases, people's priorities are unequivocal and are seamlessly translated into plans and action, evincing low conative entropy. In other cases, multiple equipotent concerns are simultaneously activated, and without a clear guide for resolving conflicts among them, people may act haphazardly, evincing conative entropy. Even at the low level of motor control, a sequence of movements may vary in the extent to which it is coordinated and smoothly executed.

In this section, I examine conative structuredness as it manifests in people's goals. I focus on goals for three reasons. First, setting a goal is by itself an act of meaning making because a goal partitions the environment into conative foreground and background, or what is relevant versus irrelevant to one's wishes, in much the same way that hypotheses partition the environment into cognitive foreground and background, or what is relevant versus irrelevant to one's hypotheses. Although the conative foreground–background partition is a rudimentary form of structuring the environment, it nevertheless reduces entropy and therefore constitutes proto-meaning making. Second, goals are regulatory structures that integrate diverse conative elements involving subjective evaluations, wishes, and plans. As such, goal structures can vary in their coherence and therefore in their meaningfulness. Third, with people holding multiple goals, one could ask whether they form a coherently structured goal system (Kruglanski, Shah, Pierro, & Mannetti, 2002). Accordingly, I first discuss coherence within goals and then coherence across goals as prime examples of conative meaning making.

Intra-Goal and Inter-Goal Coherence

Conative meaning making manifests in the coherence of the components of individual goals (*intra-goal coherence*) and the coherence across different goals (*inter-goal coherence*). Intra-goal coherence reflects the clarity and orderly interconnectedness of the different components of goal pursuit—the desired end state, the means needed to attain it, and the monitoring of progress toward the end state (e.g., Miller, Galanter, & Pribram, 1971; Carver & Scheier, 1981). For example, an individual wishing to do well in school may set a clear criterion for success, create a plan for how to succeed, and establish indicators for monitoring their academic progress. The individual goal components in this example are not only clearly specified but also organized to support an orderly deployment of means in accordance with their instrumental value for attaining the desired end state and the assessed progress toward attaining the end state (e.g., Carver & Scheier, 2012). Such goals are low-entropic entities, and constructing them constitutes conative meaning making. Conversely, a goal is structurally incoherent to the extent that the desired end state is ill-defined, the means lack instrumental value for reaching the end or contradict each other, and the monitoring of progress is loose. The pursuit of such high-entropic goals is likely to be disorderly and easily derailed by incidental distractors.

Inter-goal coherence reflects the extent to which an individual's various goals are organized or disorganized, fragmented or integrated, and consistent or contradictory. For example, one may want to work, cook, travel, read, write, hike, and socialize, without an overall scheme that interrelates the goals and organizes their pursuit. In such cases, the ensuing behavior is likely to be erratic and irregular (e.g., Hirsch, Mar, & Peterson, 2012). Meaning making serves to reduce the attendant conative entropy. This might be accomplished by organizing individual goals within a broad hierarchical structure, with high-order goals subordinating lower-order goals (Kruglanski et al., 2002). Such a structure can afford coordinated pursuit of one's goals through various strategies, including prioritization, integration, sequencing, and balancing (Fishbach, Zhang, & Koo, 2009). Through prioritization, subordinate goals that are incompatible with high-order goals can elicit counteractive control processes (e.g., Fishbach & Trope, 2008; Fishbach & Wang, this volume; Fishbach, Zhang, & Trope, 2010) and control readiness processes (Kleiman, this volume; Kleiman, Hassin, & Trope, 2014; Kleiman, Trope, & Amodio, 2016) that boost the commitment to one's high-order goals. These processes reduce the entropy in one's goals by embedding them within a coherent goal system.

Cognitive–Conative Coherence

Meaning making may also involve constructing bidirectional connections between cognition and conation. A general form of such connections manifests when expectations derived from one's beliefs inform one's goals and behavior. For example, making choices in accordance with the expected value of the choice options connects cognition (expectations) to conation (value of options) (Atkinson, 1957; Edwards, 1954; Ajzen & Fishbein, 1975; Trope, 1975; Tversky & Kahneman, 1974; Weiner, 1985). Recent work on metamotivation suggests another mechanism through which cognition affects conation—namely, people's beliefs about the types of tasks that can benefit from different motivational states, which in turn enable people to flexibly instantiate different motivation states across different task demands (Carnevale & Fujita, this volume; Fujita, Scholer, Miele, & Nguyen, 2019; Scholer, Miele, Murayama, & Fujita, 2018).

Correspondingly, conation may shape cognition. For example, people's goals may influence their expectations and perceptions, so committing to a goal may make it seem more attainable (Brickman, Dunkel-Schetter, & Abbey, 1987; Fishbach & Trope, 2008; Heckhausen & Gollwitzer, 1987; Kuhl, 1981) and may make goal-relevant objects more salient (Ferguson, 2008). In general, motivated cognition, whereby preferences influence inferences (Kruglanski, 1989; Kunda, 1990; Landy & Balcetis, this volume; Taylor & Brown, 1994; Trope & A. Lieberman, 1996; Trope & Ferguson, 2000), connects conation to cognition. A simple signal-detection mechanism that can connect preferences to inferences involves the subjective cost of falsely rejecting a possibility (error of omission) versus the cost of falsely accepting it (error of commission). When the possibility under consideration is desirable, the cost of an error of omission might be greater than that of an error of commission. This in turn can lower the evidential threshold for accepting rather than rejecting the desired possibility (Trope & A. Lieberman, 1996; Kareev & Trope, 2011). For example, the number of successes at a task needed to conclude that one has the prerequisite ability would be smaller than the number of failures needed to reject this possibility.

Importantly, the bidirectional connections people form between cognition and conation illustrate that meaning making does not necessarily increase accuracy. Meaning making integrates people's beliefs, desires, and actions and thus affords what has been variously called an *unequivocal behavior orientation* (Jones & Gerard, 1967; Harmon-Jones & Harmon-Jones, 2002; Kuhl, 1981), *flow* (Csikszentmihalyi, 1990), and *activity engagement* (Higgins, 2006; Higgins & Trope, 1990; Nakkawita & Higgins, this volume). However, there is no guarantee that these integrations will yield accurate predictions, valid judgments, or successful outcomes.

Interim Summary

The preceding discussion illustrates the pervasiveness of meaning-making processes. These processes are domain general: They apply to cognition and conation, to the self, other individuals, and groups. Meaning making also applies to the representation of the physical world, as a large amount of research on perception and cognition has shown (e.g., Bar, 2004; Bruner, 1993). Meaning making is often deliberate, effortful, and slow, but it can also be spontaneous, effortless, and fast (Ferguson & Hassin, this volume; Gilbert & Malone, 1995; Hassin, Uleman, & Bargh, 2005; Chaiken & Trope, 1999; Sherman, Gawronski, & Trope, 2014; Trope, 1986). In other words, meaning making does not necessarily depend on processing mode (e.g., automatic or controlled, conscious or unconscious, fast or slow, effortful or effortless), nor does it necessarily depend on the processing conditions that give rise to the different processing modes (e.g., time pressure, attentional resources) (Gawronski, Sherman, & Trope, 2014). Meaning making can manifest in different cognitive operations, from perception and memory to interpretation and reasoning. The organization of the perceptual field into figure and ground during early information processing is an act of meaning making. Even the passive process of memory consolidation, a process that can operate when we are unawake, involves meaning making, as stored information is organized within increasingly more schematic structures (e.g., Bartlett, 1932; Dudai, 2004). As suggested by the predictive coding framework, these knowledge structures give rise to expectancies that, through top-down processing, profoundly shape the most basic aspects of our perceptions (Bar, 2004; Clark, 2013; Friston, 2005; Ludwin-Peery & Trope, 2023). Meaning making also manifests in various aspects of conation, from evaluation and goal setting to action planning and execution. In all its manifestations, meaning making reduces mental entropy by transforming irregular and disconnected elements into coherent, interconnected, and stable cognitive and conative structures.

III. MEANING MAKING IS FOR EXPANDING REGULATORY SCOPE

What is meaning making for? What purpose does it serve? Is it for promoting a sense of predictability, control, agency, or self-worth? There doesn't seem to be a single answer to this question. It could be any one such purpose, all of them, or none. It is possible that meaning making is simply an end in and of itself rather than a means to some end, as implied by Earl Hunt's (1963) contention that motivation is intrinsic to information processing and action. Although these possibilities are plausible, it is proposed here that meaning making supports a more general function for individuals and collectives. Specifically, building on construal-level theory (CLT; Liberman & Trope, 2008; Liberman, this volume; Trope & Liberman, 2010) and the related regulatory scope theory (Fujita, Trope, & Liberman, 2025; Trope, Ledgerwood, Liberman, & Fujita, 2021), it is argued in the following section that meaning making enables individuals and collectives to expand the scope of their cognition and conation, or regulatory scope, across psychological distance beyond the here and now.

Regulatory Scope

As an illustration of the notion of regulatory scope, imagine watching a fast-motion audiovisual playback of your life from infancy to adulthood. You will see many changes. You will see yourself starting to change your lying position, then crawling, sitting, standing up, and eventually walking and running, all the time getting taller and bigger and, ultimately, depending on your age, wrinkling and graying. These and numerous other changes in you are likely vivid and palpable. But if you stop looking only at yourself and pay attention to your surroundings, you will notice something more subtle than the changes in yourself but nevertheless remarkable. You will see that the range of people you interact with keeps expanding over time. Initially, your interactions are confined to your immediate family members, those who literally bear a "family resemblance" to you (and who are quick to point it out). Gradually, your social interactions extend further to include other caregivers, teachers, peers, friends, acquaintances, and total strangers. The scope of social relations broadens as the people you interact with become increasingly more numerous and diverse.

In parallel, you will see that while you initially respond mostly to people and events in your immediate locale, over time, your interactions span increasingly greater spatial distances, crossing neighborhoods, towns, cities, and states to reach remote and new places across the globe.

Watching the playback more carefully and listening to what you are saying or doing, you will notice a concomitant change from reacting to the present situation to taking action in light of what happened in the past and what might happen in the increasingly more distant future. From infancy to adulthood, the scope of the targets of your actions encompasses increasingly broader swaths of temporal distance, prospective and retrospective. It may even include hypothetical "what if" possibilities and counterfactual scenarios.

How general is this pattern? Does it hold for some individuals and not for others? Does it manifest in some cultures yet is absent in others? To address these questions, it is instructive to zoom out from the ontogenetic time scale to larger historic and phylogenetic scales. At these time scales, our imaginary playback spans many thousands of individual lifetimes and advances at a speed that is accordingly much faster than that at the ontogenetic scale. Nevertheless, even a cursory inspection of the playback will reveal to you phylogenetic and historical patterns of expanding scope—social, spatial, temporal, and hypothetical—that are analogous to your own personal pattern of changes. You will see that our genus *Homo* ancestors primarily interact with others within small, insular, and homogenous bands. They tend to inhabit a specific physical locale, and while their artifacts suggest an expanding temporal scope, they still primarily respond to what is present and imminent. You will see that gradually, human groups increase in size and diversity from bands, clans, and tribes to cities, nations, and united nations. Their social interactions come to span across increasingly larger swaths of land, across continents, reaching out to our human conspecifics in outer space and to other intelligent beings across the universe. Concomitantly, they act more and more with reference to distant past, future, and hypothetical events.

These observations tell us that over ontogeny, history, and phylogeny, humans have expanded the scope of people, objects, and events they seek to engage, predict, and control. Two important qualifications should be noted here. The first is that the expansion of scope is not uniform. It takes a fast playback to accentuate the overall trend and discount deviations from it. A slow playback that allows a more granular scrutiny will reveal local fluctuations, including periods of contraction of scope. Such a playback of your own life will show times when you secluded yourself from others, retreated to your own little private space, immersed yourself in solitary activities, and suspended consideration of what awaits you outside of your own confines.

Analogous periods of contractive scope also manifest in history and phylogeny. The trend of human society toward increasing exploration, forward-looking, and far-flung social exchange is sometimes broken by eras of insularity, confinement to a local habitat, social uniformity, and truncated exploration. Phases of expansive scope may be intermixed with phases of contractive scope. These variations in scope, like those at the ontogenetic level, are not just random perturbations. As we will see later, they may reflect underlying mental and social processes that give rise to a lawful alternation between expansive and contractive scope.

The second qualification is that the overall trend toward expanding scope does not necessarily mean that it leads to greater harmony with our social and natural environment. We may look far into the future, explore distant habitats, and learn about remote cultures with the intent to dominate, exploit, and even exterminate them. Our intent might be benevolent, or at least not explicitly malevolent, but it might nevertheless lead to conflict, harm, and adverse outcomes for our fellow humans and the natural environment. Expansive scope is not the same as unidirectional progress toward a better world (Pinker, 2012).

The Role of Meaning Making in Expanding Scope

The point of the preceding discussion is that although our direct experience of the world is confined to what is present, our thoughts and actions extend to other times, places, minds, and hypothetical possibilities. In other words, as our scope expands, we bring to bear increasingly more psychologically distant considerations on our current predictions, preferences, and actions. This begs the question of what enables us to expand our scope. The present approach to this question is rooted in the observation that the challenge of expanding scope stems from the variability, change, and uncertainty it entails (Hubbard, Kalkstein, Liberman, & Trope, 2021). More things become possible if one considers not only what might happen today but also what might happen this week, this month, and so on. In principle, it is just a matter of sufficient expansion of scope that any event, even the most idiosyncratic and previously unknown, is eventually bound to be encountered. In other words, *expanding scope entails greater informational entropy.*

Now, meaning making, as argued earlier, compresses the variability of objects and thus reduces their informational entropy. This suggests a functional relationship between meaning making and regulatory scope. Regulatory scope theory (Fujita et al., 2025; Trope et al., 2021) is specifically about this relationship. In brief, CLT (Liberman & Trope, 2008; Trope & Liberman, 2010; Liberman, this volume) focuses on how people respond to an event at a given point that is either psychologically near or distant from the self (e.g., 2 weeks from now). Regulatory scope theory extends CLT by examining how people respond to events spanning a range across psychological distance from the self (e.g., the next

2 weeks). Both theories suggest that the meaning of events is associated with their level of construal (see also Wegner, Vallacher, Kiersted, & Dizadji, 1986). To use Heider and Simmel's cartoon experiment as an example, construing the cartoon in terms of the geometric figures' individual movements—a low-level construal—has little meaning because these movements remain entropic, that is, disjointed and unstructured. In contrast, construing the cartoon in terms of the goals or traits of the geometric figures—a high-level construal—carries more meaning because it connects the individual movements to underlying dispositions and to an overarching low-entropic narrative. Changing the intentions or traits of the geometric figures would likely change the meaning of the cartoon more than would changing any of the figures' individual movements. Importantly, construing the cartoon in terms of the figures' goals, traits, or overarching narrative expands the scope of prediction to include how the cartoon might unfold across longer time segments or even how a sequel to the original cartoon might look. In contrast, the less meaningful construal of the cartoon in terms of individual movements contracts the scope of prediction, allowing only moment-to-moment predictions within short time segments of the original cartoon.

In general, by integrating specific details within an overarching structure, high-level construals reduce the entropy of the available information and make it more meaningful. Specific details can mutate without changing the overarching structure (Gilead, Trope, & Liberman, 2020). Construing an activity (e.g., "exercise") in terms of its goal ("getting in shape") allows how the activity is carried out ("biking," "jogging," or "swimming") to vary without changing the meaning of the activity. This enables the meaning of an object to be robust to the variation that expansive scope entails and thus enables people to transcend the particularities of the here and now and expand their regulatory scope to psychologically distant objects.

Notably, meaning making allows people to go beyond the self and connect with others, and as such, it is key to human sociality. For example, classic work on cognitive tuning suggests that people construe information in a more structured, less entropic way when they expect to communicate the information to others than when they merely need to comprehend it (Zajonc, 1960). Likewise, when communicating information, people tend to construe objects in terms of general rather than idiosyncratic categories (Krauss, Vivekananthan, & Weinheimer,, 1968). More recent research has shown that people orient to more meaningful high-level construal of information when they share it with distant or diverse others (Amit et al., 2019; Amit, Wakslak, & Trope, 2013; Joshi & Wakslak, 2014; Joshi, Wakslak, Raj, & Trope, 2016; Wakslak, this volume), when they compare themselves with distant others (Yudkin, Liberman, Wakslak, & Trope, 2020), when they engage in goods exchange with distant others (Baskin, Wakslak, Trope, & Novemsky, 2014), when they emulate or learn from distant others (Kalkstein, Kleiman, Wakslak, Liberman, & Trope, 2016; Genschow, Hansen Wanke, & Trope, 2019; Hansen, Alves, & Trope, 2016), and when they self-project onto distant others (Bin-Meshar & Trope, 2025). Together, these findings support the idea that meaningful low-entropic construals, being comparable across individuals' idiosyncratic circumstances, enable us to expand the scope of our social relations.

IV. COLLECTIVE MEANING MAKING AND REGULATORY SCOPE

Analogous to the way individuals' meaning making supports the expansion of their scope, collective meaning making supports the expansion of the collective's scope. A collective's scope may be confined to its local physical habitat, to similar people, to the present or near future, and to facts known with certainty. The scope of such collectives is spatially, socially, temporally, and hypothetically contractive. Collective scope expands to the extent that it encompasses a broader physical environment, more socially diverse people, the distant past and future, and hypothetical possibilities (Trope et al., 2021). For example, an organization's scope expands when its recruitment policies apply to job applicants from geographically distant places, to applicants from socially diverse backgrounds, and to future or hypothetical applicants. Companies may differ in whether their products are designed for local and homogeneous users or for geographically distant and heterogeneous users, for present uses or for future uses, for known users or for hypothetical ones (Wiesenfeld, Reyt, Brockner, & Trope, 2017). Countries may forge geographically local ties or global ties, connect to culturally and demographically similar countries or to dissimilar countries, and orient to current concerns or to future concerns.

Collective meaning making consists of constructing collective cognitive systems (e.g., shared beliefs, expectations, and identity) and conative systems (e.g., shared values, goals, and practices). A collective becomes less meaningful when its beliefs and identity are incoherent, its values and goals are fragmented, and its practices are ill-defined and uncoordinated. These features characterize the state of affairs Durkheim (1893) called *anomie* and the group dynamics Lewin, Lippitt, and White (1939) called *laissez-faire*. Taken to the extreme, this is the state of affairs described in the biblical Tower of Babel story of God subverting postdiluvian humans' ambition to build a tower that could reach the sky by confounding their speech so that they could no longer understand each other (Genesis 11:1–9). More recently, Kafka's *The Trial* presents one of the most vivid literary depictions of how opaque and bewildering the expectations, rules, and practices of modern bureaucracy can be for the layperson.

In the present terms, such collectives are socially entropic entities. Collective meaning making acts to reduce social entropy by integrating the collective's beliefs, expectations, and identities within an overarching shared worldview, as well as by integrating the collective's values, goals, and norms within a higher-order ideology and using them as guides for collective action. These social constructions enable collectives to expand their scope despite the greater variability that an expansive scope necessarily entails. This is apparent in the structure of superordinate and subordinate roles that typically evolves in groups and organizations. For example, the administration of a university is hierarchically organized, with a president in the most central and superordinate role and various directors and managers in a series of more specific, subordinate roles. Subordinate roles are associated with concrete goals and tasks that help the group regulate in the here and now. In contrast, superordinate roles are associated with more abstract, general, and enduring aspects of the group and thus serve to expand its regulatory scope. For example, the role of a leader as a "gate keeper" (Lewin, 1943), which requires an outward orientation, may derive from the high-level construal of this role. Perhaps the complementary function of a leader's role as expanding the scope of the group might be called "gate opener."

On the larger societal scale, the expansion of regulatory scope entails greater social entropy as a result of increased societal diversity, complexity, and variability. Historical trends of expanding collective scope may have nevertheless been made possible by transitions to new forms of collective meaning making. Three such transitions are noteworthy. *First*, the transition from oral communication to written communication may have enabled an expansive scope of information exchange across greater spatial, temporal, and social distances. *Second*, the transition from a barter economy to a monetary economy may have enabled an expansive scope of goods exchange that is unbound by local needs and possessions and capable of forging global interdependence. *Third*, the transition from polytheistic religions with multiple concrete gods to monotheistic religions with one abstract, moralizing God may have enabled an expansive scope of trust and cooperation across diverse people (see, e.g., Purzycki et al., 2016, on the transition from polytheism to monotheism being associated with increasing social complexity). Oral communication, barter economies, and embodied gods are concrete and may therefore be suitable for a contractive scope of information exchange; local goods exchange, and trust within small, homogeneous, and stable social environments. In contrast, written communication, monetary economies, and monotheism are abstract and might therefore accommodate larger, more diverse, and less predictable social environments.

V. IMPLICATIONS AND AMPLIFICATIONS

The present chapter conceives of meaning making as a ubiquitous, domain-general process and thus paints a picture of humans as tireless meaning-making agents. It is argued that meaning making characterizes the cognitive and conative functioning of both individuals and collectives—from individuals seeking coherent explanations for surface-level behavioral cues and forming means–ends hierarchies as guides for their personal goal pursuit to groups developing a role structure with a division of labor and synchronizing individuals' actions to achieve the group goals. Common to all its manifestations, meaning making reduces the entropy of mental and social systems by transforming their irregular and disconnected components into coherent, integrated, and stable structures.

Because meaning making applies both to individuals and collectives, it may provide a common substrate for the interrelation between the two. It is, so to speak, where the social meets the psychological. Understanding their interrelation is the *raison d'être* of social psychology and, as such, has indeed inspired a great deal of research. However, this research has typically examined the effect of collectives on individuals in particular domains: Cultural psychology has mostly focused on dimensions such as individualism–collectivism (Triandis, 2001) and independence–interdependence (Markus & Kitayama, 1991), and group psychology has explored the effect of groups on a range of specific perceptions, beliefs, attitudes, and decisions.

The preset perspective brings to the fore different and more general questions concerning the reciprocal influences collectives and individuals might exert on each other. Are the collective and individual forms of meaning making structurally aligned even when they pertain to different content domains? Does *cognitive entropy* at the group level correlate with cognitive entropy at the individual level? For example, is the coherence of a group identity correlated with the coherence of its members' self-construal? Can members of a group with a coherent social identity have incoherent self-construal? And vice versa: Can members of a group with an incoherent identity have coherent self-construal?

Similarly, we may ask whether the amount of *conative entropy* at the group level is correlated with the amount of the corresponding entropy at the individual level. For example, is the structuredness of a group's social roles associated with the structuredness of the individual members' goals? Is the state of *anomie* of a social system associated with poor self-control by its individual members? Is the abstractness of group goals correlated with the abstractness of the members' personal goals? Does the scope of the group goals correlate with the scope of members' personal goals? For example, is a group that orients to its distant future and diverse people likely to have members who are future oriented and open to social diversity in their personal lives? Are a collective's entropy-related dysfunctions concordant with the individuals' entropy-related dysfunctions? And if so, can entropy provide a transdiagnostic substrate onto which both social disorder and personal disorder can be mapped? What are the consequences of misaligned social and personal meanings? Might a misalignment trigger changes at either level to align the meanings of the two levels? These questions suggest challenging but promising avenues for conceptual and methodological advances in our understanding of individuals in society.

REFERENCES

Abelson, R. P. (1986). Beliefs are like possessions. *Journal for the Theory of Social Behaviour, 16*(3), 223–250.

Abelson, R. P., Aronson, E., McGuire, W. J., Newcomb, T. M., Rosenberg, M. J., & Tannenbaum, P. H. (Eds.). (1968). *Theories of cognitive consistency: A sourcebook.* Rand-McNally.

Ajzen, I. (1977). Intuitive theories of events and the effects of base-rate information on prediction. *Journal of Personality and Social Psychology, 35*(5), 303–314.

Ajzen, I., & Fishbein, M. (1975). A Bayesian analysis of attribution processes. *Psychological Bulletin, 82*(2), 261–277.

Amit, E., Rim, S., Halbeisen, G., Priva, U. C., Stephan, E., & Trope, Y. (2019). Distance-dependent memory for pictures and words. *Journal of Memory and Language, 105*, 119–130.

Amit, E., Wakslak, C., & Trope, Y. (2013). The use of visual and verbal means of communication across psychological distance. *Personality and Social Psychology Bulletin, 39*(1), 43–56.

Asch, S. E. (1946). Forming impressions of personality. *Journal of Abnormal and Social Psychology, 41*(3), 258–290.

Asch, S. E., & Zukier, H. (1984). Thinking about persons. *Journal of Personality and Social Psychology, 46*(6), 1230–1240.

Atkinson, J. W. (1957). Motivational determinants of risk-taking behavior. *Psychological Review, 64*(6, Pt.1), 359–372.

Aviezer, H., Hassin, R., Bentin, S., & Trope, Y. (2008). Putting facial expressions back in context. In N. Ambady & J. J. Skowronski (Eds.), *First impressions* (pp. 255–286). Guilford Press.

Aviezer, H., Trope, Y., & Todorov, A. (2012). Body cues, not facial expressions, discriminate between intense positive and negative emotions. *Science, 338*(6111), 1225–1229.

Bar, M. (2004). Visual objects in context. *Nature Reviews Neuroscience, 5*(8), 617–629.

Bartlett, F. C. (1932). *Remembering: A study in experimental and social psychology.* Cambridge University Press.

Baskin, E., Wakslak, C. J., Trope, Y., & Novemsky, M. (2014). Why feasibility matters more to gift receivers than to givers: A construal-level approach to gift giving. *Journal of Consumer Research, 41*(1), 169–182.

Bin-Meshar, M., & Trope, Y. (2025). *Expansive and contractive scope of projection* [Unpublished manuscript]. New York University.

Brickman, P., Dunkel-Schetter, C., & Abbey, A. (1987). The development of commitment. In P. Brickman (Ed.), *Commitment, conflict, and caring* (pp. 145–221). Prentice-Hall.

Bruner, J. (1993). Do we "acquire" culture or vice versa? *Behavioral and Brain Sciences, 16*(3), 515–516.

Cameron, J. A., & Trope, Y. (2004). Stereotype-biased search and processing of information about group members. *Social Cognition, 22*(6), 650–672.

Cartwright, D., & Harary, F. (1956). Structural balance: A generalization of Heider's theory. *Psychological Review, 63*(5), 277–293.

Carver, C. S., & Scheier, M. F. (1981). The self-attention-induced feedback loop and social facilitation. *Journal of Experimental Social Psychology, 17*(6), 545–568.

Carver, C. S., & Scheier, M. F. (2012). Cybernetic control processes and the self-regulation of behavior. In R. M. Ryan (Ed.), *The Oxford handbook of human motivation* (pp. 28–42). Oxford University Press.

Chaiken, S., & Trope, Y. (Eds.). (1999). *Dual-process theories in social psychology.* Guilford Press.

Clark, A. (2013). Whatever next? Predictive brains, situated agents, and the future of cognitive science. *Behavioral and Brain Sciences, 36*(3), 181–204.

Csikszentmihalyi, M. (1990). *Flow: The psychology of optimal experience.* Harper & Row.

Dennett, D. (2003). *Freedom evolves.* Viking Books.

Dudai, Y. (2004). *Memory from A to Z: Keywords, concepts, and beyond.* Oxford University. Press.

Durkheim, E. (1983). *Pragmatism and sociology.* Cambridge University Press.

Edwards, W. (1954). The theory of decision making. *Psychological Bulletin, 51*(4), 380–417.

Eibach, R. P., Libby, L. K., & Gilovich, T. D. (2003). When change in the self is mistaken for change in the world. *Journal of Personality and Social Psychology, 84*(5), 917–931.

Ferguson, M. J. (2008). On becoming ready to pursue a goal you don't know you have: Effects of nonconscious goals on evaluative readiness. *Journal of Personality and Social Psychology, 95*(6), 1268–1284.

Festinger, L. (1957). *A theory of cognitive dissonance.* Stanford University Press.

Fishbach, A., & Trope, Y. (2008). Implicit and explicit counteractive self-control. In J. Y. Shah & W. L. Gardner (Eds.), *Handbook of motivation science* (pp. 281–294). Guilford Press.

Fishbach, A., Zhang, Y., & Koo, M. (2009). The dynamics of self-regulation. *European Review of Social Psychology, 20*(1), 315–344.

Fishbach, A., Zhang, Y., & Trope, Y. (2010). Counteractive evaluation: Asymmetric shifts in the implicit value of conflicting motivations. *Journal of Experimental Social Psychology, 46*(1), 29–38.

Fiske, S. T. (1998). Stereotyping, prejudice, and discrimination. In D. T. Gilbert, S. T. Fiske, & G. Lindzey (Eds.), *The handbook of social psychology* (4th ed., pp. 357–411). McGraw Hill.

Frankl, V. E. (1962). *Man's search for meaning: An introduction to logotherapy.* Beacon Press. (Original work published 1946)

Freeman, J. B., & Ambady, N. (2011). A dynamic interactive theory of person construal. *Psychological Review, 118*(2), 247–279.

Friston, K. (2005). A theory of cortical responses. *Philosophical Transactions of the Royal Society B: Biological Sciences, 360*(1456), 815–836.

Fujita, K., Scholer, A. A., Miele, D. B., & Nguyen, T. (2019). On metamotivation: Consumers' knowledge about the role of construal level in enhancing task performance. *Journal of the Association for Consumer Research, 4*(1), 57–64.

Fujita, K., Trope, Y., & Liberman, N. (2025). Understanding self-control as a problem of regulatory scope. *Psychological Review, 132*(1), 50–75.

Gawronski, B., Sherman, J. W., & Trope, Y. (2014). Two of what. In B. Gawronski & G. V. Bodenhausen (Eds.), *Dual-process theories of the social mind* (pp. 3–19). Guilford Press.

Gawronski, B., & Strack, F. (Eds.). (2012). *Cognitive consistency: A fundamental principle in social cognition.* Guilford Press.

Genschow, O., Hansen, J., Wänke, M., & Trope, Y. (2019). Psychological distance modulates. goal-based versus movement-based imitation. *Journal of Experimental Psychology: Human Perception and Performance, 45*(8), 1031–1048.

Gergen, K. J., & Gergen, M. M. (1988). Narrative and the self as relationship. In L. Berkowitz (Ed.), *Advances in experimental social psychology* (Vol. 21, pp. 17–56). Academic Press.

Gilbert, D. T., & Malone, P. S. (1995). The correspondence bias. *Psychological Bulletin, 117*(1), 21–38.

Gilead, M., Trope, Y., & Liberman, N. (2020). Above and beyond the concrete: The diverse representational substrates of the predictive brain. *Behavioral and Brain Sciences, 43*, Article e121.

Ginossar, Z., & Trope, Y. (1987). Problem solving in judgment under uncertainty. *Journal of Personality and Social Psychology, 52*(3), 464–474.

Hamilton, D. L., & Sherman, S. J. (1996). Perceiving persons and groups. *Psychological Review, 103*(2), 336–355.

Hamilton, L. C., Hartter, J., & Saito, K. (2015). Trust in scientists on climate change and vaccines. *Sage Open, 5*(3).

Hansen, J., Alves, H., & Trope, Y. (2016). Psychological distance reduces literal imitation: Evidence from an imitation-learning paradigm. *Journal of Experimental Psychology: Human Perception and Performance, 42*(3), 320–330.

Harmon-Jones, E., & Harmon-Jones, C. (2002). Testing the action-based model of cognitive dissonance: The effect of action orientation on postdecisional attitudes. *Personality and Social Psychology Bulletin, 28*(6), 711–723.

Hassin, R., & Trope, Y. (2000). Facing faces: Studies on the cognitive aspects of physiognomy. *Journal of Personality and Social Psychology, 78*(5), 837–852.

Hassin, R. R., Uleman, J. S., & Bargh, J. A. (Eds.). (2005). *The new unconscious.* Oxford University Press.

Hastie, R., Ostrom, T. M., Ebbesen, E. B., Wyer, R. S., Jr., Hamilton, D. L., & Carlston, D. E. (1980). *Person memory: The cognitive basis of social perception.* Erlbaum.

Heckhausen, H., & Gollwitzer, P. M. (1987). Thought contents and cognitive functioning in motivational versus volitional states of mind. *Motivation and Emotion, 11*(2), 101–120.

Heider, F. (1958). *The psychology of interpersonal relations.* Wiley.

Heider, F., & Simmel, M. (1944). An experimental study of apparent behavior. *American Journal of Psychology, 57*(2), 243–259.

Higgins, E. T. (2006). Value from hedonic experience and engagement. *Psychological Review, 113*(3), 439–460.

Higgins, E. T., & Trope, Y. (1990). Intrinsic motivation as a relational concept: Motivational consequences of multiple identifications of activities. In E. T. Higgins & R. M. Sorrentino (Eds.), *The handbook of motivation and cognition: Foundations of social behavior* (Vol. 2, pp. 229–264). Guilford Press.

Hirsh, J. B., Mar, R. A., & Peterson, J. B. (2012). Psychological entropy: A framework for understanding uncertainty-related anxiety. *Psychological Review, 119*(2), 304–320.

Hubbard, A. D., Kalkstein, D. A., Liberman, N., & Trope, Y. (2021). Construal processes. *Annual Review of Psychology, 72*, 365–394.

Hunt, J. McV. (1963). Motivation inherent in information processing and action. In O. J. Harvey (Ed.), *Motivation and social interaction: Cognitive determinants* (pp. 35–94). Ronald Press.

Jones, E. E. (1979). The rocky road from acts to dispositions. *American Psychologist, 34*(2), 107–117.

Jones, E. E., & Davis, K. E. (1965). From acts to dispositions: The attribution process in person perception. In L. Berkowitz (Ed.), *Advances in experimental social psychology* (Vol. 2, pp. 219–266). Academic Press.

Jones, E. E., & Gerard, H. (1967). *Foundations of social psychology.* Wiley.

Joshi, P. D., & Wakslak, C. J. (2014). Communicating with the crowd: Speakers use abstract messages when addressing larger audiences. *Journal of Experimental Psychology: General, 143*(1), 351–362.

Joshi, P. D., Wakslak, C. J., Raj, M., & Trope, Y. (2016). Communicating with distant others: The functional use of abstraction. *Social Psychological and Personality Science, 7*(1), 37–44.

Kahneman, D., & Tversky, A. (1979). Prospect theory: An analysis of decision under risk. *Econometrica, 47*(2), 263–291.

Kalkstein, D. A., Kleiman, T., Wakslak, C. J., Liberman, N., & Trope, Y. (2016). Social learning across psychological distance. *Journal of Personality and Social Psychology, 110*(1), 1–19.

Kareev, Y., & Trope, Y. (2011). Correct acceptance weighs more than correct rejection: A decision bias induced by question framing. *Psychonomic Bulletin & Review, 18*(1), 103–109.

Kelley, H. H. (1967). Attribution theory in social psychology. *Nebraska Symposium on Motivation, 15*, 192–238.

King, L. A., & Hicks, J. A. (2021). The science of meaning in life. *Annual Review of Psychology, 72*, 561–584.

Kleiman, T., Hassin, R. R., & Trope, Y. (2014). The control-freak mind: Stereotypical biases are eliminated following conflict-activated cognitive control. *Journal of Experimental Psychology: General, 143*(2), 498–503.

Kleiman, T., Trope, Y., & Amodio, D. M. (2016). Cognitive control modulates attention to food cues: Support for the control readiness model of self-control. *Brain and Cognition, 110*, 94–101.

Krauss, R. M., Vivekananthan, P. S., & Weinheimer, S. (1968). Inner speech and "external speech": Characteristics and communication effectiveness of socially and nonsocially encoded messages. *Journal of Personality and Social Psychology, 9*(4), 295–300.

Kruglanski, A. W. (1989). The psychology of being "right": The problem of accuracy in social perception and cognition. *Psychological Bulletin, 106*(3), 395–409.

Kruglanski, A. W., & Cohen, M. (1973). Attributed freedom and personal causality. *Journal of Personality and Social Psychology, 31*(2), 245–250.

Kruglanski, A. W., Shah, J. Y., Pierro, A., & Mannetti, L. (2002). When similarity breeds content: Need for closure and the allure of homogeneous and self-resembling groups. *Journal of Personality and Social Psychology, 83*(3), 648–662.

Kuhl, J. (1981). Motivational and functional helplessness: The moderating effect of state versus action orientation. *Journal of Personality and Social Psychology, 40*(1), 155–170.

Kunda, Z. (1990). The case for motivated reasoning. *Psychological Bulletin, 108*(3), 480–498.

Kunda, Z., & Thagard, P. (1996). Forming impressions from stereotypes, traits, and behaviors: A parallel-constraint-satisfaction theory. *Psychological Review, 103*(2), 284–308.

Lewin, K. (1936). *A dynamic theory of personality: Selected papers*. McGraw Hill.

Lewin, K. (1943). Forces behind food habits and methods of change. *Bulletin of the National Research Council, 108*(1043), 35–65.

Lewin, K., Lippitt, R., & White, R. K. (1939). Patterns of aggressive behavior in experimentally created social climates. *Journal of Social Psychology, 10*, 271–301.

Liberman, N., & Trope, Y. (2008). The psychology of transcending the here and now. *Science, 322*(5905), 1201–1205.

Ludwin-Peery, E., & Trope, Y. (2023). Predictive coding of objects and persons. In E. Balcetis & G. Moskowitz (Eds.), *Handbook on impression formation: A social psychological approach.* Routledge.

Markus, H. R., & Kitayama, S. (1991). Culture and the self: Implications for cognition, emotion, and motivation. *Psychological Review, 98*(2), 224–253.

Mead, G. H. (1934). *Mind, self, and society: From the standpoint of a social behaviorist.* University of Chicago Press.

Miller, G. A., Galanter, E., & Pribram, K. H. (1971). The unit of analysis. In *Good reading in psychology* (p. 211). Prentice-Hall.

Moscovici, S., & Zavalloni, M. (1969). The group as a polarizer of attitudes. *Journal of Personality and Social Psychology, 12*(2), 125–135.

Newcomb, T. M. (1959). Individual systems of orientation. In S. Koch (Ed.), *Psychology: A study of a science* (Vol. 3, pp. 384–422). McGraw Hill.

Nisbett, R. E., & Valins, S. (1971). Perceiving the causes of one's own behavior. In E. E. Jones, D. E. Kanouse, H. H. Kelley, R. E. Nisbett, S. Valins, & B. Weiner (Eds.), *Attribution: Perceiving the causes of behavior.* General Learning Press.

Oosterhof, N. N., & Todorov, A. (2008). The functional basis of face evaluation. *Proceedings of the National Academy of Sciences, 105*(32), 11087–11092.

Passini, F. T., & Norman, W. T. (1966). A universal conception of personality structure? *Journal of Personality and Social Psychology, 4*(1), 44–49.

Pinker, S. (2012). *The better angels of our nature.* Penguin.

Purzycki, B. G., Apicella, C., Atkinson, Q., Cohen, E., McNamara, R. A., Willard, A. K., et al. (2016). Moralistic gods, supernatural punishment and the expansion of human sociality. *Nature, 530*(7590), 327–330.

Read, S. J., & Urada, D. I. (2003). A neural network simulation of the outgroup homogeneity effect. *Personality and Social Psychology Review, 7*(2), 146–169.

Rosenberg, S., & Sedlak, A. (1972). Structural representations of implicit personality theory. In L. Berkowitz (Ed.), *Advances in experimental social psychology* (Vol. 6, pp. 235–297). Academic Press.

Sartre, J.-P. (1943). *L'Être et le néant* [Being and nothingness]. Éditions Gallimard.

Schneider, D. J. (1973). Implicit personality theory: A review. *Psychological Bulletin, 79*(5), 294–309.

Scholer, A. A., Miele, D. B., Murayama, K., & Fujita, K. (2018). New directions in self-regulation: The role of metamotivational beliefs. *Current Directions in Psychological Science, 27*(6), 437–442.

Sedikides, C., Hong, E. K., & Wildschut, T. (2023). Self-continuity. *Annual Review of Psychology, 74*, 333–361.

Shannon, C. E., & Weaver, W. (1949). *The mathematical theory of communication.* University of Illinois Press.

Sherman, J. W., Gawronski, B., & Trope, Y. (Eds.). (2014). *Dual-process theories of the social mind.* Guilford Press.

Steiner, I. D. (1970). Perceived freedom. In L. Berkowitz (Ed.), *Advances in experimental social psychology* (Vol. 5, pp. 187–248). Academic Press.

Taylor, S. E., & Brown, J. D. (1994). Positive illusions and well-being revisited: Separating fact from fiction. *Psychological Bulletin, 116*(1), 21–27.

Thornton, M. A., & Tamir, D. I. (2021). People accurately predict the transition probabilities. between actions. *Science Advances, 7*(9), Article eabd4995.

Todorov, A. (2017). *Face value: The irresistible influence of first impressions.* Princeton University Press.

Triandis, H. C. (2001). Individualism-collectivism and personality. *Journal of Personality, 69*(6), 907–924.

Trope, Y. (1974a). Inferential processes in the forced compliance situation: A Bayesian analysis. *Journal of Experimental Social Psychology, 10*(1), 1–16.

Trope, Y. (1974b). *Probabilistic information processing analysis of attribution phenomena* [Unpublished doctoral dissertation]. University of Michigan.

Trope, Y. (1975). Seeking information about one's ability as a determinant of choice among tasks. *Journal of Personality and Social Psychology, 32*(6), 1004–1013.

Trope, Y. (1978). Inferences of personal characteristics on the basis of information retrieved. from one's memory. *Journal of Personality and Social Psychology, 36*(2), 93–106.

Trope, Y. (1979). Uncertainty-reducing properties of achievement tasks. *Journal of Personality and Social Psychology, 37*(9), 1505–1518.

Trope, Y. (1983). Self-assessment in achievement behavior. In J. Suls & A. G. Greenwald (Eds.), *Psychological perspectives on the self* (Vol. 2, pp. 93–121). Erlbaum.

Trope, Y. (1986). Identification and inferential processes in dispositional attribution. *Psychological Review, 93*(3), 239–257.

Trope, Y. (1989a). Levels of inference in dispositional judgment. *Social Cognition, 7*(3), 296–314.

Trope, Y. (1989b). Stereotypes and dispositional judgment. In D. Bar-Tal, C. F. Graumann, A. W. Kruglanski, & W. Stroebe (Eds.), *Stereotypes and prejudice: Changing conceptions* (pp. 133–139). Springer-Verlag.

Trope, Y., & Bassok, M. (1982). Confirmatory and diagnosing strategies in social information gathering. *Journal of Personality and Social Psychology, 43*(1), 22–34.

Trope, Y., & Bassok, M. (1983). Information-gathering strategies in hypothesis-testing. *Journal of Experimental Social Psychology, 19*(6), 560–576.

Trope, Y., Bassok, M., & Alon, E. (1984). The questions lay interviewers ask. *Journal of Personality, 52*, 90–106.

Trope, Y., & Ben-Yair, E. (1982). Task construction and persistence as means for self-assessment of abilities. *Journal of Personality and Social Psychology, 42*(4), 637–645.

Trope, Y., & Brickman, P. (1975). Difficulty and diagnosticity as determinants of choice among tasks. *Journal of Personality and Social Psychology, 31*(5), 918–925.

Trope, Y., & Burnstein, E. (1975). Processing the information contained in another's behavior. *Journal of Experimental Social Psychology, 11*(5), 439–458.

Trope, Y., & Burnstein, E. (1977). A disposition behavior congruity model of perceived freedom. *Journal of Experimental Social Psychology, 13*, 357–368.

Trope, Y., & Burnstein, E. (1979). Inferences about others from their reports about themselves. *European Journal of Social Psychology, 9*(3), 291–305.

Trope, Y., & Cohen, O. (1989). Perceptual and inferential determinants of behavior-correspondent attributions. *Journal of Experimental Social Psychology, 25*(2), 142–158.

Trope, Y., & Ferguson, M. (2000). Wishful thinking: When preferences influence inferences. In U. Neisser (Ed.), *Uncovering the mysteries of social life: Feschtrift in the honor of Robert Zajonc* (pp. 217–244). American Psychological Association.

Trope, Y., & Gaunt, R. (2000). Processing alternative explanations of behavior: Correction or integration? *Journal of Personality and Social Psychology, 79*(3), 344–357.

Trope, Y., Ledgerwood, A., Liberman, N., & Fujita, K. (2021). Regulatory scope and its mental and social supports. *Perspectives on Psychological Science, 16*(2), 204–224.

Trope, Y., & Liberman, A. (1996). Social hypothesis testing: Cognitive and motivational mechanisms. In E. T. Higgins & A. W. Kruglanski (Eds.), *Social psychology: Handbook of basic principles* (pp. 239–270). Guilford Press.

Trope, Y., & Liberman, N. (2010). Construal-level theory of psychological distance. *Psychological Review, 117*(2), 440–463.

Trope, Y., & Mackie, D. M. (1987). Sensitivity to alternatives in social hypothesis-testing. *Journal of Experimental Social Psychology, 23*(6), 445–459.

Trope, Y., & Thompson, E. P. (1997). Looking for truth in all the wrong places? Asymmetric search of individuating information about stereotyped group members. *Journal of Personality and Social Psychology, 73*, 229–241.

Tversky, A., & Kahneman, D. (1974). Judgment under uncertainty: Heuristics and biases. *Science, 185*(4157), 1124–1131.

Vinokur, A., & Burstein, E. (1974). Effects of partially shared persuasive arguments on group-induced shifts: A group-problem-solving approach. *Journal of Personality and Social Psychology, 29*(3), 305–315.

Vinokur, A., Trope, Y., & Burnstein, E. (1975). A decision-making analysis of persuasive argumentation and the choice shift effect. *Journal of Experimental Social Psychology, 11*(2), 127–148.

Wegner, D. M., Vallacher, R. R., Kiersted, G. W., & Dizadji, D. (1986). Action identification in the emergence of social behavior. *Social Cognition, 4*(1), 18–38.

Weiner, B. (1985). An attributional theory of achievement motivation and emotion. *Psychological Review, 92*(4), 548–573.

Wiesenfeld, B. M., Reyt, J. N., Brockner, J., & Trope, Y. (2017). Construal level theory in organizational research. *Annual Review of Organizational Psychology and Organizational Behavior, 4*(1), 367–400.

Winter, L., & Uleman, J. S. (1984). When are social judgments made? Evidence for the spontaneousness of trait inferences. *Journal of Personality and Social Psychology, 47*(2), 237–252.

Yudkin, D. A., Liberman, N., Wakslak, C., & Trope, Y. (2020). Better off and far away: Reactions to others' outcomes depend on their distance. *Organizational Behavior and Human Decision Processes, 156*, 13–23.

Zajonc, R. B. (1960). The process of cognitive tuning in communication. *Journal of Abnormal and Social Psychology, 61*(2), 159–167.

Index

Note. t, f, or *n* following a page number indicates a table, a figure, or a note.